Veterinary Immunology

Veterinary Immunology

Editor: Kalus Wagner

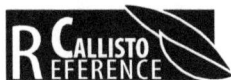

R CALLISTO
REFERENCE

www.callistoreference.com

Callisto Reference,
118-35 Queens Blvd., Suite 400,
Forest Hills, NY 11375, USA

Visit us on the World Wide Web at:
www.callistoreference.com

ISBN: 978-1-64116-639-3 (Hardback)

Cataloging-in-Publication Data

Veterinary immunology / edited by Kalus Wagner.
    p. cm.
Includes bibliographical references and index.
ISBN 978-1-64116-639-3
1. Veterinary immunology. 2. Immunologic diseases in animals. 3. Veterinary medicine. I. Wagner, Kalus.
SF757.2 .V48 2022
636.089 607 9--dc23

Table of Contents

Preface

Immunology is a discipline of biology that deals with the study of immune system in organisms. Veterinary immunology is the domain of biomedical sciences that focuses on the study of all aspects of immune system in animals. It is involved in measuring, contextualizing and charting the physiological functions, malfunctions, and the physical, chemical and physiological characteristics of the components of the immune system. The key aspects of veterinary immunology focus on how the immune system functions, how diseases are prevented and why vaccines sometimes do not work and lead to adverse reactions. This book provides comprehensive insights into the field of veterinary immunology. It also presents researches and studies performed by experts across the globe. The extensive content of this book provides the readers with a thorough understanding of the subject.

Various studies have approached the subject by analyzing it with a single perspective, but the present book provides diverse methodologies and techniques to address this field. This book contains theories and applications needed for understanding the subject from different perspectives. The aim is to keep the readers informed about the progresses in the field; therefore, the contributions were carefully examined to compile novel researches by specialists from across the globe.

Indeed, the job of the editor is the most crucial and challenging in compiling all chapters into a single book. In the end, I would extend my sincere thanks to the chapter authors for their profound work. I am also thankful for the support provided by my family and colleagues during the compilation of this book.

Editor

A descriptive pilot study of cytokine production following stimulation of ex-vivo whole blood with commercial therapeutic feline hydrolyzed diets in individual healthy immunotolerant cats

Aarti Kathrani[1,3]* , Jennifer A. Larsen[2], Gino Cortopassi[2], Sandipan Datta[2] and Andrea J. Fascetti[2]

Abstract

Background: Hydrolyzed diets are used in companion animals for the diagnosis and treatment of adverse food reaction. Similarly, hydrolyzed formulas are used in human infants with severe inflammatory bowel disease or milk allergy, and these must meet the standard of hypoallergenicity through rigorous testing. Unfortunately, no standards are currently applied to hydrolyzed veterinary therapeutic diets, and data for the immunogenicity of feline diets is also not available. Therefore, the main aim of this pilot study was to determine if ex-vivo whole blood stimulation assays could be used to characterize the cytokine response to hydrolyzed commercial diets in a small number of individual healthy immunotolerant cats. This approach has also been used to investigate cytokine production in response to cow milk protein in humans and currently similar studies do not exist in companion animals. Nine healthy cats previously eating the same basal diet were divided into groups and fed one of three hydrolyzed diets exclusively for 6 weeks. Heparinized whole blood was collected from each cat before and after the feeding trial. Ex-vivo whole blood stimulation assays were performed using crude extracts of the basal diet as a positive control, as this diet contained the same proteins present in the hydrolyzed diet but were intact, saline as a negative control, and each cat's respective hydrolyzed diet. Supernatants were collected and analyzed for tumor necrosis factor-alpha, interleukin-10 (IL-10), and interleukin-4 using enzyme-linked immunosorbant assay.

Results: Seven cats produced detectable amounts of the anti-inflammatory cytokine IL-10 upon stimulation with the basal diet. Two cats produced detectable amounts of IL-10 upon stimulation with a hydrolyzed soy-based diet and one cat produced a detectable amount of IL-10 upon stimulation with a hydrolyzed chicken-based diet (>125 pg/mL).

Conclusions: Results from this pilot study suggest that in some healthy immunotolerant cats, some hydrolyzed diets may elicit a similar cytokine response compared to their basal diet, which contained the same proteins intact. Therefore, animals may be able to recognize and react to some hydrolyzed forms of tolerated proteins, and may also suggest IL-10 as a target for investigation as a potential marker for dietary tolerance in cats, however further studies would be necessary to corroborate this. Further studies are also needed to determine if this would also be the same in immunologically naïve, sensitized and clinically hypersensitized cats.

Keywords: Feline, Hydrolyzed diet, Cytokine, Ex-vivo

* Correspondence: ak16730@bristol.ac.uk
[1]Veterinary Medical Teaching Hospital, School of Veterinary Medicine, University of California-Davis, Davis, CA 95616, USA
[3]Present address: School of Veterinary Sciences, University of Bristol, Langford House, Langford, Bristol BS40 5DU, UK
Full list of author information is available at the end of the article

Background

Hydrolyzed diets contain peptides created from chemically or enzymatically treated proteins; these peptides are small enough to theoretically avoid a type 1 hypersensitivity immune response, by preventing cross-linking of two immunoglobulin E antibody receptors on a mast cell. A peptide of 10 kDa or less is considered adequate to avoid this response; however there is evidence to suggest that the size needed may actually be smaller than three to five kDa [1]. Hydrolyzed diets are used in companion animals to diagnose and treat cutaneous and gastrointestinal adverse food reactions (AFR) [2]. Likewise, hydrolyzed baby formulas are used commonly in infants with severe inflammatory bowel disease or cow milk allergy [3]. These formulas must meet the standard of hypoallergenicity through testing using in vitro and in vivo animal models as well as clinical assessment [4, 5]. As similar standards are not currently applied to hydrolyzed pet foods, the proteins in these diets may still retain their antigenic potential. This was demonstrated in one study, which indicated that a significant proportion (21%) of dogs sensitized to the intact protein still reacted adversely to the hydrolyzed diet [6]. Therefore, the most significant clinical problem with veterinary hydrolyzed diets may be the retention of antigenicity leading to continued clinical signs. Consequently, studies are needed to verify the immunological potential of these diets.

The current pilot study aimed to describe the immunological effects of 3 available feline hydrolyzed dry diets in individual healthy immunotolerant cats before and 6-weeks after consuming a hydrolyzed diet compared to a basal diet containing these proteins intact, by measuring cytokine production using an ex-vivo whole blood stimulation assay. This assay has been used to investigate cytokine release in response to various antigens such as cow milk protein in humans [7]. Although this ex-vivo protocol has been described in dogs using bacterial ligands as a stimulant [8–10]; to the authors' knowledge this is the first pilot study to use commercial pet foods as a stimulant in companion animal studies. We assessed 3 cytokines known to be commonly modified in adverse immunological responses to food. An increase in the Th2 cytokine, IL4 and a decrease in the Th2 cytokine, IL10 have been shown to play an important role in the pathogenesis of food-induced gastrointestinal disorders in humans and mice [11–13]. Similarly, an increase in the Th1 cytokine TNF-alpha plays a role in cow-milk allergy in children and experimental food allergy in mice [14, 15]. The results of this study will help to describe the immunological response to hydrolyzed therapeutic diets in individual healthy immunotolerant adult cats; the results can be subsequently compared to immunologically naïve, sensitized and clinically hypersensitized cats in order to help characterize the pathogenesis of feline AFR and the role of hydrolyzed diets in the treatment of this disease.

Methods

Cats

Nine healthy intact female, specific pathogen free cats, residing in an existing colony at the University of California, Davis were used in this study. No abnormalities were noted on the basis of pre-study physical examinations. Mean age was 1.3 years (range 1 to 1.5 years), mean body weight was 3.6 kg (range 3.0 to 4.4 kg), and mean body condition score was 5/9 [16] (range 4/9 to 6/9). A standardized complete physical examination was completed on all cats prior to study initiation. All study cats were born to queens consuming the same commercial feline dry diet throughout gestation and lactation suitable for all life stages based on feeding trials.[1] Following weaning, study cats were then fed the same dry diet suitable for maintenance[2] (basal diet) until study initiation. This basal diet contained the same proteins present in the three hydrolyzed diets used in this study but intact.

Cats were group-housed by dietary treatment and received daily attention through activities such as petting and brushing, as well as access to numerous toys and scratching posts for behavioral enrichment. The facility maintains room temperatures between 18 and 24 °C, and has a 14 h light/10 h dark cycle. This experimental protocol was reviewed and approved by the Institutional Animal Care and Use Committee (IACUC) of the University of California, Davis (USA) (Animal Welfare Assurance Number A3433–01).

Study protocol

The cats were allocated to three groups (n = 3) using a random number generator and were housed by dietary treatment throughout the study. Cats were adapted to their respective dietary treatment group while continuing to be fed the basal diet for 7 days prior to the start of the study (day –7 to 0). All cats had free access to food and water throughout the study.

At day 0, the basal diet was discontinued and three cats received a hydrolyzed chicken based diet[3] (hydroC group), three cats received a hydrolyzed soy and chicken based diet[4] (hydroSC group), and the remaining three cats received a hydrolyzed soy based diet[5] (hydroS group). The hydrolyzed test diets were fed exclusively for 6 weeks. This duration was based on resolution of clinical signs in dogs in this time period when treated for food responsive enteropathy with a hydrolyzed diet [17]. Body weights and body condition scores were assessed by the same evaluator (AK) weekly and stool quality was monitored daily. On days 0 and 43 (at the start of the study and after the 6-week study period), six milliliters of blood were collected from each cat via jugular venipuncture into heparinized tubes following a 12 hour fast.

Preparation of diets for use in ex-vivo whole blood stimulation assays

Ten grams of each dry food (the basal diet and each of the 3 hydrolyzed diets)[2,3,4,5] collected from a new unopened bag was ground with sterile water using a clean pestle and mortar. The mixture was then transferred to a 50 ml sterile tube[6] and incubated overnight at 4-degrees on a rotator. The tube was centrifuged at 8000 rpm for 1 minute at room temperature and the supernatant was filtered using a 0.22-µm polyethersulfone sterile filter[7] in a sterile tissue culture hood.[8] The protein content in each of the filtrates was determined using the Bradford assay.[9] Working solutions of 500 µg/mL and 50 µg/mL were prepared for each of the dietary filtrates using phosphate buffered saline.[10] These concentrations were chosen based on results of studies using lymphocyte proliferative assays to various milk allergens [18, 19].

Blood analysis

Fresh heparinized whole blood, collected within 1 h before analysis, was mixed with 18 ml of RPMI[11] containing penicillin/streptomycin[l] and 1 ml plated in a 24 well plate.[12] A negative control consisting of 111 uL of phosphate buffered saline[10] and a positive control of 111 uL of 50 µg/mL and 500 µg/mL of basal diet and 111 uL of 50 µg/mL and 500 µg/mL of the respective hydrolyzed diet consumed by that cat during the 6 week study period were added to each well. All samples were analyzed in triplicates for a total of 18 wells. All plates were incubated at 37 degrees centigrade at 5% carbon dioxide for 24 h.[13] The plates were spun at 2000 x g for 4 min and the supernatant harvested and stored at −80 °C until analyzed.

The Feline TNF-alpha DuoSet ELISA,[14] Feline IL-10 DuoSet ELISA,[15] and Feline IL-4 DuoSet ELISA[16] were used to measure TNF-alpha, IL-4, and IL-10 production in the supernatants according to the manufacturers' instructions. The triplicate cell culture wells were assayed individually. The optical density was measured at 450 nm with a 540 nm wavelength correction using a Bio-Tek Synergy H1 Multi-Mode,[17] Absorbance Reader within 30 min and the data were analyzed using Gen5 Microplate Reader and Imager Software.[18] All assays were performed in duplicate. The lower limit of detection of the assays was 15.6 pg/mL for TNF-alpha, 125 pg/mL for IL-10 and 62.5 pg/mL for IL-4.

Data analysis

The mean of each of the duplicate cytokine concentrations was calculated. The mean of these values from the triplicate wells in the ex-vivo whole blood stimulation assay was then calculated for each of the diets and standardized to phosphate buffered saline by subtraction.

Differences in age, body weight, and body condition score between the three groups at inclusion was analyzed using the Mann-Whitney U test. A Wilcoxon signed-rank test was used to compare IL-10 concentrations following stimulation with the basal diet before and after the 6-week diet trial. Unfortunately, due to the small number of cats consuming each of the three hydrolyzed commercial diets, statistical analysis on cytokine production could not be performed among groups. Analyses were performed using IBM SPSS Statistics Version 23. Significance was defined as $P \leq 0.05$.

Results

Cats

There were no significant differences in age, body weight, or body condition score between the three groups ($P > 0.05$). All cats remained weight stable and maintained normal stool quality throughout the 6 week study period. All cats completed the study.

Ex-vivo whole blood stimulation assays

Numbers of cats that produced detectable amounts of IL-10, IL-4 and TNF-alpha following stimulation with 50 µg/mL or 500 µg/mL of the basal diet and the respective hydrolyzed diet before and after 6 weeks of consumption of hydrolyzed diets are presented in Table 1.

Stimulation with basal diet

On day 0 prior to starting the hydrolyzed diet, 5/9 cats produced detectable amounts of IL-10 on stimulation with 500 µg/mL of the basal diet (Fig. 1: mean 340.8 pg/mL, range 187.5–457.2 pg/mL). This number increased to 7/9 cats after consuming their assigned hydrolyzed diet for 6 weeks (Fig. 1: mean 355.6 pg/mL, range 212.7–503.7 pg/mL). Although two of the seven cats had lower IL-10 concentrations after 6 weeks compared to baseline (Fig. 1), there was no significant difference in IL-10 concentrations before and after 6 weeks ($P > 0.05$). No cat had detectable IL-10 concentration at baseline that was then undetectable at 6 weeks (Fig. 1). The two remaining cats that did not produce detectable levels of IL-10 following consumption of their respective hydrolyzed diet (hydroSC) produced TNF-alpha when stimulated with 50 µg/mL of the basal diet (65.8 pg/mL and 34.4 pg/mL respectively), but not on stimulation with 500 µg/mL of the basal diet.

Stimulation with hydrolyzed diets

One of the three cats in the hydroC group produced a detectable amount of IL-10 when stimulated with 500 µg/mL of the hydrolyzed chicken based diet both prior to and after 6 weeks of consumption (Fig. 2: 230.5 pg/mL and 185.5 pg/mL respectively).

None of the three cats in the hydroSC group produced detectable amounts of IL-10 following stimulation with the hydrolyzed soy and chicken based diet prior to or after 6 weeks of consumption (Fig. 2; <125 pg/mL).

Table 1 Number of cats producing detectable concentrations of cytokines in ex-vivo whole blood stimulation assays

Cytokine	Timepoint	Basal diet		Respective hydrolyzed diet	
		50 µg/mL	500 µg/mL	50 µg/mL	500 µg/mL
IL-10	Day 0	0/9	5/9	0/9	2/9
	Day 43	0/9	7/9	0/9	3/9
IL-4	Day 0	0/9	0/9	0/9	0/9
	Day 43	0/9	0/9	0/9	0/9
TNF-alpha	Day 0	0/9	0/9	0/9	0/9
	Day 43	2/9	0/9	0/9	0/9

Number of cat blood samples producing detectable concentrations of interleukin-10 (IL-10), interleukin-4 (IL-4), and tumor necrosis factor-alpha (TNF-alpha) following ex-vivo whole blood stimulation assay with 50 µg/mL or 500 µg/mL of pre-study basal diet and the respective hydrolyzed diet, before and after a 6-week feeding trial of one of 3 hydrolyzed diets (n = 3 cats per group). No samples produced detectable cytokines following stimulation with the negative saline control

One of the three cats in the hydroS group produced a detectable amount of IL-10 when stimulated with 500 µg/mL of the hydrolyzed soy based diet, prior to starting the diet trial (Fig. 2: 192.2 pg/mL). This same cat and a second cat produced detectable amounts of IL-10 when stimulated with 500 µg/mL of the hydrolyzed soy based diet after 6 weeks of consumption (Fig. 2: 380.5 pg/mL and 162.9 pg/mL).

Prior to starting and after 6 weeks of consumption of their assigned hydrolyzed dietary treatment, no cats in any group produced detectable amounts of TNF-alpha or IL-4 following stimulation with their respective hydrolyzed diet (<15.6 pg/mL and <62.5 pg/mL, respectively).

Discussion

In this pilot study, an ex-vivo whole blood stimulation assay was used to describe cytokine production following stimulation with three commercially available feline hydrolyzed dry diets before and after feeding exclusively for 6 weeks compared to a basal diet containing these proteins intact in a small number of individual healthy immunotolerant cats with known diet histories. Whole blood was used in the stimulation assays rather than peripheral blood mononuclear cells (PBMCs) in order to mimic the natural environment of the cells, to prevent phenotypic changes that may occur with isolation of cells, and to reduce the volume of blood needed. This technique has been shown to be comparable with the use of PBMCs [20]. Although whole blood stimulation assays have been performed using different stimulants [8, 9] in companion animals, to the authors' knowledge, commercial pet foods have not been previously utilized. Therefore, this pilot study described for the first time, the cytokine response of feline whole blood when stimulated with different commercial diets.

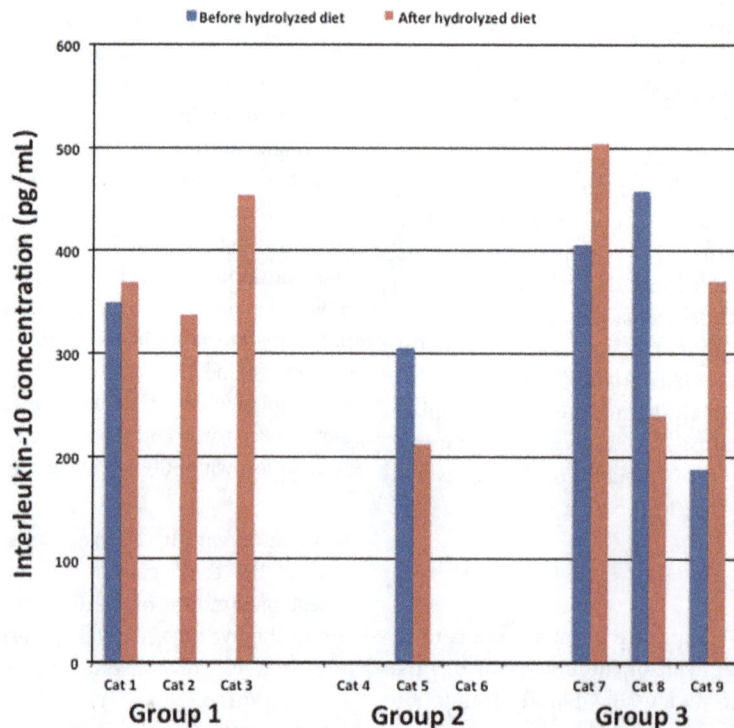

Fig. 1 Comparison of interleukin-10 in supernatants from ex-vivo whole blood stimulation assays using the basal diet. Bar graph of interleukin-10 concentration in supernatant following ex-vivo whole blood stimulation assay for all cats using 500 µg/mL of Purina Cat Chow Complete Formula dry food, before and after 6 weeks of consuming the respective hydrolyzed diet (group 1 – hydroC, group 2 – hydroSC, and group 3 – hydroS)

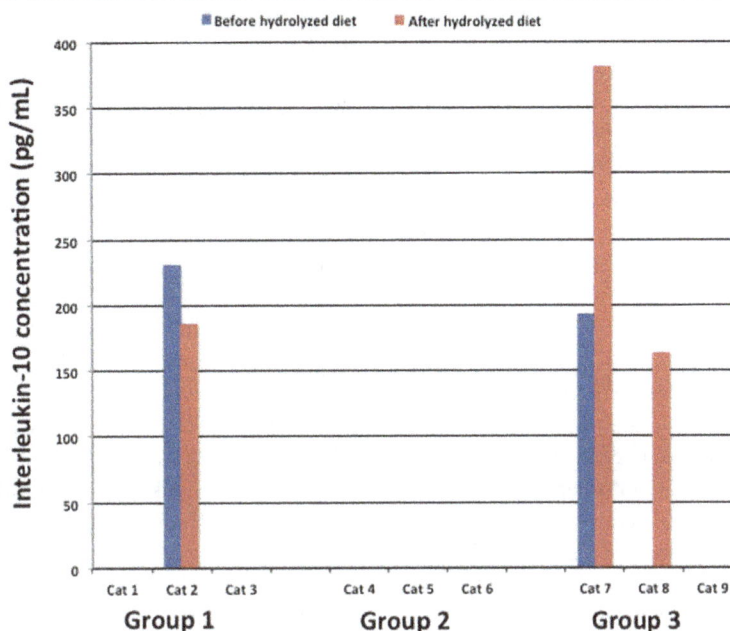

Fig. 2 Comparison of interleukin-10 in supernatants from ex-vivo whole blood stimulation assays using hydrolyzed dry diets. Bar graph of interleukin-10 concentration in supernatant following ex-vivo whole blood stimulation assay for all cats using 500 µg/mL of hydrolyzed diet, before and after 6 weeks of consuming the respective hydrolyzed diet (group 1 – hydroC, group 2 – hydroSC and group 3 – hydroS)

This study demonstrated that the majority of cats produced detectable amounts of IL-10 when their whole blood was directly stimulated with the basal diet. This may suggest that at least 1 of the mechanisms for immunological tolerance to diet in cats may occur via the production of IL-10. However, further studies utilizing a negative control that contains protein that the cats have never been sensitized to, such as sterile human albumin would be needed to confirm that the IL-10 responses seen in our study is specific to the dietary antigens present in the tested diets and therefore may be representative of immunological tolerance. Interleukin-10 is an anti-inflammatory cytokine produced by both the innate and adaptive immune system and IL-10 is able to inhibit both Th-1 and Th-2 cytokines, as well as the expression of autoimmune and pro-inflammatory conditions [21]. One study in humans reported that natural tolerance to foods was associated with increased amounts of IL-10 producing peripheral blood mononuclear cells [22]. A second study proposed a role for serum IL-10 as a useful marker in the diagnosis of food tolerance in humans [23]. However, further studies will be needed to determine if IL-10 can be used as a marker for dietary immunotolerance in companion animals.

Interestingly, this study documented at least a 4-fold difference in individual IL-10 concentrations when ex-vivo whole blood was stimulated with the basal diet. This may be due to differences in peripheral lymphocyte concentrations between the cats. Unfortunately, the peripheral lymphocyte count was not determined and therefore the numbers per well for each cat could not be standardized. Therefore, future studies should focus on standardizing the number of lymphocytes per well for each cat as this may then allow for direct comparisons between individual cats to be made. In addition, healthy cats have serum antibodies to food proteins [24], therefore any antigen specific immunoglobulins in whole blood from the cats used in our study may have bound to dietary antigens, resulting in a lower or higher cytokine response depending on the characteristics of the antibody. This may have also resulted in the variation of IL-10 concentrations seen in our study. Therefore, future studies should also focus on the correlation of cytokine production with dietary antigen specific immunoglobulins to determine the effects of these antibodies on subsequent cytokine production.

Although this study documented that there was no significant difference in IL-10 concentrations following stimulation with the basal diet before and after 6 weeks of the hydrolyzed diet (Fig. 1), two of the seven cats had a lower IL-10 concentration after the 6 weeks compared to before. These temporal differences in IL-10 concentrations in individual cats may have been due to differences in lymphocyte numbers per well and dietary antigen specific immunoglobulins at the two time points. Therefore, future studies should account for the possibility of variation in lymphocyte counts and dietary antigen specific immunoglobulins when interpreting temporal differences in cytokine concentrations in individual cats.

Some of the immunotolerant cats in this study produced detectable IL-10 when stimulated with the hydrolyzed diets; one cat to the hydrolyzed chicken based diet and two cats to the hydrolyzed soy based diet. Two of these cats, one from each dietary group produced detectable IL-10 prior to consuming the hydrolyzed diet. All nine cats in this study had been sensitized to chicken and soy, as both ingredients were present intact in the previously fed diets, including the basal diet. This may suggest that if an animal was allergic to chicken or soy, then they may be able to recognize and react to the hydrolyzed forms of these proteins. This has been shown in one study, where 21% of dogs sensitized to the intact protein still reacted adversely to the hydrolyzed diet [6]. One possible cause for the persistence of clinical signs could be due to retention of larger sized or intact proteins in the hydrolyzed diet. Therefore, determining not just the average but also the range of sizes of hydrolyzed proteins in these diets and correlating this to the production of IL-10 in these cats may be beneficial to help predict tolerance.

None of the three cats in the hydroSC group produced detectable amounts of TNF-alpha, IL-10, or IL-4 when stimulated with their respective hydrolyzed soy and chicken based diet, prior to or after 6 weeks of consumption. It is possible that this hydrolyzed diet did not elicit a cytokine response due to the size and nature of the hydrolyzed proteins. However, according to the manufacturer of this diet, the average size of the dietary protein is 12 kDa, whereas the other two hydrolyzed diets are reported to have an average size of 10 kDa or less. However, the range of protein sizes for each diet was unspecified. If larger proteins persisted after hydrolysis, this might explain the discrepancy between the average protein size of the hydrolyzed diet and the respective cytokine response. Also, this study was conducted over a 6-week period and therefore it is possible that with a longer duration of consumption of the hydrolyzed soy and chicken based diet a cytokine response may have been seen. In addition, the individual differences in production of IL-10 to different hydrolyzed diets could also be explained by potential differences in peripheral lymphocyte count and the presence of dietary antigen specific immunoglobulins.

Interestingly, two of three of the cats in the hydroSC group produced TNF-alpha when stimulated with the basal diet following the 6-week diet trial. These were the only cats that produced no detectable IL-10 when their ex-vivo whole blood was stimulated with the basal diet following 6-weeks of hydrolyzed diet. The exact reason for this result is unknown, but the lack of IL-10 production may have prevented dampening of the TNF-alpha response that normally occurs following IL-10 production. In addition, although the dietary stimulants used in the ex-vivo whole blood stimulation assays had been filtered using a 0.22 μm filter, it is possible that bacterial remnants that are known to stimulate pattern recognition receptors (PRR) such as lipopolysaccharide (LPS) may have been present and could have resulted in the TNF-alpha response in these two cats. However, as the same batch of dietary extract was used for all nine cats and the majority of cats did not produce TNF-alpha on stimulation with these extracts, it is unlikely that LPS or other PRR ligands were present in significant amounts. However, specific measurement of PRR ligands should have been performed in order to refute this possibility.

The aim of this pilot study was to describe the immunological effects of three commercially available feline hydrolyzed dry diets before and after feeding exclusively for 6 weeks compared to a basal diet containing these proteins intact in individual healthy immunotolerant cats using ex-vivo whole blood stimulation assays. A small number of cats were enrolled in this pilot study in an effort to reduce the number of animals used in a research study with an unknown outcome. In addition, only healthy immunotolerant cats were used. Several studies have shown that various non-allergic animal models can be used to assess immunogenicity of human hydrolyzed milk or rice formulas [25–28]. In addition, one study in healthy cats demonstrated immunogenicity to dietary proteins when fed as either aqueous suspensions or as part of canned diets [24]. Therefore, future studies will focus on the use of this assay in a larger number of immunologically naïve, sensitized or clinically hypersensitized cats to determine if the cytokine response to hydrolyzed diets is similar to their basal diets containing the same proteins intact. This study focused on ex-vivo whole blood incubation for 24 h as this time frame was shown to result in measurable cytokine secretion in healthy immunotolerant children following whole blood stimulation with milk antigen, after which time lower levels were detected due to degradation [7]. Although our study was able to detect measurable amounts of IL-10 protein in the supernatants of the majority of cats following stimulation with their basal diet and in some cats following stimulation with some hydrolyzed commercial diets after 24 h, a longer incubation time may have been needed to fully assess lymphocyte derived cytokine production. Therefore, future studies will aim to focus on different incubation times to help confirm an optimum time for cytokine production following incubation with dietary antigens. In addition, future studies will also focus on the use of ex-vivo intestinal biopsy stimulation assays to determine the correlation of cytokine production between whole blood and intestinal mucosa to confirm if whole blood can be used as a surrogate for intestinal tissue when stimulated with diet.

Conclusion

In conclusion, this pilot study for the first time showed that the majority of cats produced IL-10 to their basal diet using an ex-vivo whole blood stimulation assay. Similarly, some cats produced IL-10 to certain hydrolyzed therapeutic diets. This may suggest that in some healthy immunotolerant cats, some hydrolyzed diets may elicit a similar cytokine response compared to their basal diet, which contained the same proteins intact, however studies using a larger number of cats and addressing some of the limitations of the current study would be needed to corroborate this. In addition, further studies are needed to determine the immunological response to basal and hydrolyzed diets in immunologically naïve, sensitized or clinically hypersensitized cats.

Endnotes

[1]Whiskas® Kitten Dry with Chicken. Mars Incorporated, Fairfax County, VA. Main ingredients: poultry by-product meal, corn gluten meal, soybean meal, brewers rice, ground yellow corn, ground wheat, animal fat, and natural chicken and turkey flavors.

[2]Purina Cat Chow® Complete Formula® dry cat food. Nestle Purina PetCare Company, St Louis, MO. Ingredients: poultry by-product meal, corn meal, corn gluten meal, ground whole wheat, brewers rice, soy flour, animal fat preserved with mixed-tocopherols, fish meal, animal liver flavor, and meat and bone meal.

[3]Hill's Prescription Diet Feline z/d dry food. Hill's Pet Nutrition Inc., Topeka, KS. Ingredients: brewers rice, hydrolyzed chicken liver, soybean oil, powdered cellulose, and chicken liver flavor.

[4]Purina Pro Plan Veterinary Diets Feline HA dry food. Ingredients: rice starch, hydrolyzed soy protein isolate, partially hydrogenated canola oil, hydrolyzed chicken liver, tricalcium phosphate, powdered cellulose, corn oil, and hydrolyzed chicken.

[5]Royal Canin Veterinary Diet Feline Hydrolyzed Protein dry food. Royal Canin Inc. St. Charles, MO. Ingredients: brewers rice, hydrolyzed soy protein, and chicken fat.

[6]50 ml Sterile Centrifuge Tubes. Corning®. Corning Incorporated, Corning, NY.

[7]Millex ® GP Filter Unit, PES Membrane. Merck Millipore Ltd. Tullagreen, Co. Cork, IRL.

[8]Sterile culture hood, Class II Type S/B3.

[9]Bradford Reagent. Amresco, Solon, OH.

[10]PBS. Hyclone Laboratories, South Logan, UT.

[11]RPMI with L-glutamine, Corning Cellgro ®. Mediatech, Inc. Manassas, VA.

[12]Corning Costar ®24 Well Plate, individually wrapped, sterile.

[13]Hera Cell Incubator. Thermo Fischer Scientific Inc. Waltham, MA.

[14]Feline TNF-alpha DuoSet ELISA. R&D Systems, Inc. Minneapolis, MN.

[15]Feline IL-10 DuoSet ELISA. R&D Systems, Inc.

[16]Feline IL-4 DuoSet ELISA. R&D Systems, Inc.

[17]Bio-Tek Synergy H1 Multi-Mode Reader. Bio-Tek Instruments Inc. Winooski, VT.

[18]Gen5 Microplate Reader and Imager Software. Bio-Tek Instruments Inc.

Abbreviations
AFR: Adverse food reaction; HydroC: Hydrolyzed chicken based diet; HydroS: Hydrolyzed soy based diet; HydroSC: Hydrolyzed soy and chicken based diet; IL: Interleukin; TNF: Tumor necrosis factor; RPMI: Roswell Park Memorial Institute; PBS: Phosphate buffered saline; PBMC: Peripheral blood mononuclear cells

Acknowledgements
The authors thank Deborah Bee, Maria Montano, Dr. Birgit Puschner, and Dr. Pamela Lein for technical assistance.

Funding
This work was supported by the Center for Companion Animal Health, School of Veterinary Medicine, University of California-Davis and the Sommer Endowment.

Authors' contributions
AK, SD and GC were involved in hypothesis generation and experimental design. AK, AF and JL were involved in organizing and conducting the experiments. AK was involved in interpreting and analyzing the results and was a major contributor in writing the manuscript. All authors contributed, read and approved the final manuscript.

Consent for publication
Not applicable.

Competing interests
The authors declare that they have no competing interests.

Author details
[1]Veterinary Medical Teaching Hospital, School of Veterinary Medicine, University of California-Davis, Davis, CA 95616, USA. [2]Department of Molecular Biosciences, School of Veterinary Medicine, University of California-Davis, Davis, CA 95616, USA. [3]Present address: School of Veterinary Sciences, University of Bristol, Langford House, Langford, Bristol BS40 5DU, UK.

References
1. van Beresteijn EC, Meijer RJ, Schmidt DG. Residual antigenicity of hypoallergenic infant formulas and the occurrence of milk-specific IgE antibodies in patients with clinical allergy. J Allergy Clin Immunol. 1995; 96(3):365–74.
2. Cave NJ. Hydrolyzed protein diets for dogs and cats. Vet Clin N Am-Small. 2006;36(6):1251–68. vi

3.   Vandenplas Y, De Greef E, Devreker T. Treatment of Cow's milk protein allergy. Pediatr Gastroenterol Hepatol Nutr. 2014;17(1):1–5.

4.   Hill DJ, Murch SH, Rafferty K, Wallis P, Green CJ. The efficacy of amino acid-based formulas in relieving the symptoms of cow's milk allergy: a systematic review. Clin Exp Allergy. 2007;37(6):808–22.

5.   Bindslev-Jensen C, Ballmer-Weber BK, Bengtsson U, Blanco C, Ebner C, Hourihane J, Knulst AC, Moneret-Vautrin DA, Nekam K, Niggemann B, et al. Standardization of food challenges in patients with immediate reactions to foods–position paper from the European academy of Allergology and clinical immunology. Allergy. 2004;59(7):690–7.

6.   Jackson HA, Jackson MW, Coblentz L, Hammerberg B. Evaluation of the clinical and allergen specific serum immunoglobulin E responses to oral challenge with cornstarch, corn, soy and a soy hydrolysate diet in dogs with spontaneous food allergy. Vet Dermatol. 2003;14(4):181–7.

7.   Benlounes N, Candalh C, Matarazzo P, Dupont C, Heyman M. The time-course of milk antigen-induced TNF-alpha secretion differs according to the clinical symptoms in children with cow's milk allergy. J Allergy Clin Immunol. 1999;104(4 Pt 1):863–9.

8.   Kathrani A, Holder A, Catchpole B, Alvarez L, Simpson K, Werling D, Allenspach K. TLR5 risk-associated haplotype for canine inflammatory bowel disease confers hyper-responsiveness to flagellin. PLoS One. 2012;7(1):e30117.

9.   Schmitz S, Henrich M, Neiger R, Werling D, Allenspach K. Stimulation of duodenal biopsies and whole blood from dogs with food-responsive chronic enteropathy and healthy dogs with toll-like receptor ligands and probiotic Enterococcus faecium. Scand J Immunol. 2014;80(2):85–94.

10. Schmitz S, Henrich M, Neiger R, Werling D, Allenspach K. Comparison of TNFalpha responses induced by toll-like receptor ligands and probiotic Enterococcus faecium in whole blood and peripheral blood mononuclear cells of healthy dogs. Vet Immunol Immunopathol. 2013;153(1–2):170–4.

11. Dang TD, Tang ML, Koplin JJ, Licciardi PV, Eckert JK, Tan T, Gurrin LC, Ponsonby AL, Dharmage SC, Allen KJ. Characterization of plasma cytokines in an infant population cohort of challenge-proven food allergy. Allergy. 2013;68(10):1233–40.

12. Shandilya UK, Kapila R, Singh S, Dahiya D, Kapila S, Kansal VK. Induction of immune tolerance to caseins and whey proteins by oral intubation in mouse allergy model. J Anim Physiol Anim Nutr (Berl). 2014;98(3):467–75.

13. Brown P, Nair B, Mahajan SD, Sykes DE, Rich G, Reynolds JL, Aalinkeel R, Wheeler J, Schwartz SA. Single nucleotide polymorphisms (SNPs) in key cytokines may modulate food allergy phenotypes. Eur Food Res Technol. 2012;235(5):971–80.

14. Semeniuk J, Wasilewska J, Kaczmarski M. Serum interleukin–4 and tumor necrosis factor alpha concentrations in children with primary acid gastroesophageal reflux and acid gastroesophageal reflux secondary to cow's milk allergy. Adv Med Sci. 2012;57(2):273–81.

15. Dourado LP, Noviello Mde L, Alvarenga DM, Menezes Z, Perez DA, Batista NV, Menezes GB, Ferreira AV, de Souza DG, Cara DC. Experimental food allergy leads to adipose tissue inflammation, systemic metabolic alterations and weight loss in mice. Cell Immunol. 2011;270(2):198–206.

16. Laflamme D. Development and validation of a body condition score system for cats: a clinical tool. Feline Pract. 1997;25:13–8.

17. Schmitz S, Glanemann B, Garden OA, Brooks H, Chang YM, Werling D, Allenspach K. A prospective, randomized, blinded, placebo-controlled pilot study on the effect of Enterococcus faecium on clinical activity and intestinal gene expression in canine food-responsive chronic enteropathy. J Vet Intern Med. 2015;29(2):533–43.

18. Hoffman KM, Ho DG, Sampson HA. Evaluation of the usefulness of lymphocyte proliferation assays in the diagnosis of allergy to cow's milk. J Allergy Clin Immunol. 1997;99(3):360–6.

19. Shek LP, Bardina L, Castro R, Sampson HA, Beyer K. Humoral and cellular responses to cow milk proteins in patients with milk-induced IgE-mediated and non-IgE-mediated disorders. Allergy. 2005;60(7):912–9.

20. Deenadayalan A, Maddineni P, Raja A. Comparison of whole blood and PBMC assays for T-cell functional analysis. BMC Res Notes. 2013;6:120.

21. Saraiva M, O'Garra A. The regulation of IL-10 production by immune cells. Nat Rev Immunol. 2010;10(3):170–81.

22. Qamar N, Fishbein AB, Erickson KA, Cai M, Szychlinski C, Bryce PJ, Schleimer RP, Fuleihan RL, Singh AM. Naturally occurring tolerance acquisition to foods in previously allergic children is characterized by antigen specificity and associated with increased subsets of regulatory T cells. Clin Exp Allergy. 2015;45(11):1663–72.

23. Alonso R, Pineda F, Enrique E, Tella R, Cistero-Bahima A. Usefulness of serum interleukin-10 in determining food tolerance. Allergy. 2007;62(6):710–1.

24. Cave NJ, Marks SL. Evaluation of the immunogenicity of dietary proteins in cats and the influence of the canning process. Am J Vet Res. 2004;65(10):1427–33.

25. Duan C, Yang L, Li A, Zhao R, Huo G. Effects of enzymatic hydrolysis on the allergenicity of whey protein concentrates. Iran J Allergy Asthma Immunol. 2014;13(4):231–9.

26. Peng HJ, Su SN, Wu KG, Ho CK, Kuo HL. Effect of ingestion of cow's milk protein hydrolysate formulas on alpha-casein-specific immunoglobulin E and G1 antibody responses in naive and sensitized mice. J Pediatr Gastroenterol Nutr. 2005;41(4):438–44.

27. Piacentini GL, Vicentini L, Bodini A, Mazzi P, Peroni DG, Maffeis C, Boner AL. Allergenicity of a hydrolyzed rice infant formula in a guinea pig model. Ann Allergy Asthma Immunol. 2003;91(1):61–4.

28. Granati B, Marioni L, Rubaltelli FF. Evaluation in guinea pigs of the allergenic capacity of two infant formulae based on hydrolyzed milk proteins. Biol Neonate. 1985;48(2):122–4.

2

A novel *Salmonella* strain inactivated by a regulated autolysis system and expressing the B subunit of Shiga toxin 2e efficiently elicits immune responses and confers protection against virulent Stx2e-producing *Escherichia coli*

Gayeon Won[†], Tae Hoon Kim[†] and John Hwa Lee[*]

Abstract

Background: *Salmonella* Typhimurium (*S.* Typhimurium) inactivated by a regulated autolysis system was genetically engineered to express the homo-pentameric B subunit of Shiga toxin 2e (Stx2eB) on its surface. To prepare a strain able to yield autolyzed *Salmonella* bearing Stx2eB, the plasmid pJHL184 harboring *stx₂ₑB* gene was transformed into the attenuated *S.* Typhimurium strain, JOL1454. Stx2eB subcloned into the antigen delivery cassette of the plasmid was expressed as fusion protein with the outer membrane protein

Results: The expression of Stx2eB fused to the signal peptide in JOL1454 was validated by immunoblot analysis. To determine the immunogenicity of JOL1454, female BALB/c mice were intramuscularly injected with 1×10^8 CFU of the inactivated cells at weeks 0 and 2. Significantly elevated levels of IgG and IgA specific to Stx2eB was observed at weeks 4 and 6 post-immunization (PI) ($P < 0.05$). Proportion of CD3⁺CD4⁺ T lymphocyte subpopulation was also significantly augmented in in vivo stimulated splenocytes relative to that in the control group. The increased titers of IgG1 and IgG2a, and of immunomodulatory cytokines indicated that the immunization elicited Th1 and Th2 immune responses. Further, immunomodulatory cytokine genes (IL-6, IL-17A, IL21 and JOL1454) efficiently upregulated in naïve porcine peripheral blood mononuclear cells (PBMCs) pulsed with JOL1454. At week 6 PI, following the challenge with a virulent Stx2e-producing *Escherichia coli* in the mice, all immunized mice survived whereas approximately 30% of the mice in the control group died.

Conclusions: JOL1454 provided superior immunogenicity and effective protection against challenge with a sublethal dose, which demonstrates its potential as a candidate vaccine against edema disease.

Keywords: Shiga toxin, Edema disease, Bacterial ghost, *Salmonella* typhimurium

* Correspondence: johnhlee@jbnu.ac.kr
[†]Equal contributors
College of Veterinary Medicine, Chonbuk National University, Iksan campus, Gobong-ro 79, Iksan 54596, Republic of Korea

Background

Among Shiga toxin-producing *Escherichia coli* (STEC) strains, Stx2e is the second most common subtype of *stx₂* found in isolates from environmental sources [1]. Although STEC harboring the *stx2e* gene has only rarely been detected in human feces, causing mild diarrhea [2], *stx2e* is the most frequently encountered variant of *stx* gene in STEC isolated from porcine feces [3], and STEC harboring the *stx2e* gene has been reported to contribute to the virulence of edema disease (ED) in weaned piglets [4]. Shiga toxin 2e, encoded by the *stx2e* gene, inhibits protein biosynthesis by ribosome inactivation, which is chiefly responsible for the clinical signs and lesions of ED, including subcutaneous and submucosal edema. In addition, brain vascular injury caused by endothelial cell edema can elicit fatal neurological disorders and sudden deaths [4]. Binding of the non-toxic pentamer B subunits of Stx2e (Stx2eB) to the cell surface globotetraosylceramide (Gb4Cer) receptor allows the toxic A subunit of Stx2e (Stx2eA) to enter the cytoplasm, where cytotoxic effects occur [5]. Prevention of Stx2eB binding to the relevant receptors located on the intestines and cerebral endothelial cells thus represents a possible mechanism to prevent the transmission of this pathogen. Hence, Stx2eB may represent a practical target for the generation of neutralizing antibodies that could contribute to impairing the interaction between Stx2eB and cell surface receptors on intestines, thereby inhibiting the subsequent cytotoxic effects on epithelial cells that are mediated by Shiga toxin [5].

ED causes significant economic losses due to sudden deaths of infected pigs. The factors affecting the prevalence of ED are not clearly understood, despite mortality rates due to ED as high as 50 to 90% [6], with substantial variance among countries and farming units, and depending on the health status of the infected pigs. Elaborate efforts have been made in an attempt to reduce disease burden and economic loss in the swine industry. In particular, the need for optimal vaccination strategies against ED has increased, as frequently reported incidences of antimicrobial-resistant STEC in swine farms worldwide become progressively more burdensome to public health [7]. In addition, the administration of antibiotics appears to come too late to treat diseased pigs, since even when antibiotics are administered at the onset of visible clinical signs, severe neurological symptoms subsequently develop. Accordingly, several vaccine strategies based on targeting Shiga toxin have arisen. Active and passive immunization of piglets with an Stx2e toxoid has been reported to provide protection against challenge with Stx2e toxin [6]. However, those results did not imply that the toxoid would protect piglets against virulent STEC infection. Live attenuated STEC carrying genetically modified Stx2e has been constructed

that confers somewhat effective protection against a challenge with a lethal dose [6], although a high degree of reactogenicity remained. Thus, despite the continuous effort to improve vaccines against ED, no commercial vaccine is currently available.

A virulent strain of *Salmonella* Typhimurium has been successfully prepared for use in expressing a broad range of homologous antigens, to induce enhanced immune responses against them [8]. To minimize the risk of live attenuated *Salmonella* reverting to a virulent strain, autolyzed ghost strains derived from *Salmonella enterica*, including *S.* Enteritis [9], *S.* Gallinarum [10], and *S.* Typhi [11] have been genetically engineered for use as candidate vaccines or vaccine delivery carriers. Inactivated bacterial ghosts retaining the entire surface antigenic features of the original bacteria can efficiently target antigen-presenting cells and induce strong immunological responses [12].

A particular form of autolyzed bacteria generated via PhiX174 *E* gene-mediated lysis, so-called "bacterial ghosts" (BGs), are non-living gram-negative bacterial cell envelopes that lack cytoplasmic contents, yet conserve all the surface components of their parental bacteria [12, 13]. BGs have induced strong immunological immune responses against retained surface antigenic determinants, such as lipopolysaccharide and peptidoglycan [14]. The capacity of BGs as a presentation system for heterologous antigens has been evaluated in previous studies [15, 16]. Foreign target proteins presented by BGs have been successfully expressed as outer membrane proteins via fusion with signal sequences, or been translocated into the periplasmic space [16]. *Salmonella* ghost strains have been widely used as vehicles for antigen delivery due to their ability to induce adjuvant effects by invading host immune systems [15]. In the present study, an attenuated *S.* Typhimurium strain harboring a recombinant plasmid carrying a lysis gene permitting induction of bacterial autolysis, as well as the *stx₂eB* gene, was constructed. Lysis of *S.* Typhimurium was mediated by the PhiX174 *E* gene under the control of the face-to-face promoter system to generate *S.* Typhimurium ghost cells [17]. During lysis, Stx2eB protein fused with the outer membrane protein A signal peptide (*ompA* ss) is expressed, which enables Stx2eB to be exported across membranes of autolyzed cells. The immunogenicity of *S.* Typhimurium ghosts expressing Stx2eB was evaluated in a mouse model, and protective efficacy was also examined by challenging immunized mice with virulent STEC.

Methods

Bacterial strains and culture conditions

All bacteria strains and plasmids used in this study are described in Table 1. The *S.* Typhimurium mutant

Table 1 Bacterial strains and plasmids used in this study

Strain/plasmid	Description	Reference/source
Bacterial strains		
E. coli		
BL21(DE3)pLysS	F⁻ ompT hsdSB (rB⁻ mB⁻) dcm galλ(DE3) pLysS Cmr	Promega
JOL232	F⁻ λ⁻ φ80 Δ(lacZYA-argF) endA1 recA1 hadR17 deoR thi-1 glnV44 gyrA96 relA1 ΔasdA4	Lab stock
JOL606	Wild-type LT⁺, K99⁺, F6⁺,F18⁺, stx_2^+, stx_{2e}^+ STEC isolate from pig	Lab stock
JOL654	Wild-type LT⁺,F18⁺,STa⁺, stx_2^+, stx_{2e}^+ STEC isolate from pig	Lab stock
S. Typhimurium		
JOL912	Δlon ΔcpxR Δasd, a derivative of S. Typhimurium	[20]
JOL 1400	JOL912 harboring pJHL184	This study
JOL 1454	JOL912 harboring pJHL184-stx_{2eB}	This study
Plasmids		
pET28a	IPTG-inducible expression vector; Kmʳ	Novagen
pET28a-stx_{2eB}	pET28a derivative containing stx_{2eB}	This study
pJHL184	asd^+ vector, pBR ori plasmid carrying ss ompA/His₆, multiple cloning site, cI857/λPR promoter, araC P$_{araBAD}$, phiX174 lysis gene E	[47]
pJHL184-stx_{2eB}	pJHL184 harboring stx_{2eB} gene	This study

strains, Δasd Δlon ΔcpxR JOL912 and Δasd Escherichia coli χ6212, were grown in either Luria-Bertani (LB) broth or LB agar at 37 °C with 50 μg/ml of diaminopimelic acid (DAP) (Sigma-Aldrich, St. Louis, MO). The bacterial strains harboring the ghost plasmid were grown at 28 °C in nutrient broth (NB) containing 0.2% L-arabinose. All bacterial strains were stored at −80 °C in growth medium containing 20% glycerol.

Construction of *Salmonella* ghosts bearing Stx2eB

The S. Typhimurium mutant strain Δasd Δlon ΔcpxR, JOL912, was prepared by allelic exchange methods as previously described [18]. The ghost plasmid, pJHL184, carries a pBR origin, a multiple cloning site (MCS), a C-terminal His-tag, and a ghost cassette [19]. The stx_{2eB} gene was amplified by polymerase chain reaction (PCR) from wild-type STEC JOL606 isolated from pig diarrhea, using the primer pair, S1: 5'-ccgccaattcaagaagatgtt-tatggcg-3' and S2: 5'-ccgcaagcttgtcattattaaactgcac-3'. The thermal cycle parameters of the PCR reaction consisted of an initial denaturation at 94 °C for 5 mins, followed by 30 cycles of 95 °C for 15 s, 54 °C for 15 s, and 72 °C for 30 s, with a final extension step of 7 mins at 72 °C. The gene fragment was designed to produce an EcoRI restriction endonuclease site at the 5' end and a HindIII site at the 3' end. The resultant PCR products were

subcloned into the overexpression plasmid pET28a, thus generating pET28a-stx_{2eB}. The E. coli BL21 (DE3) pLysS strain was transformed with pET28a-stx_{2eB}. Stx2eB protein was purified as described previously [19]. The stx_{2eB} gene-containing DNA fragments derived from pET28a-stx_{2eB} were subcloned into EcoRI/HindIII-digested pJHL184 to generate the recombinant plasmid pJHL184-stx_{2eB} [17]. Stx2eB secretion into the periplasmic space is achieved by fusion with the signal sequence of E. coli outer membrane protein OmpA, which was subcloned into the MCS of pJHL184. pJHL184-stx_{2eB} was initially transformed into E. coli χ6212 (JOL232) to maintain the stability of the plasmid in the absence of antibiotics, and the plasmid subsequently was introduced into JOL912 by electroporation. The resultant strain was designated as JOL1454. The Δasd Δlon ΔcpxR S. Typhimurium strain JOL1400, carrying pJHL184, was used as a vector control.

Production of *Salmonella* ghosts bearing Stx2eB

A single colony of JOL1454 was inoculated into nutrient broth containing 0.2% L-arabinose, and the inoculum was incubated at 28 °C with agitation at 120 rpm until mid-logarithmic growth phase to achieve mass production of the strain. The cells were collected and washed twice with nutrient broth (NB) to remove L-arabinose. The cells were resuspended in 100 ml NB and incubated at 42 °C in a shaking incubator at 200 rpm to induce E gene-mediated lysis over the course of 48 h. After lysis, the ghost cells were harvested via centrifugation at 13,000 rpm for 15 min, washed twice with sterile phosphate-buffered saline (PBS) (pH 7.4), and stored at −70 °C.

Stx2eB expression in JOL1454

Western blot analysis was performed to verify the expression of Stx2eB antigen from JOL1454, as previously described [19]. Bacterial ghosts expressing the target antigen, and hyperimmune rabbit serum raised against Stx2eB, were prepared as previously described [19]. Protein lysates of the prepared ghost cells (5 μl) were subjected to sodium dodecyl sulfate-polyacrylamide gel electrophoresis (SDS-PAGE) on 15% gels. Resolved proteins were transferred onto polyvinylidene fluoride membranes (Millipore, Billerica, MA, USA), immunoblot analysis was performed, and immunoreactive bands were detected as previously described using hyperimmune rabbit serum raised against Stx2eB (1:5,000) and a HRP-labeled goat anti-rabbit IgG (1:8,000) [19]. JOL1400, JOL912 carrying pJHL184 and the purified Stx2eB protein were utilized as negative and positive controls, respectively. Subsequently, the amount of Stx2eB expressed in JOL1454 was relatively quantified in a calibration standard using indirect enzyme-linked immunosorbent assays (ELISA) [21]. Stx2eB containing $6 \times$ His-tag at the C-terminal end in JOL1454 were purified by Ni–NTA spin columns (Ni–NTA Spin Kit, Qiagen) according to the manufacturer's instruction. The His-tagged Stx2eB protein in a volume of 5 ml of the prepared ghost cell (1×10^8 cfu per ml) were eluted from the column with 2 ml of elution buffer (7 M urea: 7 M urea; 0.1 M sodium dihydrogen phosphate; 0.01 M Tris·Cl; pH 8.0). A calibration standard was generated by using twofold serial dilutions of Stx2eB protein extracted from BL21 harboring pET28a-stx_{2eB}. The diluted protein samples ranging from 1 μg to 31.25 ng, and the purified His-tagged protein as antigen were coated in the ELISA plate (Greiner) and incubated at 4 °C overnight. After the incubation, the hyperimmune rabbit serum raised against Stx2eB (1:300) and a HRP-labeled goat anti-rabbit IgG (1:5,000) were used as primary and secondary antibodies, respectively as previously described [19]. The concentration of the His-tagged Stx2eB protein expressed in JOL1454 were calculated by the known concentration of the purified Stx2eB corresponding to values of optical density at 490 nm in the calibration standard. The final concentration of the protein presented was based on the number of cells in initial bacterial culture.

Animal experiments

Eighteen female BALB/c mice were randomly assigned to two groups at five weeks of age. The mice in group A were intramuscularly immunized with 1×10^8 JOL1454 ghost cells at weeks zero and two. PBS was injected into the mice in group B, which served as a non-immunized control group. For measurement of total serum immunoglobulin (Ig) G, as well as of IgG1 and IgG2a, serum samples were collected, and for measurement of secretory IgA (sIgA), vaginal wash samples were collected, as previously described [20], at weeks 0, 2, 4 and 6. All samples were stored at –70 °C until used. For immunological assays using the primed splenocytes, additional 10 mice (5 mice per group) were inoculated at week 0 using the same protocol described above. Further, although ED results from oral transmission of the pathogen in natural infections, we found that ED did not occur in BALB/C model mice orally challenged with JOL654. However, intraperitoneal injection with the challenge strain efficiently induced symptoms in mice similar to those of ED such as hemorrhage in small intestine and bloody diarrhea. At week 7, non-immunized and immunized mice were intraperitoneally challenged with wild type STEC JOL654 isolated from porcine diarrhea (Table 1). The murine sublethal dose (2×10^7 CFU) was determined by the Reed-Muench method [22] following a protocol used in a previous study [10]. Mice were

monitored daily for mortality, clinical signs, and body weight for one week after inoculation.

Humoral and cellular immunological response

Stx2eB-specific titers of total IgG, the IgG1 and IgG2a isotypes, and secretory IgA (IgA) in sera or vaginal washes, as appropriate, were measured by ELISA [19] on 96-well plates with 500 ng of purified Stx2eB protein coating each well. Fluorescence-activated cell sorting (FACS) was used to assay changes in T cell subpopulations induced by immunization. Splenocytes were aseptically isolated from mice at day seven post-immunization, and single-cell suspensions were prepared. One million cells were stained by combining them with anti-mouse CD3a-PE and anti-mouse CD4-perCP-vio700 antibodies (Miltenyi Biotec, Bergisch Gladbach, Germany) and incubating for 20 min. After washing twice with FACS buffer (Miltenyi Biotec, Bergisch Gladbach, Germany), changes in $CD3^+$ and $CD4^+$ T cell subpopulations were determined using a MACSQuant® analyzer (Miltenyi Biotec, Bergisch Gladbach, Germany). Splenocyte proliferation following antigen stimulation in vitro was assessed by incorporation of MTT (3-(4,5-dimethylthiazol-2-yl)-2,5-diphenyltetrazolium bromide), which is only converted to blue formazan dye by actively proliferating cells [23]. Splenocytes were isolated from the immunized group at week two post-immunization (PI). Suspensions of 1×10^6 single cells were cultured in triplicate with 500 ng/ml of stx2eB antigen in RPMI 1640 medium (GIBCO, cat. no.11875093) containing 5% FCS (GIBCO, cat. no. 10099141), at 37 °C in a 5% CO_2 incubator for 72 h. Following stimulation, the cells were incubated with MTT (1 mg/ml) for another 4 h. The precipitated blue formazan in each well was solubilized in dimethyl sulfoxide, and colorimetric absorbance was measured as optical density (OD) at 570 nm with a spectrophotometer. The results are presented as a stimulation index, calculated as the mean OD value of the wells stimulated with antigen, divided by the mean OD value of the unstimulated wells.

Cytokine measurement

Induction of expression at the mRNA level of the cytokines, interleukin-4 (IL-4) and interferon-γ (IFN-γ), induced by immunization of the mice was measured by reverse transcription real-time PCR. At week 2 PI, splenocytes were isolated from immunized and non-immunized mice. Viable cells (1×10^6) stimulated with 500 ng/ml of Stx2eB protein were incubated in a 96-well cell culture plate with RPMI 1640 medium supplemented with 20% fetal bovine serum (FBS) in a humidified 5% CO_2 atmosphere for 72 h. Total RNA from the cultured cell suspensions was isolated using a GeneAll®

Hybrid-R™ kit (GeneAll Biotechnology, Seoul, Korea) and converted into cDNA with a ReverTra Ace® qPCR RT Kit (FSQ-101, TOYOBO, Japan). Levels of IL-4 and IFN-γ mRNA expression were quantified by real-time reverse transcription polymerase chain reaction (RT-PCR). The sequences of the primer pairs used to amplify IL-4, IFN-γ and β-actin (used as an internal standard) were those described by Lut et al. [24]. The mRNA expression levels of the cytokines were determined by the threshold method, using Cycle threshold (ΔC_T) values calculated based on the internal standard. The fold change of the mRNA levels compared to those of the non-immunized group is expressed as $2^{-(\Delta\Delta CT)}$ [25].

Cytokine profiles assessed in porcine PBMC pulsed with JOL1454

To determine the extent of porcine lymphocyte activation following stimulation of the lysed *S.* Typhimurium expressing Stx2eB, immunomodulatory cytokines were measured in mRNA level in naïve porcine peripheral blood mononuclear cells (PBMC) pulsed in vitro with JOL1454. Naïve porcine PBMCs were obtained from 2 ml of blood samples of five non-vaccinated pigs (15-18 kg, 6 weeks of age) raised at an experimental animal farm of the college by density gradient centrifugation using Histopaque-1077® solution (Sigma, St. Louis, MO) following the manufacturer's instruction. After the PBMC isolation, the cells were placed in RPMI 1640 medium supplemented with 1% fetal bovine serum and 1% glutamine/penicillin/streptomycin (Thermo Scientific), and then plated at a density of 5×10^6 per well in 96 well cell culture plate. Subsequently, the resuspended cells were treated with the lysed JOL1454 with 10 multiplicity of an infection (MOI), and were incubated for 48 h at 37 °C in a humidified atmosphere of 5% CO_2. Following the incubation, the pulsed cells were lysed directly in 500ul of Trizol reagent for RNA extraction. The preparation of RNA and cDNA were carried out as described above and 2 μl synthesized cDNA were added as qRT-PCR template. Cytokine (IL-6, IL-17A, IL-21, IFN-γ) mRNA expressions were determined by using the primer pairs [26–28] with SYBR® Green Realtime PCR Master Mix (QPK-201, TOYOBO, Japan) following the manufacturer's instruction. Porcine glyceraldehyde-3-phosphate dehydrogenase (GADPH) and 60s ribosomal protein L19 (RPL-19) genes were used as reference genes for normalization [29]. ΔC_T values were standardized by the average Ct values of two internal controls and non-stimulated cells. Relative fold changes were determined by $2^{-\Delta\Delta CT}$ method [25].

Statistical analysis

Data are presented as mean ± standard deviation (s.d.). One-way ANOVA test was used to evaluate significant differences in immune responses between the immunized and non-immunized groups. Statistical differences were considered significant when *P* values were <0.05.

Results

Construction of *Salmonella* ghosts expressing Stx2eB

The *Stx2eB* gene was cloned under control of a constitutive promoter in the pJHL184 plasmid, which contains a convergent promoter system tightly regulating the induction of the *E* lysis gene and consequent lysis of JOL1454. To constitutively express stx_{2eB}, JOL1454 cells were grown at 42 °C for 48 h in the absence of L-arabinose. Lysis of JOL1454 was confirmed by the inviability of cells plated from JOL1454 cultures grown at 42 °C. No viable cells were observed on LB plates after overnight incubation under conditions wherein the *E* gene was repressed (data not shown). The Stx2eB protein fused to ompA expressed in JOL1454 was verified by western blot analysis. The distinct immuno-reactive band of Stx2eB fused with OmpA was observed at ~24 kDa (Fig. 1; lane 1). Considering that the size of Stx2eB protein is ~13 kDa, we speculated that OmpA ss were properly fused with the target protein. In the lane 1 of Fig. 1 in which the lysed JOL1400 was loaded, the band corresponding to the size of Stx2eB was not shown. For the positive control, Stx2eB fused to 6xHis purified from pET28a-*stx2eB* in BL21 was loaded where immuno-reactive band was detected (Fig. 1; lane 3). The relative amount of Stx2eB protein expressed in JOL1454 was estimated by the linear regression standard curve showing a fit of $R^2 = 0.971$. Concentration of the His-

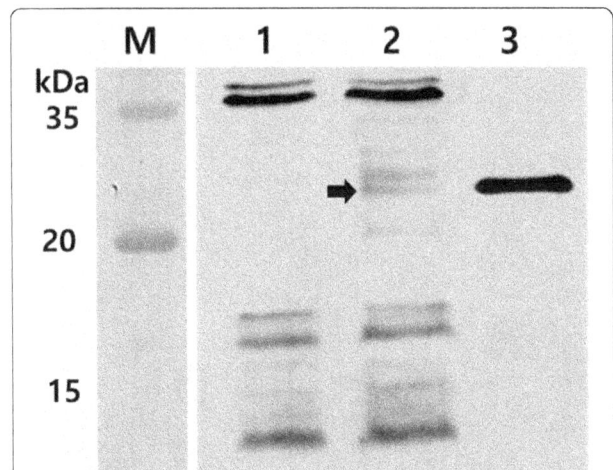

Fig. 1 Western blot analysis of Stx2eB protein expressed in JOL1454 cells. The Stx2eB protein expressed and secreted by JOL1454 cells was detected by western blotting with rabbit anti-Stx2eB antibody. The arrow indicates the expected size of the fusion protein. JOL1400, consisting of JOL912 cells containing the empty vector pJHL184 and purified Stx2eB were used as a negative and positive control, respectively. Lane M, size marker; lane 1: vector control; lane 2: JOL1454; lane 3: purified Stx2eB

tagged Stx2eB was approximately 909.18 ng per 10^8 cfu of JOL1454.

Humoral and mucosal immune responses raised by immunization

The immunogenicity induced by JOL1454 immunization of the mice was assessed by measuring Stx2eB-specific serum IgG and sIgA titers. The sIgA and IgG titers specific to the Stx2eB antigen were significantly elevated ($P <0.05$) in the JOL1454 group compared to those in the control group (Fig. 2). The IgG titers significantly increased at week 4 ($P <0.05$, 2.59-fold) and week 6 post-immunization (PI) ($P <0.001$, 2.79-fold) compared to those measured in the negative control. The concentration of sIgA was moderately increased at week 2 PI and was significantly raised in comparison to those in the negative control at week 4 and 6 PI ($P <0.05$). Furthermore, the ratio of the IgG1 to IgG2a (IgG1/IgG2a) immunoglobulin isotypes, markers of T helper 2 (Th2) and T helper1 (Th1) lymphocytes, respectively, was calculated from the titers of the individual isotypes. JOL1454 immunization induced IgG1 to a greater degree than it

did IgG2a (Fig. 3). The level of IgG1 was consistently higher than that of IgG2a throughout the entire observation period (Fig. 3).

T lymphocyte proliferation induced by immunization

Changes in splenic T cell fractions at week one post-immunization were assessed by measuring expression of the T cell surface markers CD3 and CD4 using flow cytometry. Both the $CD3^+$ T cell population and $CD3^+CD4^+$ T cell subpopulations were significantly elevated ($P <0.05$, respectively) in JOL1454-immunized mice (Fig. 4a), leading to significant average increases of 3.52% and 2.6% in the $CD3^+$ and $CD3^+CD4^+$ T cell subpopulations, respectively, compared to the non-immunized group. In the MTT cell viability assay, the JOL1454-immunized mice showed a significant increase ($P <0.05$) in stimulation index (SI) at week 2 PI, resulting in a significantly increased mean SI of 2.54 ± 0.49 in the immunized group, compared to 1.26 ± 0.29 in the PBS control group (Fig. 4b).

Cytokine measurement

To evaluate immunomodulatory cytokines secreted by the stimulated splenic lymphocytes, mRNA copy numbers of the IL-4 and IFN-γ cytokines were analyzed by qPCR. Fold changes were normalized against the murine β-actin gene. In vitro stimulation of splenic T cells with JOL1454 resulted in marked changes in relative fold values for the IFN-γ ($P <0.05$) and IL-4 ($P = 0.01$) cytokines in the immunized group compared to those in the control group (Fig. 5). These results indicated that the expression of IL-4 and IFN-γ in the immunized group were significantly upregulated compared to the control group, following stimulation of splenic T cells with Stx2eB.

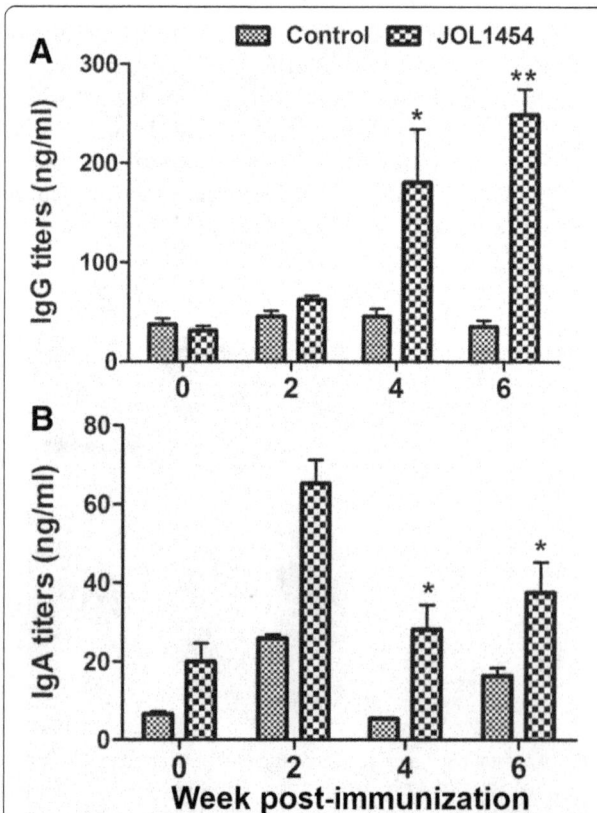

Fig. 2 Stx2eB antigen-specific humoral immune responses in immunized and non-immunized mice. Titers of **a** serum IgG, and **b** secretory IgA in ng/ml. Data are presented as the means of all mice in each group ($n = 9$), and error bars indicate s.d. *, $P < 0.05$ and **, $P < 0.001$ vs. control group at each week post-immunization

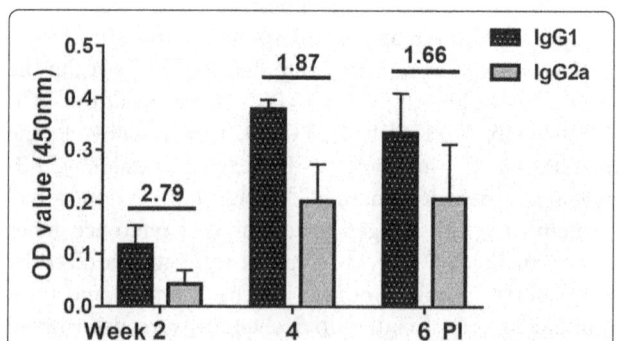

Fig. 3 The levels of two IgG isotypes, IgG1 and IgG2a, elicited by JOL1454 immunization. The values indicate the means of optical density at 450 nm from sera collected from immunized mice ($n = 9$), and error bars indicate standard deviation (s.d). The numbers above the bars indicate the IgG1/IgG2a ratios. PI: post-immunization

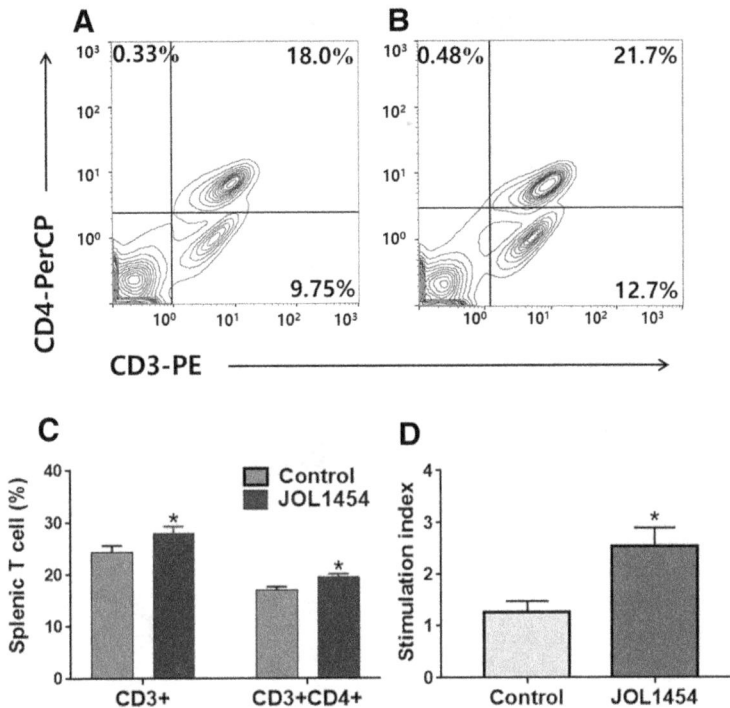

Fig. 4 T cell-related immune responses elicited in JOL1454-immunized mice. Representative flow cytometry scatter dot plots for CD3+ and CD3 + CD4+ splenic T cell populations of non-immunized mice (**a**) and the immunized mice (**b**). The subpopulations are presented as a percentage of gated cells. CD3+ and CD3 + CD4+ T lymphocyte populations in immunized and non-immunized mice (**c**) and stimulation index (SI) values of splenic T cells of the purified Stx2eB protein-immunized group, determined by MTT assay (**d**). The values are expressed as the mean ± s.d. of five individual values. *, $P < 0.05$

Immunomodulatory cytokines measured in the activated porcine PBMC

In vitro stimulation of porcine PBMCs with JOL1454 induced upregulation of immunomodulatory cytokine gene expressions (Fig. 6). The expression of IFN-γ, one of Th1-specific cytokine [29] and IL-6 promoting Th2 responses [30] increased up to 28.9 ± 8.5 and 15.13 ± 3.7 fold, respectively. Gene expression of IL-17A involving with differentiation of Th17 cells [31], were predominantly upregulated in the stimulated PBMC (71.88 ± 12.29-fold). Concomitantly, a moderate increase of expression of IL-21 produced by Th17 cells [32, 33] (6.07 ± 1.73-fold) were also observed in the pulsed PBMCs.

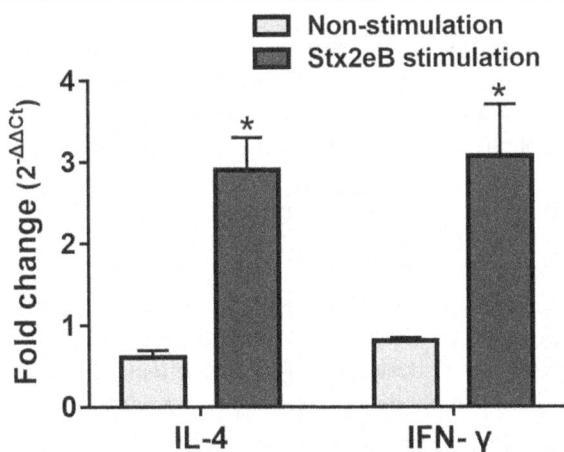

Fig. 5 Cytokine mRNA transcript levels in stimulated and unstimulated splenic T cells isolated from JOL1454-immunized mice. The mRNA transcript levels of cytokines were evaluated by performing RT q-PCR with gene-specific primers. Each fold change value represents the mean ± standard error of the mean (SEM) of five individual values. *$P < 0.05$ when values were compared with the control group

Protective efficacy conferred by JOL1454

To assess the protective efficacy conferred by JOL1454 immunization, all immunized mice were intraperitoneally injected with a sublethal dose of virulent STEC JOL654 at week 7 PI. The survival rates and weight losses of the mice were monitored in immunized and non-immunized animals for seven days after challenge. In both the immunized and the control group mice, weight loss, which began only following the challenge, was observed through day 1 post-challenge. While the weights of the immunized animals rapidly recovered, body weight of the negative control was markedly dropped compared to the immunized mice at days 2, 3, 4 and 7 post challenge ($P < 0.05$) (Fig. 7b). All immunized mice survived during the entire observation period, but 22.2% of the non-immunized mice died within 18 h of

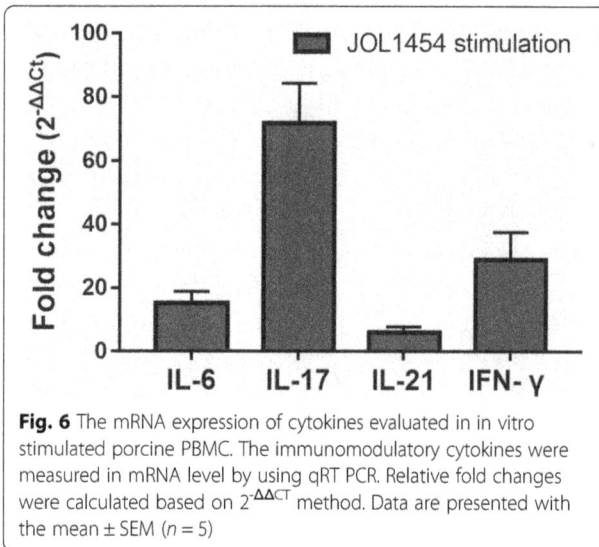

Fig. 6 The mRNA expression of cytokines evaluated in in vitro stimulated porcine PBMC. The immunomodulatory cytokines were measured in mRNA level by using qRT PCR. Relative fold changes were calculated based on $2^{-\Delta\Delta CT}$ method. Data are presented with the mean ± SEM ($n = 5$)

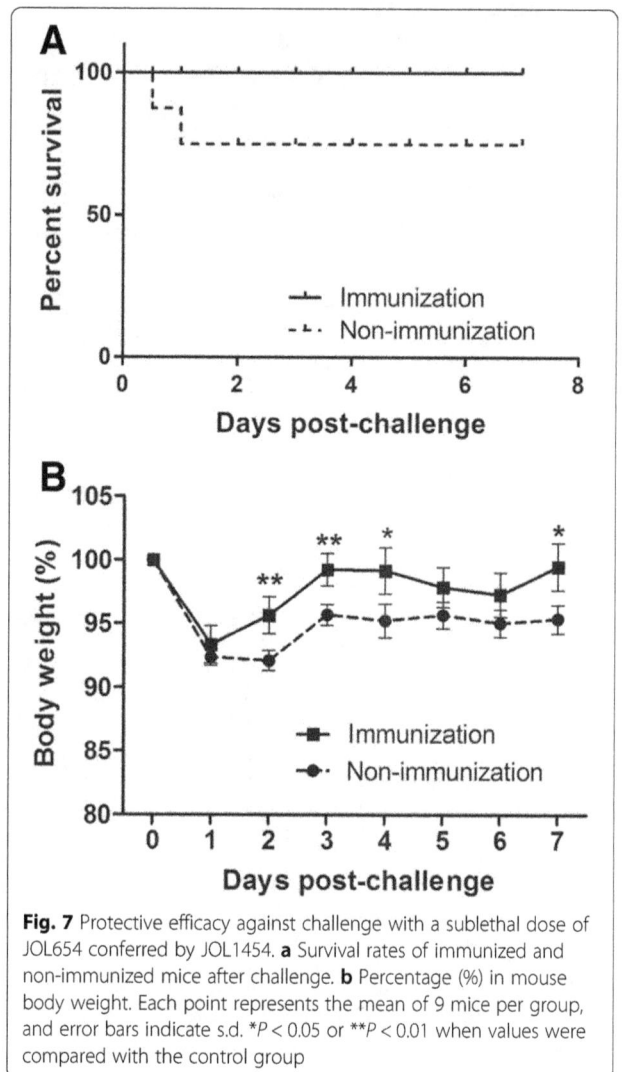

Fig. 7 Protective efficacy against challenge with a sublethal dose of JOL654 conferred by JOL1454. **a** Survival rates of immunized and non-immunized mice after challenge. **b** Percentage (%) in mouse body weight. Each point represents the mean of 9 mice per group, and error bars indicate s.d. *$P < 0.05$ or **$P < 0.01$ when values were compared with the control group

challenge (Fig. 7a). Clinical signs such as diarrhea, hunched posture, and hair election were also observed in non-immunized mice.

Discussion

Stx2eB is not only an intrinsically non-toxic and immunogenic protein of STEC but also a proven candidate vaccine antigen for prevention and control of ED in pigs [34]. In this study, we constructed an autolyzed *S.* Typhimurium strain expressing Stx2eB, which we designate as JOL1454, and confirmed the expression of Stx2eB fused with the six transmembrane domains (TMD) of the *E. coli* outer membrane protein A (OmpA) in this strain (Fig. 1). OmpA signal peptides have been successfully employed to translocate target antigens across the cytoplasmic space or insert proteins into the outer membranes of gram-negative bacteria [35]. In the present study, detection of Stx2eB protein expression in the cell pellet indicated that the OmpA signal peptide efficiently directed the expressed Stx2eB in the *Salmonella* ghosts (Fig. 1). Additionally, the relative amount of the His-tagged Stx2eB protein was measured in the lysed JOL1454. The significantly elevated levels of antibodies specific to Stx2eB in mice immunized with JOL1454 (Fig. 2) demonstrated that modified *S.* Typhimurium mediated efficient expression of Stx2eB on the outer membrane of the *Salmonella* ghosts.

In this study, immunization of mice with JOL1454 markedly elevated their titers of anti-Stx2eB IgG and sIgA (Fig. 2). The in vivo role of systemic IgG (sIgG) in neutralizing Shiga toxin has been emphasized in strategies to protect piglets against ED [36]. Stx-specific sIgG antibodies can protect immunized pigs against systemic infection with STEC, and the magnitude of protection relies on the dose of the antibodies [37]. sIgA antibodies,

however, serve as the first line of defense against infection at mucosal surfaces [38]. As the natural infection of STEC occurs via the oral route, sIgA also has an essential role in preventing adherence or attachment of pathogens [39]. These findings indicate that immunization with JOL1454 may mediate protection against ED by eliciting humoral and mucosal immune responses against Stx2eB.

The IgG isotypes, IgG1 and IgG2a, are regarded as markers of T helper (Th) 2- and Th1-type immune responses, respectively [40]. The Fc portions of the IgG1 and IgG2a antibodies primarily interact with the activatory Fc-γ receptors (FcγR) III and FcγR IV, which elicit Th2- and Th1-type immune responses, respectively [41]. The IgG1-to-IgG2a (IgG1/IgG2a) ratio has been used to determine the relative contribution of Th2- versus Th1-type immune responses to STEC infection [42]. In our current study, the IgG1/IgG2a ratio declined from 2.79 to 1.66 in response to JOL1454 immunization (Fig. 3).

The decreased ratio indicated that the contribution of IgG2a antibodies continuously increased during the observation period (Fig. 3). This implies that, despite the predominance of the Th2 subpopulation, the Th1 immune response was steadily elevated in JOL1454-immunized animals.

Naïve CD4 + T lymphocytes stimulated with an antigenic peptide differentiate into Th1 and Th2 subpopulations [43]. Th1 and Th2 cells promote cell-mediated immune responses involving antigen-specific cytotoxic effects and humoral immune responses, respectively [44]. JOL1454 immunization significantly elevated the $CD3^+CD4^+$ T cell subpopulations in mice, (Fig. 4a), indicating that JOL1454 can stimulate naïve $CD4^+$ T cell maturation. Additionally, we observed that the copy numbers of IL-4 and IFN-γ mRNA were significantly elevated in restimulated splenic lymphocytes of the immunized mice (Fig. 5). The immunomodulatory cytokines, IFN-γ and IL-4, are exclusively expressed in mature Th1 and Th2 cells, respectively [43]. Thus, this observation supports the interpretation that JOL1454 was able to efficiently stimulate CD4+ T cell differentiation into Th1 and Th2 subpopulations, which drive the induction of cellular and humoral immune responses, respectively.

Salmonella ghosts elicit robust cell-mediated immune responses (CMI), as they retain the entire surface antigenic determinants of their pre-lysed condition, in the native forms thereof [10]. We observed markedly enhanced in vitro SI in re-stimulated splenic T cells of JOL1454-immunized mice (Fig. 4B). This implies that JOL1454 can induce lymphocyte proliferation, which is a primary parameter of CMI responses. In parallel, mRNA levels of IFN-γ, a marker of CMI, were significantly elevated in splenic T cells after in vitro restimulation. In a previous report, mice immunized with purified Stx2eB protein did not show increased serum levels of IFN-γ [36]. These results support the conclusion that the Salmonella ghost system delivering Stx2eB can induce CMI responses in immunized mice.

Ren et al. constructed a plasmid expressing Stx2eB for use as a candidate vaccine, and investigated its protective efficacy using the construct in a mouse model [45]. In that study, immunized mice were intraperitoneally challenged with a virulent ED-associated E. coli, and 80% of the immunized mice survived. Immunization of mice with JOL1454 in our study also offered highly effective protection against a challenge with wild-type STEC. While no mortality occurred in any of the immunized mice, approximately 30% of the mice in the non-immunized group died. The protection conferred by JOL1454 immunization might be due to the following: JOL1454 Salmonella ghosts efficiently secreted Stx2eB in the cells due to fusion of the protein with ompA ss;

Stx2eB delivered by JOL1454 ghosts elicited circulating antibodies specific to Stx2eB, which may neutralize Shiga toxin; and Salmonella ghosts bearing Stx2eB can trigger CMI responses mediating phagocytosis and elimination of the challenge strain. Additionally, JOL1454 efficiently induced upregulated expression of immunomodulatory cytokines involved with activation of Th1, Th2 and Th17 cells in the pulsed porcine PBMC (Fig. 6), which implicated that JOL1454 may have a capacity to differentiate naïve porcine lymphocytes toward matured $CD4^+$ T cell subpopulation. Particularly, the increased expression of IL-6, IL-17A and IL-21 in the present study indicated Th17 cells was matured and activated in the pulsed porcine lymphocytes, which is crucial for intestinal mucosal host defense [46]. These preliminary data supported that JOL1454 has a potential to elicit subsequent immune responses following the cytokine production in porcine.

Conclusions

The present data indicate that Stx2eB delivered by a Salmonella ghost strain could effectively stimulate the immune system so as to confer sufficient protection to prevent ED. The results also suggest that Salmonella inactivated by E gene-mediated lysis that preserves their intact antigenic determinants may not only effectively deliver the target antigen but also provide an adjuvant property. Additionally, given the immunostimulatory effect of JOL1454 which can elicit immunomodulatory and proinflammatory cytokines in the porcine lymphocyte, this autolyzed Salmonella strain producing Stx2eB may constitute a novel alternative approach to developing an effective vaccine candidate against porcine edema disease.

Abbreviations

BGs: Bacterial ghosts; C_T: Cycle threshold; DAP: Diaminopimelic acid; ED: Edema disease; ELISA: Enzyme-linked immunosorbent assays; FACS: Fluorescence-activated cell sorting; Gb4Cer: Globotetraosylceramide receptor; Ig: Immunoglobulin; IL: Interleukin; MCS: A multiple cloning site; MTT: 3-(4,5-dimethylthiazol-2-yl)-2,5-diphenyltetrazolium bromide; NB: Nutrient broth; OD: Optical density; ompA ss: Outer membrane protein A signal peptide; PBMCs: Peripheral blood mononuclear cells; PBS: Phosphate-buffered saline; PCR: Polymerase chain reaction; PI: Post-immunization; S. Typhimurium: Salmonella Typhimurium; SDS-PAGE: Sodium dodecyl sulfate-polyacrylamide gel electrophoresis; STEC: Shiga toxin-producing Escherichia coli; Stx2eA: Toxic A subunit of Stx2e; Stx2eB: Homo-pentameric B subunit of Shiga toxin 2e

Acknowledgements

Not applicable.

Funding

This work was supported by the National Research Foundation of Korea (NRF) grant funded by the Korea government (MISP) (No. 2015R1A2A1A14001011).

Authors' contributions

GW and TK conducted the experiments and was involved in manuscript preparation. JHL conceived the study, precipitated in the design of the study and was involved in manuscript preparation. All authors read and approved the final manuscript.

Competing interests

The authors declare that they have no competing interests.

Consent for publication

Not applicable.

References

1. Sonntag AK, Bielaszewska M, Mellmann A, Dierksen N, Schierack P, Wieler LH, Schmidt MA, Karch H. Shiga toxin 2e-producing *Escherichia coli* isolates from humans and pigs differ in their virulence profiles and interactions with intestinal epithelial cells. Appl Environ Microbiol. 2005;71(12):8855–63.
2. Pierard D, Huyghens L, Lauwers S, Lior H. Diarrhoea associated with *Escherichia coli* producing porcine oedema disease verotoxin. Lancet. 1991; 338(8769):762.
3. Fratamico PM, Bagi LK, Bush EJ, Solow BT. Prevalence and characterization of Shiga toxin-producing *Escherichia coli* in swine feces recovered in the national animal health monitoring System's swine 2000 study. Appl Environ Microbiol. 2004;70(12):7173–8.
4. Marques L, Peiris J, Cryz S, O'brien A. *Escherichia coli* strains isolated from pigs with edema disease produce a variant of Shiga-like toxin II. FEMS Microbiol Lett. 1987;44(1):33–8.
5. Donohue-Rolfe A, Kondova I, Mukherjee J, Chios K, Hutto D, Tzipori S. Antibody-based protection of gnotobiotic piglets infected with *Escherichia coli* O157:H7 against systemic complications associated with Shiga toxin 2. Infect Immun. 1999;67(7):3645–8.
6. Makino S, Watarai M, Tabuchi H, Shirahata T, Furuoka H, Kobayashi Y, Takeda Y. Genetically modified Shiga toxin 2e (Stx2e) producing *Escherichia coli* is a vaccine candidate for porcine edema disease. Microb Pathog. 2001;31(1):1–8.
7. Ho WS, Tan LK, Ooi PT, Yeo CC, Thong KL. Prevalence and characterization of verotoxigenic-*Escherichia coli* isolates from pigs in Malaysia. BMC Vet Res. 2013;9:109-6148-9-109.
8. Russmann H, Shams H, Poblete F, Fu Y, Galan JE, Donis RO. Delivery of epitopes by the *Salmonella* type III secretion system for vaccine development. Science. 1998;281(5376):565–8.
9. Peng W, Si W, Yin L, Liu H, Yu S, Liu S, Wang C, Chang Y, Zhang Z, Hu S. *Salmonella* enteritidis ghost vaccine induces effective protection against lethal challenge in specific-pathogen-free chicks. Immunobiology. 2011; 216(5):558–65.
10. Chaudhari AA, Jawale CV, Kim SW, Lee JH. Construction of a *Salmonella* gallinarum ghost as a novel inactivated vaccine candidate and its protective efficacy against fowl typhoid in chickens. Vet Res. 2012;43(1):44–54.
11. Wen J, Yang Y, Zhao G, Tong S, Yu H, Jin X, Du L, Jiang S, Kou Z, Zhou Y. *Salmonella* typhi Ty21a bacterial ghost vector augments HIV-1 gp140 DNA vaccine-induced peripheral and mucosal antibody responses via TLR4 pathway. Vaccine. 2012;30(39):5733–9.
12. Lubitz W. Bacterial ghosts as carrier and targeting systems. Expert Opin Biol Ther. 2001;1(5):765–71.
13. Szostak MP, Hensel A, Eko FO, Klein R, Auer T, Mader H, Haslberger A, Bunka S, Wanner G, Lubitz W. Bacterial ghosts: non-living candidate vaccines. J Biotechnol. 1996;44(1):161–70.
14. Haslberger A, Kohl G, Felnerova D, Mayr U, Fürst-Ladani S, Lubitz W. Activation, stimulation and uptake of bacterial ghosts in antigen presenting cells. J Biotechnol. 2000;83(1):57–66.
15. Jalava K, Eko FO, Riedmann E, Lubitz W. Bacterial ghosts as carrier and targeting systems for mucosal antigen delivery. Expert Rev Vaccines. 2003; 2(1):45–51.

16. Walcher P, Mayr UB, Azimpour-Tabrizi C, Eko FO, Jechlinger W, Mayrhofer P, Alefantis T, Mujer CV, DelVecchio VG, Lubitz W. Antigen discovery and delivery of subunit vaccines by nonliving bacterial ghost vectors. Expert Rev Vaccines. 2004;3(6):681–91.
17. Jawale CV, Kim SW, Lee JH. Tightly regulated bacteriolysis for production of empty *Salmonella* enteritidis envelope. Vet Microbiol. 2014;169(3):179–87.
18. Kang HY, Srinivasan J, Curtiss R. 3rd: immune responses to recombinant pneumococcal PspA antigen delivered by live attenuated *Salmonella* enterica serovar typhimurium vaccine. Infect Immun. 2002;70(4):1739–49.
19. Jawale CV, Lee JH. *Salmonella* enterica serovar enteritidis ghosts carrying the escherichia coli heat-labile enterotoxin B subunit are capable of inducing enhanced protective immune responses. Clin Vaccine Immunol. 2014;21(6):799–807.
20. Hur J, Lee JH. Immune responses to new vaccine candidates constructed by a live attenuated *Salmonella* typhimurium delivery system expressing *Escherichia coli* F4, F5, F6, F41 and intimin adhesin antigens in a murine model. J Vet Med Sci. 2011;73(10):1265–73.
21. Nemchinov LG, Natilla A. Transient expression of the ectodomain of matrix protein 2 (M2e) of avian influenza a virus in plants. Protein Expr Purif. 2007; 56(2):153–9.
22. Reed LJ, Muench H. A simple method of estimating fifty per cent endpoints. Am J Epidemiol. 1938;27(3):493–7.
23. Denizot F, Lang R. Rapid colorimetric assay for cell growth and survival: modifications to the tetrazolium dye procedure giving improved sensitivity and reliability. J Immunol Methods. 1986;89(2):271–7.
24. Overbergh L, Valckx D, Waer M, Mathieu C. Quantification of murine cytokine mRNAs using real time quantitative reverse transcriptase PCR. Cytokine. 1999;11(4):305–12.
25. Fitzmaurice J, Glennon M, Duffy G, Sheridan J, Carroll C, Maher M. Application of real-time PCR and RT-PCR assays for the detection and quantitation of VT 1 and VT 2 toxin genes in E. coli O157: H7. Mol Cell Probes. 2004;18(2):123–32.
26. Khoufache K, Cabaret O, Farrugia C, Rivollet D, Alliot A, Allaire E, Cordonnier C, Bretagne S, Botterel F. Primary in vitro culture of porcine tracheal epithelial cells in an air-liquid interface as a model to study airway epithelium and aspergillus fumigatus interactions. Med Mycol. 2010;48(8):1049–55.
27. Wulster-Radcliffe MC, Ajuwon KM, Wang J, Christian JA, Spurlock ME. Adiponectin differentially regulates cytokines in porcine macrophages. Biochem Biophys Res Commun. 2004;316(3):924–9.
28. Kiros TG, van Kessel J, Babiuk LA, Gerdts V. Induction, regulation and physiological role of IL-17 secreting helper T-cells isolated from PBMC, thymus, and lung lymphocytes of young pigs. Vet Immunol Immunopathol. 2011;144(3):448–54.
29. Vandesompele J, De Preter K, Pattyn F, Poppe B, Van Roy N, De Paepe A, Speleman F. Accurate normalization of real-time quantitative RT-PCR data by geometric averaging of multiple internal control genes. Genome Biol. 2002;3(7):1–12.
30. Roman M, Martin-Orozco E, Goodman JS, Nguyen MD, Sato Y, Ronaghy A, Kornbluth RS, Richman DD, Carson DA, Raz E. Immunostimulatory DNA sequences function as T helper-1-promoting adjuvants. Nat Med. 1997;3(8): 849–54.
31. Rincon M, Anguita J, Nakamura T, Fikrig E, Flavell RA. Interleukin (IL)-6 directs the differentiation of IL-4-producing CD4+ T cells. J Exp Med. 1997; 185(3):461–9.
32. Korn T, Bettelli E, Oukka M, Kuchroo VK. IL-17 and Th17 Cells. Annu Rev Immunol. 2009;27:485–517.
33. Korn T, Bettelli E, Gao W, Awasthi A, Jäger A, Strom TB, Oukka M, Kuchroo VK. IL-21 initiates an alternative pathway to induce proinflammatory TH17 cells. Nature. 2007;448(7152):484–7.
34. Lencer WI, Saslowsky D. Raft trafficking of AB 5 subunit bacterial toxins. Biochim Biophys Acta Mole Cell Res. 2005;1746(3):314–21.
35. Takahara M, Hibler DW, Barr PJ, Gerlt JA, Inouye M. The ompA signal peptide directed secretion of Staphylococcal nuclease A by *Escherichia coli*. J Biol Chem. 1985;260(5):2670–4.
36. Sato T, Matsui T, Takita E, Kadoyama Y, Makino S, Kato K, Sawada K, Hamabata T. Evaluation of recombinant forms of the shiga toxin variant Stx2eB subunit and non-toxic mutant Stx2e as vaccine candidates against porcine edema disease. J Vet Med Sci. 2013;75(10):1309–15.
37. Matise I, Cornick NA, Booher SL, Samuel JE, Bosworth BT, Moon HW. Intervention with Shiga toxin (Stx) antibody after infection by Stx-producing escherichia coli. J Infect Dis. 2001;183(2):347–50.

A novel Salmonella strain inactivated by a regulated autolysis system and expressing the B subunit of Shiga...

19

38. McGhee JR, Kiyono H. New perspectives in vaccine development: mucosal immunity to infections. Infect Agents Dis. 1993;2(2):55–73.

39. Anonymous *Proceedings of the PEDIATRIC RESEARCH:* INT PEDIATRIC RESEARCH FOUNDATION, INC 351 WEST CAMDEN ST, BALTIMORE, MD 21201–2436 USA; 2002.

40. Romagnani S. Type 1 T helper and type 2 T helper cells: functions, regulation and role in protection and disease. Int J Clin Lab Res. 1992; 21(2–4):152–8.

41. Parham P. On the fragmentation of monoclonal IgG1, IgG2a, and IgG2b from BALB/c mice. J Immunol. 1983;131(6):2895–902.

42. Gupta P, Singh MK, Singh Y, Gautam V, Kumar S, Kumar O, Dhaked RK. Recombinant Shiga toxin B subunit elicits protection against Shiga toxin via mixed Th type immune response in mice. Vaccine. 2011;29(45):8094–100.

43. Hodgkin PD, Lee JH, Lyons AB. B cell differentiation and isotype switching is related to division cycle number. J Exp Med. 1996;184(1):277–81.

44. MacLeod MK, Kappler JW, Marrack P. Memory CD4 T cells: generation, reactivation and re-assignment. Immunology. 2010;130(1):10–5.

45. Ren W, Yu R, Liu G, Li N, Peng Y, Wu M, Yin Y, Li Y, Fatufe AA, Li T. DNA vaccine encoding the major virulence factors of Shiga toxin type 2e (Stx2e)-expressing escherichia coli induces protection in mice. Vaccine. 2013;31(2):367–72.

46. Conti HR, Shen F, Nayyar N, Stocum E, Sun JN, Lindemann MJ, Ho AW, Hai JH, Yu JJ, Jung JW, Filler SG, Masso-Welch P, Edgerton M, Gaffen SL. Th17 cells and IL-17 receptor signaling are essential for mucosal host defense against oral candidiasis. J Exp Med. 2009;206(2):299–311.

47. Hur J, Lee JH. A new enterotoxigenic escherichia coli vaccine candidate constructed using a *Salmonella* ghost delivery system: comparative evaluation with a commercial vaccine for neonatal piglet colibacillosis. Vet Immunol Immunopathol. 2015;164(3):101–9.

3

Humoral and cellular immune responses in mice against secreted and somatic antigens from a *Corynebacterium pseudotuberculosis* attenuated strain: Immune response against a *C. pseudotuberculosis* strain

Vera Lúcia Costa Vale[1,5*], Marcos da Costa Silva[4,5], Andréia Pacheco de Souza[5], Soraya Castro Trindade[3,5], Lília Ferreira de Moura-Costa[2], Ellen Karla Nobre dos Santos-Lima[5], Ivana Lucia de Oliveira Nascimento[2,5], Hugo Saba Pereira Cardoso[1], Edson de Jesus Marques[1], Bruno Jean Adrien Paule[5] and Roberto José Meyer Nascimento[2,5]

Abstract

Background: *Corynebacterium pseudotuberculosis* is the etiologic agent of caseous lymphadenitis (CL), a chronic disease that affects goats and sheep. CL is characterized by the formation of granulomas in lymph nodes and other organs, such as the lungs and liver. Current knowledge of CL pathogenesis indicates that the induction of humoral and cellular immune responses are fundamental to disease control. The aim of this study was to evaluate the humoral and cellular immune responses in BALB/c mice inoculated with a *C. pseudotuberculosis* strain isolated in the state of Bahia, Brazil.

Results: The lymphocyte proliferation and *in vitro* production of IFN-γ, IL-4, IL-10, IL-12 and nitric oxide by spleen cells stimulated with secreted and somatic antigens from the studied strain were evaluated. IgG subclasses were also analyzed. Results showed a significant increase of Th1-profile cytokines after 60 days post-inoculation, as well as an important humoral response, represented by high levels of IgG2a and IgG1 against *C. pseudotuberculosis*.

Conclusion: The T1 strain of *C. pseudotuberculosis* was shown to induce humoral and cellular immune responses in BALB/c mice, but, even at a dosage of 1×10^7 CFU, no signs of the disease were observed.

Keywords: *Corynebacterium pseudotuberculosis*, Cytokines, BALB/c, IgG isotypes

Abbreviations: CL, Caseous lymphadenitis; NO, Nitric oxide; OD, Optical density; Se, Secreted antigen; So, Somatic antigen.

* Correspondence: vvale@uneb.br
[1]Department of Exact and Earth Sciences, State University of Bahia, Campus II, Alagoinhas, BA CEP 48110-100, Brazil
[5]Immunology and Molecular Biology Laboratory, Health Sciences Institute, Federal University of Bahia, Av. Reitor Miguel Calmon s/n, Vale do Canela, Salvador, BA CEP 40110-100, Brazil
Full list of author information is available at the end of the article

Background

Caseous lymphadenitis (CL) is a chronic disease caused by *Corynebacterium pseudotuberculosis* that mainly affects small ruminants. Despite the economic [1, 2] and zoonotic [3] relevance of CL, a satisfactory vaccine model has not been developed [4, 5].

C. pseudotuberculosis is a facultative intracellular pathogen that can persist inside macrophages and stimulate the formation of granulomas [6, 7]. This species is distributed worldwide, but has the most severe economic impacts in Oceania, Africa and South America [8].

The pathogenesis of CL in mice was demonstrated by monitoring the progression of lesions in the skin and viscera of infected animals [9]. Moreover, the physiology, pathogenicity and virulence mechanisms of *C. pseudotuberculosis* strains have been elucidated using genomics [8, 10], transcriptomics and proteomics methodologies [11, 12].

The immune response against *C. pseudotuberculosis* has a well-known humoral component and involves a complex cellular mechanism against secreted and somatic bacterial antigens [13–15].

The cytokines Tumor necrosis factor-α (TNF-α) and interferon-γ (IFN-γ) are important to mount an immune response in mice as well as sheep, whether naturally infected or inoculated with *C. pseudotuberculosis* [16–19]. It is known that, with respect to *Mycobacterium tuberculosis*, a microorganism largely phylogenetically similar to *C. pseudotuberculosis*, these cytokines play a major role in susceptibility and regulation of associated lesions in mice [20].

El-Enbaawy *et al.* (2005) [21] demonstrated that antigens obtained from a *C. pseudotuberculosis* strain isolated from a naturally infected sheep, specifically a toxoid associated with bacterin, induce the production of IFN-γ, as well as elicit a humoral immune response in BALB/c mice. The present study employed a naturally attenuated strain of *C. pseudotuberculosis*, denominated T1, isolated from a granuloma taken from a goat in a rural region of the state of Bahia, located in northeastern Brazil. Studies previously conducted with this strain show that it grows quickly in BHI broth medium, when compared to other strains, but is incapable of inducing disease in goats [22–24].

The present study characterized the immune response in BALB/c mice, considering five animals per group, against antigens derived from the T1 strain of *C. pseudotuberculosis*. This murine model was chosen because of impaired IFN-γ production in response to antigens derived from *M. tuberculosis*, which is very closely related to *C. pseudotuberculosis* [25]. The proliferation of spleen cells was investigated, as well as the production of cytokines, nitric oxide (NO) and serum IgG subclasses to expand the understanding of humoral and cellular

immune responses against this strain, which may represent an ideal vaccine candidate against this disease.

Results

To determine the optimal inoculation dosage, four different infection dosages (5×10^5, 1×10^6, 5×10^6 and 1×10^7 CFU) of the T1 *C. pseudotuberculosis* strain were tested in BALB/c mice. ELISA results showed higher IgG levels in mice infected with the two higher dosages in comparison to the two lower levels tested ($P < 0.001$) (Fig. 1a). No significant differences in IgG levels were seen between the groups inoculated with 5×10^6 and 1×10^7 CFU, nor in the groups inoculated with 5×10^5 and 1×10^6 CFU. At 120 days post-infection, none of the animals presented any evidence of lesions characteristic of the disease under clinical examination or necropsy. Because the 1×10^7 CFU dosage was not observed to induce lesions, this experimental protocol was used to evaluate the production of IgG subclasses and cytokines.

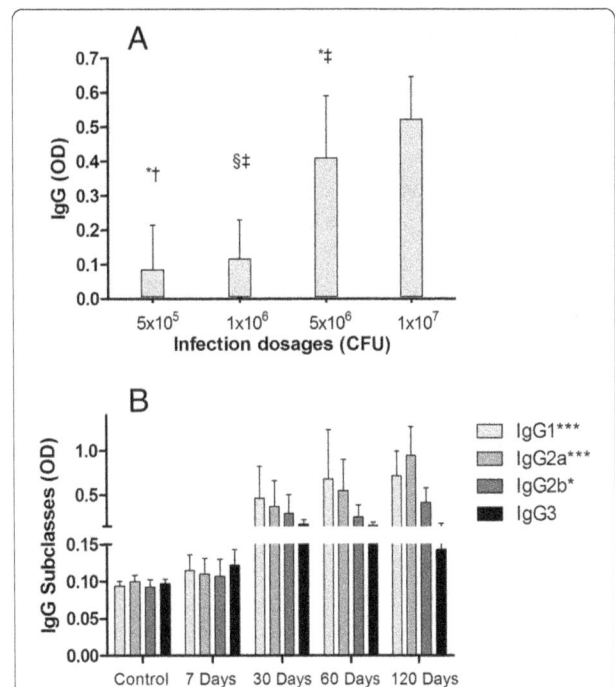

Fig. 1 Serum IgG immune response in mice inoculated with T1 *C. pseudotuberculosis* strain, as evaluated by ELISA. Graph represents means of Optical Density (OD) values found for each group ($n = 5$ animals for group). Results are representative of the mean values obtained from two experiments. **a.** BALB/c mice were inoculated with increasing dosages: 5×10^5, 1×10^6, 5×10^6 and 1×10^7 CFU. Blood was collected 120 days after inoculation. Data were analyzed by ANOVA and Tukey post-hoc tests; *, †, ‡ and § indicate pairs with statistically significant differences. **b.** IgG subclass (IgG1, IgG2a, IgG2b and IgG3) production throughout the course of the experiment: control (before infection), 7, 30, 60, and 120 days after infection. Mice were inoculated with 10^7 CFU of T1 strain of *C. pseudotuberculosis*. Data were analyzed by ANOVA. *$P < 0.05$; ***$P < 0.001$

Analysis of the humoral immune response against T1 *C. pseudotuberculosis* revealed that IgG2a production gradually increased over time, being the predominant IgG subclass at 120 days after infection ($P < 0.001$). A significant increase in IgG1 levels ($P < 0.001$) was also observed, and a discrete, yet still statistically significant, increase of IgG2b ($P < 0.05$) was seen. No statistically significant differences in IgG3 levels were detected over the course of experimentation. Control group results are representative of the mean OD readings obtained from five animals before infection (Fig. 1b).

With respect to spleen cell response to antigenic stimuli, a significant lymphoproliferative response, expressed as SI, was observed after stimulation with secreted antigen (Se) ($p < 0.05$) at 60 days post-infection in comparison to 7 and 30 days (Fig. 2). Stimulation with Se provoked a significant difference in SI in comparison to So at 60 days after inoculation.

In vitro production of interleukin-12 (IL-12) by spleen cells after stimulation with So or Se antigens is shown in Fig. 3a. Cell stimulated with both antigens had higher IL-12 concentrations at 60 and 120 days post-infection in comparison to controls ($p < 0.05$).

No differences were seen in IFN-γ concentration in the antigen-stimulated culture supernatants in comparison to controls at seven and 30 days post-infection, but there significant increases were observed at 60 days ($p < 0.05$) and 120 days ($p < 0.05$) post infection. So also induced a higher and statistical significant INF-γ production, when compared to Se stimulation (Fig. 3b) at both of these times points.

With respect to *in vitro* interleukin-10 (IL-10) production, a significant statistical difference was observed in So-stimulated cells at 60 days post-inoculation ($p < 0.05$) in comparison to the previous infection times, and also

in comparison to cells stimulated with Se at this same time point. A similar situation was observed at 120 days after inoculation (Fig. 3c). In addition, cells stimulated with So induced higher levels of IL-10 than Se throughout the experiment.

Interleukin-4 (IL-4) concentrations were very low at all experiment times evaluated with respect to both antigens. However, IL-4 production by cells stimulated with So was observed to significantly increase throughout the course of investigation ($p < 0.05$), but decreased at the 120 day time point (Fig. 3d).

Nitric oxide (NO) production measured in the supernatant of cell cultures stimulated So and Se is illustrated in Fig. 4. A significant increase ($p < 0.05$) in NO levels was seen only at 120 days post-infection in comparison to controls.

NO production by cells stimulated with So was also observed to be higher in comparison to Se, with statistical significance ($p < 0.05$) at 120 days after inoculation.

Discussion

The present study found that experimental inoculations of the attenuated T1 strain of *C. pseudotuberculosis* at a dosage of 10^7 CFU did not result in lesions in BALB/c mice, even though these animals have demonstrated susceptibility to intracellular pathogens [26, 27]. Nevertheless, a previous study has shown that a wild-type strain of *C. pseudotuberculosis* was able to induce lesions at a dosage of 10^2 [15].

In addition, cell cultures stimulated with T1 strain antigens were found to induce a proliferation of spleen cells, with secreted antigens (Se) demonstrating greater effectiveness than somatic antigens (So) two months after inoculation. A previous study showed that Se was able to enhance lymphocyte proliferation in PBMCs of an experimentally infected goat [23], which is consistent with our results. Se was found to induce a more intense proliferation than So due to the presence of phospholipase D, an exotoxin secreted by *C. pseudotuberculosis* at the beginning of infection to cleave the host cell membrane [28], which may cause a preeminent proliferation of B lymphocytes and elicit antibody production. Notably, lymphoproliferation in a murine model after stimulus with *C. pseudotuberculosis* antigens has not been described in the literature to date.

Experimental inoculation with T1 was observed to elicit high titers of IgG antibodies. The main IgG subclasses produced throughout the course of infection were IgG1 and IgG2a. As *C. pseudotuberculosis* is an intracellular pathogen that produces phospholipase D, an exotoxin with highly immunogenic properties [29, 30], the production of specific immunoglobulins is crucial to neutralize phospholipase D.

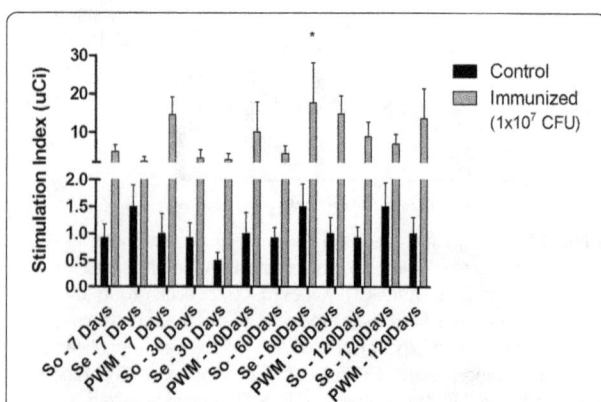

Fig. 2 Proliferation of murine spleen cells stimulated with somatic (So) and secreted (Se) antigens. Results express the stimulation index (μCi) calculated from two independent experiments using splenocytes retrieved from five non-infected (control) and five infected (inoculated) animals from each group. Data were analyzed by ANOVA and Tukey post-hoc tests; *$P < 0.05$

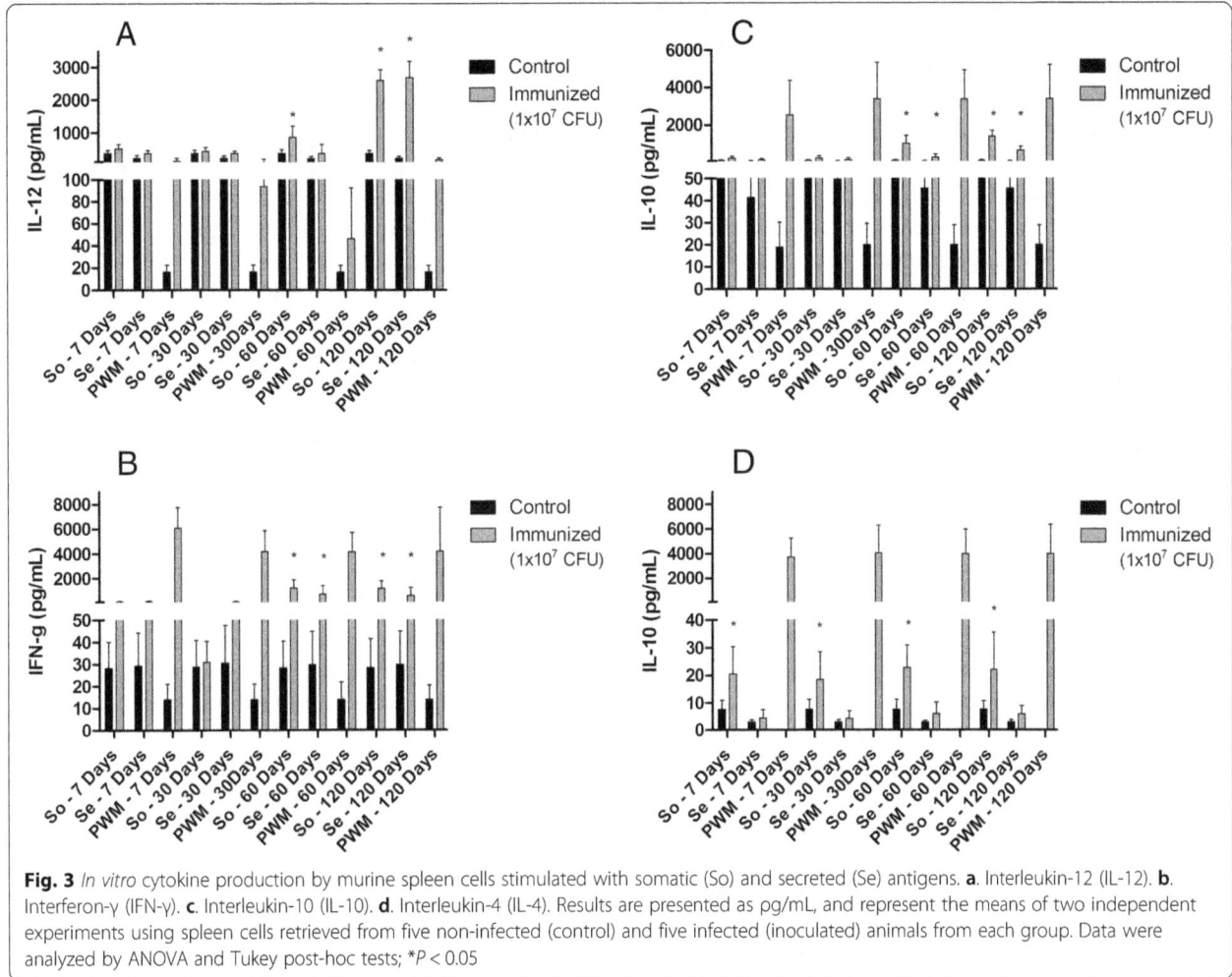

Fig. 3 *In vitro* cytokine production by murine spleen cells stimulated with somatic (So) and secreted (Se) antigens. **a**. Interleukin-12 (IL-12). **b**. Interferon-γ (IFN-γ). **c**. Interleukin-10 (IL-10). **d**. Interleukin-4 (IL-4). Results are presented as ρg/mL, and represent the means of two independent experiments using spleen cells retrieved from five non-infected (control) and five infected (inoculated) animals from each group. Data were analyzed by ANOVA and Tukey post-hoc tests; *$P < 0.05$

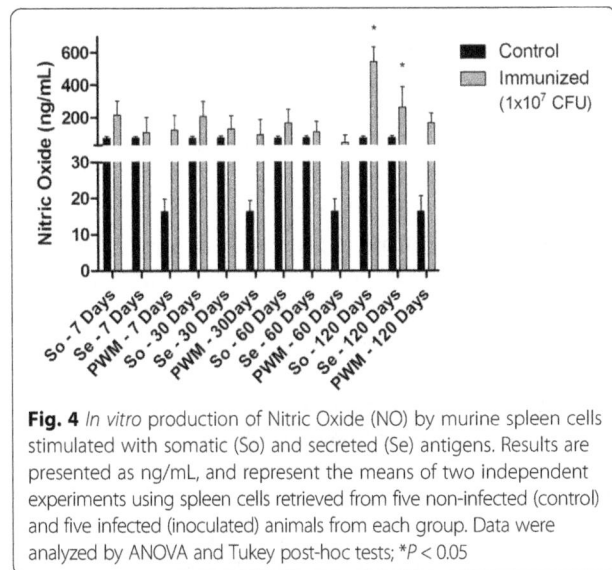

Fig. 4 *In vitro* production of Nitric Oxide (NO) by murine spleen cells stimulated with somatic (So) and secreted (Se) antigens. Results are presented as ng/mL, and represent the means of two independent experiments using spleen cells retrieved from five non-infected (control) and five infected (inoculated) animals from each group. Data were analyzed by ANOVA and Tukey post-hoc tests; *$P < 0.05$

In addition, the cellular immune response is another way of reducing the dissemination of the pathogen, which can survive and multiply inside macrophages [7, 14, 18]. Accordingly, we found a significant production of IFN-γ by spleen cells after stimulation with So or Se *C. pseudotuberculosis* antigens two months after inoculation. This situation was sustained until the end of the experiment (120 days). Elevated IL-4 production was not detected, yet, in cells stimulated with So, the production of this cytokine was four times higher in comparison to those stimulated with Se and controls. This phenomenon may possibly have occurred because So has a larger amount of structural proteins and lipid antigens than Se [31]. Relatedly, Lan *et al.* (1999) [19] found a pronounced increase in IFN-γ production starting in the third week post-inoculation in splenic cell cultures of ICR-JCL mice inoculated with ATCC 1940 strain and stimulated with formalin-killed bacterial cells, which was sustained until the eighth week. In the same experiment, no significant production of IL-4 was observed.

IL-10 and IL-12 production by spleen cells stimulated by Se or So antigens increased post-inoculation time and was sustained at all time points evaluated. So was found to induce higher levels of IL-10 than Se, probably due the structural components of So, such as cytoplasm and membrane lipoproteins [31].

IL-10 may control IFN-γ synthesis during infection, thereby avoiding Th1 over-reactivity [32]. On the other hand, IL-12 can also trigger mechanisms related to cell proliferation and IFN-γ production [33]. Some studies have showed that IFN-γ, IL-10 and IL-12 are required to control persistent infections caused by intracellular parasites [34–36]. IL-12 is a cytokine crucial to Th1 shift, which is required to prevent the dissemination of pathogens within the host in order to control infection by facultative intracellular bacteria, such as *C. pseudotuberculosis* [14]. Accordingly, we found increased IL-12 production after 60 days, probably resulting from an immune response to reduce bacterial proliferation. Higher levels of IL-12 were detected at 120 days for both So and Se antigens, probably due to the persistence of infection. It is possible that, after this time, these levels would decrease as a result of IL-10 production.

NO production was also evaluated, due to its effectiveness in regulating the growth of intracellular pathogens [37]. Proteomic analysis has identified NO-responsive extracellular proteins of *C. pseudotuberculosis* and it also demonstrated the participation of the extracytoplasmic function sigma factor σ^E in composition of *C. pseudotuberculosis* exoproteome [38]. In the present studt, while NO production by spleen cells stimulated with So and Se antigens was higher at 120 days post-infection, So resulted in higher proliferations than Se, in accordance to what was observed in IFN-γ and IL-10 production.

Conclusion

The attenuated T1 strain of *C. pseudotuberculosis* was found to induce both humoral and cellular immune responses in an experimental model of susceptible BALB/c mice. A 10^7 CFU dosage did not result in any lesions in the mice evaluated. As the present study has demonstrated that, in addition to the production of antibodies, an efficient cellular response is important to the control of CL, the T1 strain can be considered as a promising option for potential vaccine candidates.

Methods
Bacterial strain

The T1 strain of *C. pseudotuberculosis* was isolated from granulomas obtained from goats raised in the municipality of Juazeiro, located in the state of Bahia in northeastern Brazil. Isolates were stored in the Department of Microbiology collection center at the Health Sciences Institute of the Federal University of Bahia (ICS - UFBA).

The identification of the T1 strain was confirmed by several microbiological methods: Gram staining, colony morphology, synergistic hemolytic (CAMP) reactions with *Rhodococcus equi*, urease and catalase production, as well as glucose and maltose fermentation. A commercial kit was used to aid in identification (API Coryne - BioMérieux, Merci l'Etoile, France). Since the T1 strain demonstrated a less severe pattern of hemolysis during synergistic hemolysis testing in comparison to other wild strains, other authors have suggested its use as a vaccinal strain [39].

The T1 strain was cultivated in Brain/Heart Infusion (BHI) broth and incubated for 72 h at 37 °C. The bacterial suspension was washed in Phosphate Buffer Saline (PBS) and centrifuged for 30 min at 3,000 g at 4 ° C.

Somatic antigen (So)

The bacterial pellet was homogenized in PBS (pH 7.4) and sonicated at 60 Hz under 4 °C for five cycles lasting 60 s each (Branson Sonifier 450, Branson, Dunbury, CT, USA). The sample was centrifuged for 30 min at 10,000 g and, after collection, the supernatant was stored at -20 °C in aliquots until use. Protein concentration was determined by Lowry's modified method using a Bio-Rad Protein Assay (Bio-Rad, Hercules, CA, USA).

Secreted antigen (Se)

Se was obtained from the culture supernatant by saturation with 30 % ammonium sulfate (HCl) pH 4.0 and n-butanol under slow agitation at room temperature. The sample was homogenized, left undisturbed for 60 min, and then centrifuged for 10 min at 1,350 g under 4 ° C. The resulting interphase was dissolved in 20 mM of Tris buffer pH 7.4 (500 μL of buffer to 5 mL of culture supernatant), followed by dialysis in 50 mM Phosphate buffer pH 7.4 for 48 h. The sample was concentrated by ultrafiltration with a 10 kDa membrane (Millipore, Billerica, MA, USA). Protein concentration was determined by Lowry's modified method using a Bio-Rad Protein Assay (Bio-Rad, Hercules, CA, USA).

Inoculation protocol and experimental design

Prior to experimental inoculation, an optimal inoculation dose experiment was performed to obtain maximum antibody production. Eight-week-old male and female BALB/c mice, provided by the Experimental Animal Facility at the Gonçalo Moniz Research Center, Oswaldo Cruz Foundation, Salvador, Bahia-Brazil, were used to establish the inoculation protocol. The optimal dose was determined using five groups of five mice. Four groups received an intraperitoneal inoculation of $5\times10^5, 10^6, 5\times10^6$ and 10^7 colony forming units (CFU) of

C. pseudotuberculosis T1 strain diluted in sterile PBS at a final volume of 1 mL. The control group received 1 mL of sterile PBS by intraperitoneal inoculation. Blood was collected from the tail vein and the animals used for dosage experimentation were euthanized in a CO_2 chamber. ELISA was performed 120 days after inoculation to evaluate humoral immune response by identifying the highest levels of IgG and its subclasses.

After determining the optimal inoculation dosage, male and female BALB/c mice received intraperitoneal inoculations with 10^7 CFU/mL of T1 strain in 1 mL of sterile PBS, while the control group was inoculated with 1 mL of sterile PBS. After blood sampling from the tail vein, five animals from each group were euthanized in a CO_2 chamber at 7, 30, 60 and 120 days after receiving inoculation. The animals' spleens were removed for splenocyte isolation in order to perform *in vitro* lymphocyte proliferation and cytokine production assays. Blood was also collected for immunoglobulin analysis.

Indirect ELISA for analysis of IgG and its isotypes

ELISA plates (Costar, Corning Life Sciences, Lowell, MA, USA) were coated with So (1 µg in 100 µL of 50 mM Carbonate-bicarbonate buffer pH 9.6, in each well), incubated overnight at 4 °C and washed twice in 0.05 % PBS Tween-20 (PBS-T). Plates were then blocked with 200 µL of 5 % skim milk in 0.05 % PBS-T and incubated for 2 h at 37 °C. Next, the plates were washed once with PBS-T and 50 µL of diluted serum (1:50 in 1 % skim milk/PBS-T) was added to each well. Plates were then incubated for 1 h at 37 °C and washed five times with PBS-T. Next, wells were filled with 50 µL/well of HRP conjugated rabbit Ig antimouse IgG (Sigma-Aldrich, St Louis, MO, USA) at a dilution of 1:10,000 in 1 % skim milk/PBS-T to assess total IgG. To evaluate IgG1, IgG2a, IgG2b and IgG3, wells were filled with 50 µL/well of HRP conjugated rabbit Ig antimouse IgG1, IgG2a, IgG2b or IgG3 (Zymed, San Francisco, CA, USA), respectively, each diluted at 1:8.000 in 1 % skim milk/PBS-T. All plates were then incubated for 45 min at 37 °C. Each plate was washed five times in PBS-T and 50 µL/well of Citrate Phosphate Buffer pH 5.1, ortho-phenyl-diamine (Sigma, St Louis, MO, USA) and 30 % H_2O_2] were added and left for 15 min at room temperature in a dark chamber. Reactions were stopped with 25 µL/well of 4 N H_2SO_4 and Optical Density (OD) was measured at 490 nm using an ELISA Plate Reader (BIORAD, Hercules, CA, USA).

Lymphocyte proliferation assay

The spleen of each mouse was removed, washed three times with Hanks' solution, and then placed in a petri dish containing 5 mL of RPMI 1640 medium (Gibco Laboratories, North Andover, MA, USA) supplemented with penicillin and streptomycin. The spleens were then macerated and the cellular suspension was transferred to a conical tube containing 5 mL of the same medium, followed by centrifugation at 400 g for 3 min. Pellets were resuspended in 0.17 M of NH_4Cl for 5 min at 4 °C in order to lyse erythrocytes. Cells were washed 3 times with RPMI and then resuspended in RPMI enriched with 10 % bovine fetal serum.

Cell viability was determined by a Trypan Blue exclusion assay. 10^6 cells/mL were cultivated in 96-well microculture plates in RPMI-1640 medium supplemented with L-glutamine, penicillin/streptomycin, gentamicin and 10 % fetal calf serum. Cells were stimulated by So or Se *C. pseudotuberculosis* antigens (40 µg/mL), and pokeweed mitogen (2.5 µg/mL) was used as a positive control, while medium alone was used as a negative control. All plates were incubated for 120 h at 37° C under 5 % CO_2. 1 µBq/well (10 µL) of fresh [^{3}H] thymidine (GE Healthcare, Bucks, UK) was added 18 h prior to the end of the incubation time using a beta counter system (iMatic Canberra, Meriden, USA). After 120 h, plates were frozen at -20 °C and β-radiation was measured as described by Paule *et al.* (2004) [23]. Results are expressed in terms of a Stimulation Index (SI), calculated by dividing the β-radiation found for each stimulated sample by the radiation measured from its respective negative control.

ELISA for cytokines quantification

Cytokine analysis was performed in a culture supernatant obtained from cells (10^6/mL) cultivated in the same medium used for lymphoproliferation assay. Spleen cells were stimulated with So and Se *C. pseudotuberculosis* antigens (40 µg/mL), pokeweed mitogen (2,5 µg/mL) as a positive control, and the medium alone (negative control). The plates were incubated for 120 h at 37° C in 5 % CO_2 [40]. The supernatant was collected, centrifuged, and kept at -20° C until use.

Cytokine profile analysis was performed using commercial kits for IFN-γ and IL-10 (R&D Systems, Minneapolis, MN, USA), and IL-12 and IL-4 (Pharmigen, San Jose, CA, USA) according to the manufacturer instructions. Results are expressed in ρg/mL.

Nitric oxide (NO) production assay

The presence of NO in the supernatant of spleen cells cultures that were incubated for 120 h was measured by nitrite assay, based on Griess reaction [41]. Briefly, supernatant (50 µL) was mixed with 50 µL of Griess reagent (1 % sulfanilamide and 0.1 % N-(1-naphthyl)ethylenediamine, in 5 % phosphoric acid) and incubated for 10 min at room temperature. Absorbances were measured at 492 ηm using an ELISA microplate reader (BioRad, Hercules, CA, USA). The standard curve of NO_2^- was prepared by diluting nitrite stock solution (1 M $NaNO_2$

diluted in Milli-Q water) in spleen cell culture media. Results are expressed in ηg/mL.

Statistical analysis

For determination of statistical significance between experimental groups at an individual time-point, a analysis of variance (ANOVA) was performed using SPSS 12.0. (IBM Statistics, Chicago, EUA). A p value of <0.05 was considered significant.

Acknowledgements

Authors are sincerely grateful to the technical staff of the LABIMUNO/ICS for their assistance.

Funding

This study was supported by Laboratory of Immunology of Health Sciences Institute of Federal University of Bahia (Laboratório de Imunologia do Instituto de Ciências da Saúde da Universidade Federal da Bahia - LABIMUNO/ICS/UFBA) and by the Scientific and Technological Development Fund (Fundo de Desenvolvimento Científico e Tecnológico - FUNDECI) of Banco do Nordeste do Brasil S. A. (BNB).

Authors' contributions

MCS, APS and EJM carried out the immunoassays. HSPC and LFMC carried out the microbiological experiments. BJAP and SCT participated in the design of the study and performed the statistical analysis. EKNSL and ILON helped to draft the manuscript. VLCV and RJMN conceived of the study and participated in its design and coordination. All authors read and approved the final manuscript.

Competing interests

The authors declare that they have no competing interests.

Consent for publication

Not applicable.

Author details

[1]Department of Exact and Earth Sciences, State University of Bahia, Campus II, Alagoinhas, BA CEP 48110-100, Brazil. [2]Department of Biointeraction, Federal University of Bahia, Av. Reitor Miguel Calmon s/n, Vale do Canela, Salvador, BA CEP 40110-100, Brazil. [3]Department of Health, Feira de Santana State University, Avenida Transnordestina s/n, Novo Horizonte, Feira de Santana, BA CEP 44036-900, Brazil. [4]Department of Life Sciences, State University of Bahia, Rua Silveira Martins 2555, Cabula, Salvador, BA CEP 41150-000, Brazil. [5]Immunology and Molecular Biology Laboratory, Health Sciences Institute, Federal University of Bahia, Av. Reitor Miguel Calmon s/n, Vale do Canela, Salvador, BA CEP 40110-100, Brazil.

References

1. Unanian MM, Feliciano Silva AE, Pant KP. Abscesses and caseous lymphadenitis in goats in tropical semi-arid north-east Brazil. Trop Anim Health Prod. 1985;17:57–62.
2. Guimarães AS, Carmo FB, Heinemann MB, Portela RW, Meyer R, Lage AP, et al. High sero-prevalence of caseous lymphadenitis identified in slaughterhouse samples as a consequence of deficiencies in sheep farm management in the state of Minas Gerais, Brazil. BMC Vet Res. 2011;7:68.
3. Bastos BL, Dias Portela RW, Dorella FA, Ribeiro D, Seyffert N, Castro TLP, et al. Corynebacterium pseudotuberculosis: immunological responses in
4. Costa MP, McCulloch JA, Almeida SS, Dorella FA, Fonseca CT, Oliveira DM, et al. Molecular characterization of the Corynebacterium pseudotuberculosis hsp60-hsp10 operon, and evaluation of the immune response and protective efficacy induced by hsp60 DNA vaccination in mice. BMC Res Notes. 2011;4:243.
5. Bastos BL, Loureiro D, Raynal JT, Guedes MT, Vale VL, Moura-Costa LF, et al. Association between haptoglobin and IgM levels and the clinical progression of caseous lymphadenitis in sheep. BMC Vet Res. 2013;9:254.
6. Batey RG. Pathogenesis of caseous lymphadenitis in sheep and goats. Aust Vet J. 1986;63:269–72.
7. McKean S, Davies J, Moore R. Identification of macrophage induced genes of Corynebacterium pseudotuberculosis by differential fluorescence induction. Microbes Infect. 2005;7:1352–63.
8. Ruiz JC, D'Afonseca V, Silva A, Ali A, Pinto AC, Santos AR, et al. Evidence for reductive genome evolution and lateral acquisition of virulence functions in two Corynebacterium pseudotuberculosisstrains. PLoS ONE. 2011;6:e18551.
9. Batey RG. Aspects of pathogenesis in a mouse model of infection by Corynebacterium pseudotuberculosis. Aust J Exp Biol Med Sci. 1986;64:237–49.
10. Soares SC, Silva A, Trost E, Blom J, Ramos R, Carneiro A, et al. The pan-genome of the animal pathogen Corynebacterium pseudotuberculosis reveals differences in genome plasticity between the biovar ovis and equi strains. PLoS ONE. 2013;8:e53818.
11. Pacheco LGC, Slade SE, Seyffert N, Santos AR, Castro TLP, Silva WM, et al. A combined approach for comparative exoproteome analysis of Corynebacterium pseudotuberculosis. BMC Microbiol. 2011;11:12.
12. Dorella FA, Gala-Garcia A, Pinto AC, Sarrouh B, Antunes CA, Ribeiro D, et al. Progression of "OMICS" methodologies for understanding the pathogenicity of Corynebacterium pseudotuberculosis: the Brazilian experience. Comput Struct Biotechnol J. 2013;6:e201303013.
13. Cameron CM, Engelbrecht MM. Mechanism of immunity to Corynebacterium pseudotuberculosis (Buchanan, 1911) in mice using inactivated vaccine. Onderstepoort J Vet Res. 1971;38:73–82.
14. Pépin M, Seow HF, Corner L, Rothel JS, Hodgson AL, Wood PR. Cytokine gene expression in sheep following experimental infection with various strains of Corynebacterium pseudotuberculosis differing in virulence. Vet Res. 1997;28:149–63.
15. de Souza AP, Vale VLC, Silva MC, Araújo IBO, Trindade SC, Moura-Costa LF, et al. MAPK involvement in cytokine production in response to Corynebacterium pseudotuberculosis infection. BMC Microbiol. 2014;14:230.
16. Ellis JA, Lairmore MD, Otoole D, Campos M. Differential induction of Tumor Necrosis Factor Alpha in ovine pulmonary alveolar macrophages following infection with Corynebacterium pseudotuberculosis, Pasteurella haemolytica, or Lentiviruses. Infect Immun. 1991;59:3254–60.
17. Ellis JA, Russell HI, Du CW. Effect of selected cytokines on the replication of Corynebacteriurn pseudotuberculosis and ovine lentiviruses in pulmonary macrophages. Vet Immunol Immunopathol. 1994;40:31–47.
18. Lan DT, Taniguhi S, Makino S, Shirahata N, Nakane A. Role of endogenous Tumor Necrosis Factor Alpha and Gamma Interferon in resistance to Corynebacterium pseudotuberculosis infection in mice. Microbiol Immunol. 1998;42:863–70.
19. Lan DT, Makino SI, Shirahata T, Yamada M, Nakane A. Tumor necrosis factor alpha and gama interferon are required for the development of protective immunity to secondary Corynebacterium pseudotuberculosis infection in mice. J Vet Med Sci. 1999;11:1203–8.
20. Flynn JL, Chan J, Triebold KJ, Dalton DK, Stewart TA, Bloom BR. An essential role for Interferon gamma in resistance to Mycobacterium tuberculosis infection. J Exp Med. 1993;178:2249–54.
21. El-Enbaawy MI, Saad MM, Selim SA. Humoral and cellular immune responses of a murine model against Corynebacterium pseudotuberculosis antigens. Egypt J Immunol. 2005;12:13–9.
22. Paule BJ, Azevedo V, Regis LF, Carminati R, Bahia CR, Vale VL, et al. Experimental Corynebacterium pseudotuberculosis primary infection in goats: kinetics of IgG and interferon-gamma production, IgG avidity and antigen recognition by Western blotting. Vet Immunol Immunopathol. 2003;96:129–39.
23. Paule BJ, Meyer R, Moura-Costa LF, Bahia RC, Carminati R, Regis LF, et al. Three-phase partitioning as an efficient method for extraction / concentration of immunoreactive excreted-secreted proteins of Corynebacterium pseudotuberculosis. Protein Expr Purif. 2004;34:311–16. A.
24. Meyer R, Regis L, Vale V, Paule B, Carminati R, Bahia R, et al. In vitro IFN-gamma production by goat blood cells after stimulation with somatic and

(animal models and zoonotic potential. J Clin Cell Immunol. 2012;S4:005.)

secreted *Corynebacterium pseudotuberculosis* antigens. Vet Immunol Immunopathol. 2005;107:249–54.

25. Huygen K, Palfliet K. Strain variation in interferon gamma production of BCG-sensitized mice challenged with PPD II. Importance of one major autosomal locus and additional sexual influences. Cell Immunol. 1984;85:75–81.

26. Oswald IP, Afroun S, Bray D, Petit JF, Lemaire G. Low response of BALB/c macrophages to priming and activating signals. J Leukoc Biol. 1992;52:315–22.

27. Tumitan AR, Monnazzi LG, Ghiraldi FR, Cilli EM. Machado de Medeiros BM. Pattern of macrophage activation in yersinia-resistant and yersinia-susceptible strains of mice. Microbiol Immunol. 2007;51:1021–8.

28. Muckle CA, Menzies PI, Li Y, Hwang YT, van Wesenbeeck M. Analysis of the immunodominant antigens of *Corynebacterium pseudotuberculosis*. Vet Microbiol. 1992;30:47–58.

29. Eggleton DG, Haynes JA, Middleton HD, Cox JC. Immunisation against ovine caseous lymphadenitis: correlation between *Corynebacterium pseudotuberculosis* toxoid content and protective efficacy in combined clostridial-corynebacterial vaccines. Aust Vet J. 1991;68:322–5.

30. Hodgson AL, Tachedjian M, Corner LA, Radford AJ. Protection of sheep against caseous lymphadenitis by use of a single oral dose of live recombinant *Corynebacterium pseudotuberculosis*. Infect Immun. 1994;62:5275–80.

31. Paule BJA, Azevedo V, Moura-Costa LF, Freire SM, Regis LF, Vale VLC, et al. SDS-PAGE and Western blot analysis of somatic and extracellular antigens of *Corynebacterium pseudotuberculosis*. Rev Ciênc Méd Biol. 2004;3:44–52.

32. Pestka S, Krause CD, Sarkar D, Walter MR, Shi Y, Fisher PB. Interleukin-10 and related cytokines and receptors. Annu Rev Immunol. 2004;22:929–79.

33. Trinchieri G, Scott P. Interleukin-12: a proinflammatory cytokine with immunoregulatory functions. Res Immunol. 1995;146:423–31.

34. Pohl-Koppe A, Balashov KE, Steere AC, Logigian EL, Hafler DA. Identification of a T cell subset capable of both IFN-γ and IL-10 secretion in patients with chronic *Borrelia burgdorferi* infection. J Immunol. 1998;160:1804–10.

35. Trinchieri G. Regulatory role of T cells producing both interferon gamma and interleukin 10 in persistent infection. J Exp Med. 2001;194:F53–7.

36. Fortune SM, Solache A, Jaeger A, Hill PJ, Belisle JT, Bloom BR, et al. *Mycobacterium tuberculosis* inhibits macrophage responses to IFN-γ through myeloid differentiation factor 88-dependent and -independent mechanisms. J Immunol. 2004;172:6272–80.

37. Green SJ, Nacy CA, Meltzer MS. Cytokine-induced synthesis of nitrogen oxides in macrophages: a protective host response to Leishmania and other intracellular pathogens. J Leukoc Biol. 1991;50:93–103.

38. Pacheco LGC, Castro TLP, Carvalho RD, Moraes PM, Dorella FA, Carvalho NB, et al. A role for sigma factor σ^E in *Corynebacterium pseudotuberculosis* resistance to nitric oxide / peroxide stress. Front Microbiol. 2012;3:126.

39. Moura-Costa LF, Bahia RC, Carminati R, Vale VL, Paule BJ, Portela RW, et al. Evaluation of the humoral and cellular immune response to different antigens of *Corynebacterium pseudotuberculosis* in Canindé goats and their potential protection against caseous lymphadenitis. Vet Immunol Immunopathol. 2008;126:131–41.

40. Salas-Téllez E, Núñez del Arco A, Tenorio V, Díaz-Aparicio E, de la Garza M, Suárez-Güemes F. Subcellular fractions of *Brucella ovis* distinctively induce the production of interleukin-2, interleukin-4, and interferon-gamma in mice. Can J Vet Res. 2005;69:53–7.

41. Green LC, Wagner DA, Glogowski J, Skipper PL, Wishnok JS, Tannenbaun SR. Analysis of nitrite and (^{15}N) nitrate in biological fluids. Anal Biochem. 1982;126:131–8.

4

Effectiveness of regionally-specific immunotherapy for the management of canine atopic dermatitis

Jon D. Plant[1*] and Moni B. Neradilek[2]

Abstract

Background: Canine atopic dermatitis is a common pruritic skin disease often treated with allergen immunotherapy (AIT). AIT in dogs traditionally begins with attempting to identify clinically relevant environmental allergens. Current allergen testing methodologies and immunotherapy techniques in dogs are not standardized. Immunotherapy with a mixture of allergenic extracts selected based on regional aerobiology rather than intradermal tests or serum IgE assays has been described. The objective of this study was to evaluate the effectiveness of regionally-specific immunotherapy in dogs with atopic dermatitis. The medical records of a veterinary dermatology referral clinic were searched for dogs with atopic dermatitis that began regionally-specific subcutaneous immunotherapy from June, 2010 to May, 2013. An overall assessment of treatment effectiveness (excellent, good, fair, or poor) was assigned based upon changes in pruritus severity, lesion severity, and the reduction in concurrent medication(s) during a follow-up period of at least 270 days. Baseline characteristics that might predict treatment success were analyzed with the Spearman's correlation and the Kruskal-Wallis tests.

Results: Of the 286 dogs that began regionally-specific immunotherapy (RESPIT) during a 3 year period, 103 met the inclusion criteria. The overall response to RESPIT was classified as excellent in 19%, good in 38%, fair in 25%, and poor in 18% of dogs. The response classification correlated significantly with a reduction in pruritus severity ($r = 0.72$, $p < 0.001$) and lesion severity ($r = 0.54$, $p < 0.001$), but not with the dogs' baseline characteristics. Adverse reactions were reported in 7/286 (2.4%) of treated dogs.

Conclusions: Under the conditions of this study, RESPIT was safe and effective for the treatment of atopic dermatitis in dogs.

Keywords: Dog, Atopic dermatitis, Regionally-specific immunotherapy, RESPIT, Allergen, Immunotherapy, Pruritus

Background

Canine atopic dermatitis (AD) is a common inflammatory and pruritic skin disease that is frequently associated with sensitization to environmental allergens [1]. Affected dogs often exhibit pruritus of the face, pinnae, feet, axillae, and inguinal region [2]. Secondary otitis externa, staphylococcal pyoderma and *Malassezia* dermatitis frequently develop in atopic dogs.

Canine AD often requires long-term management and therapy [1]. There is substantial evidence to support the use of glucocorticoids, cyclosporine, oclacitinib, and allergen immunotherapy (AIT) for canine AD [3]. With AIT, dogs are given allergenic extracts in order to minimize flares upon subsequent natural exposure [4]. The mechanism of action of AIT is not well defined in dogs, but may include the production of blocking IgG antibodies, a shift in the cytokine balance from a predominantly T-helper (Th) 2 to a Th1 cell profile, and a regulatory T-cell response [5, 6]. Therapeutic allergens are identified through a combination of aerobiology, intradermal test (IDT) findings, serum allergen-specific IgE assays (SIA), and clinical history [2]. Allergenic extracts are administered either by subcutaneous injection or via application to the oral mucosa [3].

Allergen immunotherapy prescriptions are customized for each dog. An optimal allergenic extract mixture would

* Correspondence: jon.plant@skinvetclinic.com
[1]SkinVet Clinic, 15800 Upper Boones Ferry Road, Suite 120, Lake Oswego 97035, OR, USA
Full list of author information is available at the end of the article

contain only allergens that elicit clinical signs upon natural exposure. However, customizing an allergenic extract involves multiple subjective variables. Veterinarians choose which allergens to test for, whether to test with IDT or SIA, which laboratory's SIA to use, how to interpret borderline reactions, which positive reactions are deemed clinically relevant, what dose of each allergen to include in the ASIT prescription, and by what schedule and route it will be administered. These variables are not trivial. Within a geographic region, the allergens veterinary dermatologists evaluate with IDT vary substantially [7], as do the allergens assayed by different laboratories offering SIA [8]. The agreement between IDT and SIA findings is often poor [2]. False positive and false negative results occur with both testing methods [1]. Recently, Plant et al. found poor agreement between four SIAs, indicating that the choice of laboratories is likely to influence treatment recommendations [9]. Once allergens are selected for inclusion, the optimal dose of each is unknown in veterinary medicine. Allergen immunotherapy may, therefore, be considered a heterogeneous therapy.

Although subject to the variables described above, AIT has been found to be effective for the management of canine AD in one placebo-controlled and multiple retrospective studies [5]. Results from these studies are difficult to compare directly because they report different outcome measures, but those that defined effectiveness as a greater than 50% reduction in pruritus and lesion severity found AIT to be effective in 52–77% of dogs [5]. In most of these studies, the response to AIT was independent of the testing method, the age of onset of AD, the age at which AIT was begun, and the duration of disease prior to AIT. Mixed findings have been reported concerning the correlation of treatment success with breed, gender, and the seasonality of signs [5].

An alternative to AIT is RESPIT, allergenic extract mixtures that are formulated based on a dog's geographic location rather than individual allergy test findings. Reports on the use of non-specific AIT mixtures in dogs or humans are limited [10–12]. The aim of this study was to evaluate the effectiveness of subcutaneous RESPIT for the treatment of atopic dermatitis in 103 dogs that began therapy during a 3-year period at a veterinary dermatology clinic in the northwestern United States.

Methods

The electronic medical records (Vetport, Vetport, LLC, Milford, OH, USA) of a veterinary dermatology clinic were searched for dogs with AD for which RESPIT (RESPIT® Injectable Region 1, Respit, LLC, Lake Oswego, OR, USA) was prescribed on the same date as an initial examination between June 1, 2010 and May 31, 2013. The diagnosis of AD was made based on identifying characteristic clinical features and ruling out alternative diagnoses [13].

The following history and examination findings from the initial encounter on day 0 (D0) were exported to a spreadsheet: patient identification, date of birth, gender, breed, weight, encounter date, pruritus visual analogue scale (PVAS) [14], seasonality of signs, current medications, and lesion severity. Lesion severity was recorded with an ad hoc canine lesion severity index (LSI) with a range from 0 to 1000 (the product of lesion severity graded from 0 to 10 and estimated percent body area affected). Dogs without a D0 PVAS entry were excluded from analysis. The records of the remaining dogs were reviewed to identify those that returned for an examination after receiving RESPIT for at least 270 days. Nine to twelve months is often the duration of therapy recommended to evaluate the response to AIT in dogs [15, 16]. The date of the first examination following 270 days of RESPIT therapy (designated D270+) was recorded and the following data were further extracted from the medical records: D270+ PVAS, D270+ LSI, D270+ concurrent medication(s), and adverse reactions suspected by the pet owner. The last date that RESPIT was dispensed before July 15, 2015 was also recorded.

On the basis of the changes in the dogs' PVAS, LSI, and those concomitant systemic medications with substantial evidence of efficacy (glucocorticoids, cyclosporine, or oclacitinib) between D0 and D270+, an overall assessment score was assigned by the primary investigator as follows: 1 (poor) = no clinical change or a deterioration, 2 (fair) = improvement, but concurrent medications could not be substantially decreased, 3 (good) = greater than 50% improvement in clinical signs and reduction in medications, 4 (excellent) = complete remission without concurrent medications [17]. The percentages of dogs with D270+ PVAS in the normal (<2.0) and mild (2.0–3.5) ranges were determined.

All statistical analyses were carried out in the statistical software R: A Language and Environment for Statistical Computing (R Foundation for Statistical Computing, Vienna, Austria) version 3.1.3. Continuous and categorical characteristics were analyzed with Spearman's correlation and the Kruskal-Wallis test, respectively. A P-value of <0.05 was considered statistically significant. Trends in bivariate relationships were highlighted by local regression trend lines [18].

Results

During a 3 year period, 286 dogs with AD began RESPIT on the day of an initial examination during which the pruritus severity was recorded. Of these dogs, 103 (36%) returned for an examination after 270 days while still receiving RESPIT, thereby meeting the inclusion criteria. Most commonly, dogs were excluded due to poor compliance. Eighty-five dogs received only the initial prescription of RESPIT, an insufficient volume to last 270 days. Three of these dogs transitioned to an oromucosal formulation of RESPIT. Fifty-five dogs had their prescriptions renewed for the last time before day 200 and likely did not receive a volume sufficient to reach D270+. These 55 dogs were not examined after D270 while receiving subcutaneous RESPIT. Two of these dogs also transitioned to the oromucosal formulation of RESPIT. D270+ examinations while receiving RESPIT were not performed for 39 dogs that did have RESPIT prescriptions renewed after day 200. Four additional dogs had lengthy (7 month to 4 year) lapses in therapy before the D270+ examinations. The D0 baseline characteristics (age, weight, gender, seasonality of signs, PVAS, and LSI) of the included ($n = 103$) and excluded ($n = 183$) dogs were not significantly different ($p > 0.05$).

The overall response to RESPIT was scored as excellent in 19%, good in 38%, fair in 25%, and poor in 18% of dogs. The percentages of dogs with normal or mild pruritus at D270+ were 20 and 25%, respectively. The mean duration of therapy evaluated was 424 days (median 365, range 273–1735 days). D0 age ($r = 0.06$, $p = 0.5$), weight ($r = -0.03$, $p = 0.7$), gender ($p = 0.2$), pruritus severity ($r = 0.09$, $p = 0.4$), lesion severity ($r = 0.10$, $p = 0.3$), seasonal history ($p = 0.2$), and the calendar month of the D270+ examination ($p = 0.8$, Fig. 1) did not correlate significantly with the response classification. The number of dogs assigned to each response classification per 30-day period following D270+ is depicted in Fig. 2. Ninety percent of dogs scored as excellent and 33% of dogs scored as good were not receiving antipruritic medications at the time of the D270+ examination (Table 1). One dog scored as excellent was receiving occasional oral diphenhydramine and a second infrequent topical fluocinonide cream.

The response classification at D270+ significantly correlated with a reduction in pruritus severity (Fig. 3, $r = 0.72$, $p < 0.001$), a reduction in lesion severity (Fig. 4, $r = 0.54$, $p < 0.001$), the duration of therapy to D270+ ($r = 0.24$, $p = 0.02$)

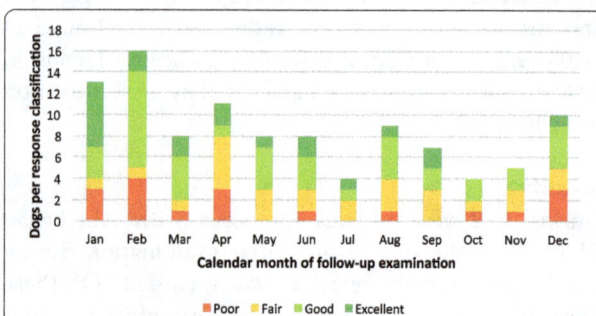

Fig. 2 Effectiveness of regionally-specific immunotherapy by duration of treatment in 97 atopic dogs. Dogs with follow-up examinations beyond 21 months (2 classified as excellent, 2 as good, and 2 as fair) are not depicted

and the total duration of therapy as of the date of the data retrieval ($r = 0.40$, $p < 0.001$).

No adverse reactions to RESPIT were reported in the 103 evaluable dogs meeting the inclusion criteria. Seven of 286 dogs initially screened (2.4%) were suspected by pet owners to have experienced adverse reactions to RESPIT, including three with increased pruritus, and one each with vomiting, blepharitis, restlessness, or urticaria. In 5/7 dogs the dose was decreased and RESPIT was continued. In one dog with increased pruritus during the induction phase, RESPIT was temporarily discontinued then resumed 1 month later following the induction schedule up to a lower maintenance dose. In the dog that reportedly developed hives after two injections, RESPIT was discontinued by the owner and the dog was lost to follow up.

Discussion

In this study, 59/103 dogs (57%) had good or excellent responses to RESPIT. Similar rates have been reported in studies evaluating AIT effectiveness [5, 15–17, 19, 20]. Therapeutic extracts are likely to be imperfectly matched with dogs' actual sensitivity with both AIT and RESPIT, perhaps accounting for the similarity in response rates.

The efficacy of immunotherapy using uniform allergen mixtures has been evaluated in two randomized controlled trials in atopic dogs, both reported only in abstract form with limited details or analysis [10, 11]. In a 12-month study of 78 dogs, Garfield found a 76% good to excellent response (>51% resolution of pruritus) to a uniform mixture of 32 aqueous allergens [10]. This was not significantly different from the response of those dogs that received either of two doses of AIT based on IDT findings. In contrast are the findings of an 8-month trial of 30 dogs in which a uniform mixture of four alum-precipitated allergens (house dust, dog dander, human dander, and grass mix) was compared to AIT.

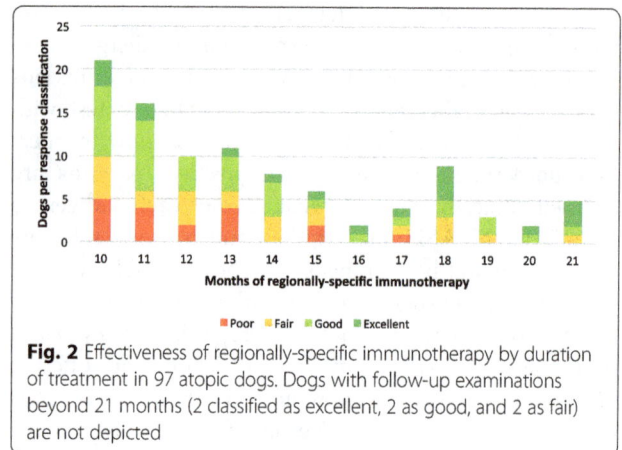

Fig. 1 Effectiveness of regionally-specific immunotherapy by calendar month of follow-up examination in 103 dogs with atopic dermatitis

Table 1 Number of dogs per response classification receiving concomitant anti-pruritic medications with RESPIT at D270+

Concomitant anti-pruritic medication	Poor $n = 18$	Fair $n = 26$	Good $n = 39$	Excellent $n = 20$
None	4 (22%)	6 (23%)	13 (33%)	18 (90%)
Oral glucocorticoid	7 (39%)	10 (38%)	17 (44%)	0 (0%)
Cyclosporine	4 (22%)	7 (27%)	7 (18%)	0 (0%)
Oclacitinib	0 (0%)	0 (0%)	2 (5%)	0 (0%)
Antihistamine	3 (17%)	5 (19%)	1 (3%)	1 (5%)
Topical glucocorticoid, including otic	1 (6%)	1 (4%)	0 (0%)	1 (5%)

5/103 dogs were receiving two classes of medications

The median improvement in clinical scores (pruritus and lesion severity) was 70% in the AIT group and 18% in the group that received the uniform mixture of allergens [11]. The discrepancy in response rates between the latter study versus those of Garfield and the present study may reflect differences in the number or type of allergens in the uniform mixtures and their formulations (alum-precipitated vs. aqueous).

Beneficial effects of immunotherapy with imperfectly matched or unrelated allergens have also been reported in cats and humans [12, 21, 22]. In a feline asthma model, eosinophilic airway inflammation responded to AIT with allergens matched to experimental sensitization, but also to immunotherapy with imperfectly matched or unrelated allergens [21]. Cats dually sensitized to both Bermuda

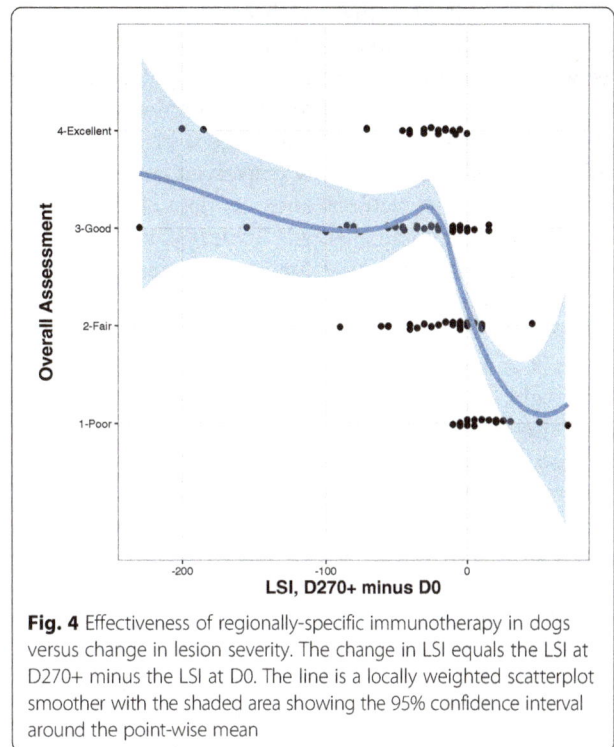

Fig. 4 Effectiveness of regionally-specific immunotherapy in dogs versus change in lesion severity. The change in LSI equals the LSI at D270+ minus the LSI at D0. The line is a locally weighted scatterplot smoother with the shaded area showing the 95% confidence interval around the point-wise mean

grass allergen and house dust mite given AIT to either allergen displayed decreased eosinophilic airway inflammation and higher levels of CD4+ CD25+ FoxP3+ Treg cells compared to placebo-treated cats. Differences were found in the immunological responses of cats given sensitivity-matched allergens versus those given unrelated allergens. Cats monosenesitized to Bermuda grass allergen displayed evidence of lymphocyte hypoproliferation during immunotherapy with Bermuda grass allergen, whereas Bermuda grass sensitized cats displayed lymphocyte hyperproliferation with house dust mite immunotherapy. The authors concluded that sensitizing allergens and those used in AIT need not be identically matched in order to provide a clinical benefit. Analogous findings have been reported in humans sensitive to both birch and grass pollen [22]. Sublingual immunotherapy with either birch or grass pollen led to clinical improvement and lower nasal eosinophil counts during both pollen seasons, although the improvement was greater when both were given.

Whereas perfectly matching an atopic dog's clinical sensitivity is the objective of AIT, the mechanism of action of RESPIT may be both allergen-specific and non-specific. Phylogenetically related allergens frequently cross react on IDT in atopic dogs [23]. About 30 major groups of cross-reactive botanical proteins have been identified [24]. The RESPIT extract used in this study contained 20 allergens representing a spectrum of botanically related allergen groups and house dust mites.

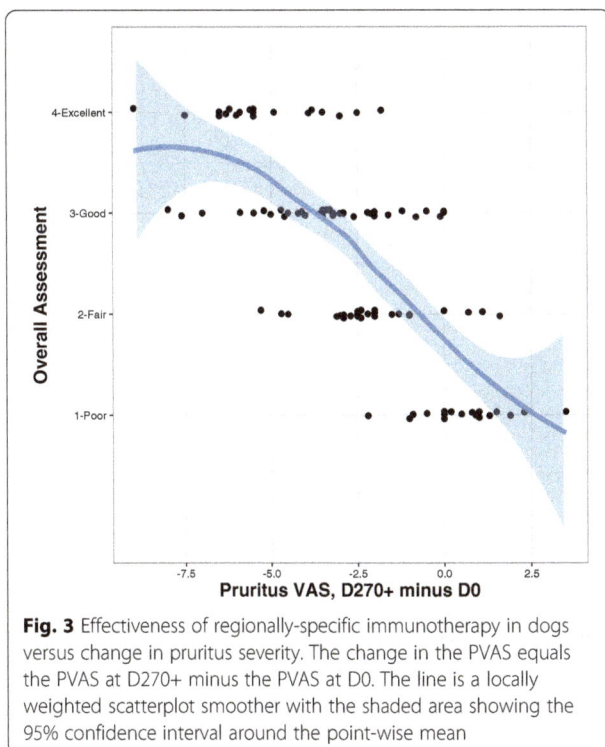

Fig. 3 Effectiveness of regionally-specific immunotherapy in dogs versus change in pruritus severity. The change in the PVAS equals the PVAS at D270+ minus the PVAS at D0. The line is a locally weighted scatterplot smoother with the shaded area showing the 95% confidence interval around the point-wise mean

RESPIT may imperfectly match an atopic dog's actual sensitivities, but include some allergen-specific epitopes as well as panallergens (e.g. profilins, polcalcins, and non-specific lipid transfer proteins) common to distinct allergen groups. Although panallergens are widely distributed in nature with highly conserved amino acid sequence regions, structures, and functions, their clinical significance in human allergy is unclear [24, 25].

In the present study, the median duration of therapy at the time of the D270+ evaluation was 12 months and the majority of D270+ evaluations (74/103) occurred between 9 and 15 months after beginning RESPIT (Fig. 2). The slight correlation between the days until D270+ and response classification, and the moderate correlation between the total length of therapy and response classification at D270+ likely reflect pet owners' higher level of compliance when satisfied with their dogs' response. The calendar month during which D270+ evaluations took place did not correlate with the response to RESPIT (Fig. 1). Taken together, these findings suggest that the possible confounding variable of seasonality did not account for the clinical improvement detected in this study.

Similar to a number of retrospective studies of AIT in atopic dogs [5], these results suggest that a dog's response to RESPIT cannot be predicted from their age, weight, gender, or from the seasonality of their signs. The relatively low number of dogs of any given breed did not allow for rigorous analysis of the possible correlation of breed and response classification. Neither D0 pruritus severity nor lesion severity significantly correlated with the response classification. The dataset did not allow for precise reporting of the duration of clinical signs prior to RESPIT therapy.

For many pet owners, pruritus is the most important burden of canine atopic dermatitis [26]. Pruritus severity was scored with the validated visual analog scale [10], however, lesion severity was scored with an ad hoc scale (LSI). The third iteration of the canine atopic dermatitis extent and severity index, the only validated lesion severity scale available when the data collection began, was not practical for routine use in a clinical setting [27].

Immunotherapy with irrelevant allergens could, in theory, lead to the development of clinical sensitivity. This outcome may occur with either RESPIT or AIT with imperfectly matched allergens. However, this study found that the prevalence of adverse reactions to RESPIT (2.4%) was at the low end of the wide range reported for AIT (5–50%) [4, 5]. In a small study, immunotherapy with irrelevant allergens did not lead to the development of clinical signs of atopic dermatitis in normal dogs [28].

In children with rhinitis or asthma who are sensitive to house dust mite, AIT may have a tolerogenic effect, preventing the sensitization to additional allergens by inducing a shift from a T_H2 to a T_H1 allergen response

[29]. Irrelevant allergens that are prescribed in either AIT or RESPIT may also confer some degree of non-specific allergen tolerance. This could explain, in part, why the reported success rates of AIT are similar when utilizing a variety of allergy testing techniques and assays that exhibit poor agreement with one another [9].

A limitation of this study was the open, retrospective design, similar to most studies on the effectiveness of AIT [5]. A placebo-controlled trial could provide a higher level of evidence concerning the efficacy of immunotherapy, but may suffer from a high rate of non-compliance during a long-term study. Forty-three percent of dogs were lost to follow up by 12 months in the prospective study of AIT by Willemse [16]. A second limitation of our study was that only 36% of the dogs initially identified met the inclusion criteria, which required a follow-up examination after 270 days of therapy. In the current study, dogs that continued to receive RESPIT prescribed by their primary care veterinarian but did not return for the D270+ examination were excluded. Allowing telephone interviews for follow-up, as have some retrospective studies of AIT [15, 20], may have resulted in excluding fewer dogs, but would not have allowed for consistent scoring of pruritus and lesion severity.

Conclusion

This retrospective study suggests that subcutaneous RESPIT is a safe and effective alternative to AIT in atopic dogs with the advantage of avoiding the subjectivity involved in allergy testing and AIT formulation.

Abbreviations

AD: Atopic dermatitis; AIT: Allergen immunotherapy; D0: Day 0; D270+: Days from the initial examination to the first examination to occur at least 270 days later; IDT: Intradermal test; LSI: Canine lesion severity index (an ad hoc 0–1000 scale equal to the product of lesion severity graded from 0 to 10 and the estimated percent body area affected); PVAS: Pruritus visual analogue scale; RESPIT: Regionally-specific immunotherapy; SIA: Serum allergen-specific IgE assay

Acknowledgements

Not applicable.

Funding

SkinVet Clinic, llc funded the statistical analysis performed by The Mountain-Whisper-Light Statistics, Inc., MN's employer.

Authors' contributions

JP conceived of the study, participated in its design and implementation, and drafted the manuscript. MN participated in the design of the study and performed the statistical analysis. Both authors read and approved the final manuscript.

Competing interests

JP has an ownership interest in Respit, LLC and SkinVet Clinic, LLC.

Consent for publication

Not applicable.

Author details

[1]SkinVet Clinic, 15800 Upper Boones Ferry Road, Suite 120, Lake Oswego 97035, OR, USA. [2]The Mountain-Whisper-Light Statistics, 1827 23rd Avenue East, Seattle 98112, WA, USA.

References

1. Miller WH, Griffin CE, Campbell KL, Muller GH, Scott DW. Muller & Kirk's small animal dermatology. 7th ed. St. Louis: Elsevier; 2013. p. 376–80.
2. Hensel P, Santoro D, Favrot C, Hill P, Griffin C. Canine atopic dermatitis: detailed guidelines for diagnosis and allergen identification. BMC Vet Res. 2015;11:196.
3. Olivry T, DeBoer DJ, Favrot C, Jackson HA, Mueller RS, Nuttall T, et al. Treatment of canine atopic dermatitis: 2015 updated guidelines from the International Committee on Allergic Diseases of Animals (ICADA). BMC Vet Res. 2015;11:210.
4. Griffin CE, Hillier A. The ACVD task force on canine atopic dermatitis (XXIV): allergen-specific immunotherapy. Vet Immunol Immunopathol. 2001;81: 363–83.
5. Loewenstein C, Mueller RS. A review of allergen-specific immunotherapy in human and veterinary medicine. Vet Dermatol. 2009;20:84–98.
6. Jutel M, Agache I, Bonini S, Burks AW, Calderon M, Canonica W, et al. International consensus on allergen immunotherapy II: mechanisms, standardization, and pharmacoeconomics. J Allergy Clin Immunol. 2016;137:358–68.
7. Hensel P. Differences in allergy skin testing among dermatologists within the same geographical region in the USA. Vet Dermatol. 2012;23 Suppl 1:60.
8. Thom N, Favrot C, Failing K, Mueller RS, Neiger R, Linek M. Intra- and interlaboratory variability of allergen-specific IgE levels in atopic dogs in three different laboratories using the Fc-epsilon receptor testing. Vet Immunol Immunopathol. 2010;133:183–9.
9. Plant JD, Neradelik MB, Polissar NL, Fadok VA, Scott BA. Agreement between allergen-specific IgE assays and ensuing immunotherapy recommendations from four commercial laboratories in the USA. Vet Dermatol. 2014;25:15-e6.
10. Garfield R. Injection immunotherapy in the treatment of canine atopic dermatitis: comparison of 3 hyposensitization protocols. Montreal: Annual members' meeting AAVD & ACVD; 1992. p. 7–8.
11. Anderson RK, Sousa CA. Workshop report 7: in vivo vs in vitro testing for canine atopy. In: Ihrke P, Mason IS, White SD, editors. Advances in veterinary dermatology, proceedings of the 2nd world congress of veterinary dermatology. Montreal: Pergamon Press; 1993. p. 425–7.
12. Song CH, Heiner DC. Successful replacement of allergen-specific immunotherapy by allergen-mixture therapy. Ann Allergy Asthma Immunol. 1995;75:402–8.
13. Favrot C, Steffan J, Seewald W, Picco F. A prospective study on the clinical features of chronic canine atopic dermatitis and its diagnosis. Vet Dermatol. 2010;21:23–31.
14. Hill PB, Lau P, Rybnicek J. Development of an owner-assessed scale to measure the severity of pruritus in dogs. Vet Dermatol. 2007;18:301–8.
15. Nuttall TJ, Thoday KL, van den Broek AH, Jackson HA, Sture GH, Halliwell RE. Retrospective survey of allergen immunotherapy in canine atopy. Vet Rec. 1998;143:139–42.
16. Willemse A, Van den Brom WE, Rijnberk A. Effect of hyposensitization on atopic dermatitis in dogs. J Am Vet Med Assoc. 1984;184:1277–80.
17. Schnabl B, Bettenay SV, Dow K, Mueller RS. Results of allergen-specific immunotherapy in 117 dogs with atopic dermatitis. Vet Rec. 2006;158:81–5.
18. Cleveland WS, Devlin SJ. Locally-weighted regression: an approach to regression analysis by local fitting. J Am Stat Assoc. 1988;83:596–610.
19. Mueller R, Bettenay S. Long-term immunotherapy of 146 dogs with atopic dermatitis–a retrospective study. Aust Vet Pract. 1996;26:128–32.
20. Zur G, White SD, Ihrke PJ, Kass PH, Toebe N. Canine atopic dermatitis: a retrospective study of 169 cases examined at the University of California, Davis, 1992–1998. Part II. Response to hyposensitization. Vet Dermatol. 2002;13:103–11.
21. Reinero C, Lee-Fowler T, Chang CH, Cohn L, Declue A. Beneficial cross-protection of allergen-specific immunotherapy on airway eosinophilia using unrelated or a partial repertoire of allergen(s) implicated in experimental feline asthma. Vet J. 2012;192:412–6.
22. Marogna M, Spadolini I, Massolo A, Zanon P, Berra D, Chiodini E, et al. Effects of sublingual immunotherapy for multiple or single allergens in polysensitized patients. Ann Allergy Asthma Immunol. 2007;98:274–80.
23. Buckley L, Schmidt V, McEwan N, Nuttall T. Cross-reaction and co-sensitization among related and unrelated allergens in canine intradermal tests. Vet Dermatol. 2013;24:422–7.
24. Hauser M, Roulias A, Ferreira F, Egger M. Panallergens and their impact on the allergic patient. Allergy, Asthma Clin Immunol. 2010;6:1.
25. Asero R, Jimeno L, Barber D. Preliminary results of a skin prick test-based study of the prevalence and clinical impact of hypersensitivity to pollen panallergens (polcalcin and profilin). J Investig Allergol Clin Immunol. 2010;20:35–8.
26. Linek M, Favrot C. Impact of canine atopic dermatitis on the health-related quality of life of affected dogs and quality of life of their owners. Vet Dermatol. 2010;21:456–62.
27. Plant JD, Gortel K, Kovalik M, Polissar NL, Neradilek MB. Development and validation of the canine atopic dermatitis lesion index, a scale for the rapid scoring of lesion severity in canine atopic dermatitis. Vet Dermatol. 2012;23:515-e103.
28. Codner E, Lessard P. Effect of hyposensitization with irrelevant antigens on subsequent allergy test results in normal dogs. Vet Dermatol. 1992;3:209–14.
29. Inal A, Altintas DU, Yilmaz M, Karakoc GB, Kendirli SG, Sertdemir Y. Prevention of new sensitizations by specific immunotherapy in children with rhinitis and/or asthma monosensitized to house dust mite. J Investig Allergol Clin Immunol. 2007;17:85–91.

5

Plasma markers of inflammation and hemostatic and endothelial activity in naturally overweight and obese dogs

R. Barić Rafaj[1], J. Kuleš[2]* ⓘ, A. Marinculić[3], A. Tvarijonaviciute[4], J. Ceron[4], Ž. Mihaljević[5], A. Tumpa[1] and V. Mrljak[6]

Abstract

Background: Obesity is one of the most prevalent health problems in the canine population. While haemostatic parameters and markers of endothelial function have been evaluated in various disease conditions in dogs, there are no studies of these markers in canine obesity. This study was designed to evaluate the effect of naturally gained weight excess and obesity on inflammatory, hemostatic and endothelial biomarkers in dogs. A total of 37 overweight and obese dogs were compared with 28 normal weight dogs.

Results: Overweight and obese dogs had significantly elevated concentrations of serum interleukin-6 (IL-6) and C-reactive protein (hsCRP). Number of platelets, activity of factor X and factor VII were significantly higher, while activated partial thromboplastine time (aPTT) and soluble plasminogen activator receptor (suPAR) were significantly decreased. Statistical analysis of high mobility group box – 1 protein (HMGB-1), soluble intercellular adhesive molecule -1 (sICAM-1) and plasminogen activator inhibitor type 1 (PAI-1) concentrations did not show significant differences between the total overweight and obese group and the normal weight group of dogs.

Conclusions: Analytical changes in the dogs in our study reflects that weight excess in dogs can be associated with a chronic low degree of inflammation and a hypercoagulable state, where primary and secondary hemostasis are both affected. However obesity is not associated with impairment of endothelial function in dogs.

Keywords: Canine, IL-6, HsCRP, Clotting factors, Platelets

Background

Obesity is a widespread health problem in dogs living in developed countries. The incidence of canine obesity is increasing in parallel with human obesity [1]. Current estimates indicate that more than 30% of dogs are overweight or obese, and canine obesity should be a serious concern both for veterinarians as well as for pet owners due to the high number of diseases that can be associated with this condition [1–3].

Although there are controversial results for dogs, a link between obesity and inflammation has been established in human obesity, and increases in interleukin-6 (IL-6) in obese humans were observed [4, 5]. Interleukin -6 is a pleiotropic cytokine with a wide range of biological activities in immune regulation, inflammation, and whole-body energy homeostasis [6–8]. One of the main effects of IL-6 is activation of hepatocytic receptors, resulting in increased synthesis of certain proteins [9]. This includes induction of hepatic C-reactive protein (CRP) and fibrinogen (FIB) production, which are known to be acute phase proteins in dogs [10] and major risk markers of cardiovascular complications in humans [11].

Inflammation and coagulation are closely linked, both in health and disease, and share common activation and regulation systems [12]. Various mediators that induce a chronic inflammatory state in obesity are closely connected with haemostatic disturbances and recent studies have shown that the obesity state is characterised by prothrombotic state in humans [13–15], rodents [16], cats [17] and pigs [18]. Obesity induces alterations of both intrinsic and extrinsic pathways increasing the activities of vitamin K-dependent clotting factors [15]. There is also evidences that primary hemostasis is affected by weight excess, characterised by increased

* Correspondence: jkules@vef.hr
[2]ERA Chair team VetMedZg, Internal Diseases Clinic, Faculty of Veterinary Medicine, University of Zagreb, Heinzelova 55, 10 000 Zagreb, Croatia
Full list of author information is available at the end of the article

platelet number in circulation in humans [14] and dogs [19]. In addition, impaired fibrinolysis due to increased concentrations of plasminogen activator inhibitor-1 (PAI-1), and the soluble form of plasminogen activator receptor (suPAR) could occur as a consequence of weight excess [20, 21]. While the mechanisms linking human obesity with prothrombotic changes, including upregulation of procoagulant factors, downregulation of anticoagulants and inhibition of fibrinolysis are beginning to be understood and explained [13, 15], haemostatic balance in canine overweight/obesity conditions remains uninvestigated.

Endothelial dysfunction is a complication described in human obesity and other species including mice [22, 23]. Disturbances in endothelial function can be assessed by two serum biomarkers, high mobility group box – 1 protein (HMGB – 1) and intercellular adhesive molecule -1 (ICAM - 1) [24, 25]. Fiuza et al. [26] demonstrated that HMGB-1 induces a proinflammatory change in human microvascular endothelial cells in vitro, being considered as a marker of endothelial function. ICAM -1 is also considered as a marker of endothelial activation [25] and is elevated in a broad array of disease states, including obesity [25]. Both biomarkers are increased in human obesity and are also related, since HMGB-1 induces a proinflammatory change in human microvascular endothelial cells in vitro, characterized by up-regulation of ICAM-1 and production of proinflammatory cytokines [26].

Haemostatic parameters and markers of endothelial function have been evaluated in numerous disease conditions in humans and mices, including obesity [25, 27], although there are no studies of these markers in canine weight excess. The aim of the present study was to establish whether naturally gained canine weight excess could produce changes in primary and secondary haemostasis as well as in markers of endothelial function.

Methods

Study population

This was a prospective study in which two groups were established: lean dogs and overweight and obese dogs. Clients from the University Veterinary Hospital were contacted and were asked whether they had dogs that would fulfill the criteria of admission to the study that consisted of being free of illness, and of vaccination or medication administration within 2 months prior to sample collection. In case of overweight and obese dogs, they should have been in this state for at least one year and not participated in a weight-loss program at the time of enrolment. If the dog fullfilled the inclusion criteria, its owner was asked to bring the dog to the hospital for a systematic examination, which included detailed clinical inspection and routine hematological and biochemical analysis.

All lean dogs ($n = 28$) were deemed healthy based on a detailed normal history, clinical inspection, hematological and biochemical laboratory results and that were all in the reference range. Mixed different breeds were represented. The lean group was matched in age and sex to the group of dogs with weight excess.

Each owner of overweight and obese ($n = 41$) dogs was questioned about the duration of weight excess. Various breeds were represented. The overweight and obese group of dogs consisted of 10 crossbreeds, 7 golden retrievers, 7 labradors, 2 pekingese, 2 belgian shepherds, 2 beagles, 1 bernese mountain dog, 1 pug-dog, 1 tornjak, 1 dalmatian dog, 1 great dane, 1 mexican hairless dog and 1 stafford. The normal weight group of dogs consisted of 7 crossbreeds, 6 golden retrievers, 4 labradors and 10 mixed breeds. In four overweight and obese dogs we determined two metabolic underlying conditions that could have been related to weight excess - hypothyroidism (2 dogs) and diabetes mellitus (2 dogs). These dogs were excluded from the study, so the total number of overweight and obese dogs was 37. The assessment of the nutritional condition was based on a 5-point body condition scoring (BCS) system [28]. A single investigator assigned the dog to either lean (BCS 3), overweight (BCS 4) or obese (BCS 5). In addition, the weight of the dogs was compared with the standard weight for the breed. The weight of overweight dogs was 15 – 30% above ideal and the weight of obese dogs was > 30% above ideal [29] Table 1.

Basic hematological and biochemical parameters of two groups of the dogs are shown in Table 2.

Laboratory measurements

The dog owners were asked to fast their dogs for 12 h prior to presentation for blood sampling. A sample of 6 ml of peripheral venous blood was drawn into EDTA or citrate tubes (Becton Dickinson, Rutherford, NJ, USA). Plasma was separated from blood cells by centrifugation at 1200 g for 15 min. Two 0.5 ml aliquots of EDTA and citrate plasma were separated and transferred to -80 °C within 1 h of collection and stored until analysis. The hematological, biochemical and hormonal analysis were performed immediately after the venipuncture.

Table 1 Characterization of the study population

	Normal weight	Overweight and obese
Number of dogs	28	37
Number of males and females (%)	40, 60	40, 60
Neutered/spayed	3	4
Age (years, range)	6.5 (2–14)	7.5 (2–15)
Weight excess (%, range)	0	28 (15–54)
Body condition score	3	4 and 5

Table 2 Basic hematological and biochemical parameters in normal weight and overweight/obese dogs

Group	RBC (x10^12/L)	RDW (fl)	MCV (fl)	MCH (pg)	MCHC (g/l)	HB (g/l)	HTC (%)
N	6.0 5.3–8.5	14 11–16	72 65–77	23 20–26	328 309–369	162 135–193	49 38–58
O	7.0 5.5–9.2	14 11–16	71 60–76	23 21–31	329 179–457	170 121–233	50 37–62
Ref.	5.5–8.5	11–16	60–77	19–23	320–360	120–180	37–55
	WBC (x10^9/L)	NEU (%)	MO (%)	LY (%)	EO (%)	NS (%)	Ba (%)
N	9.4 5.4–17.4	60 39–77	1 0–8	34 17–55	4 0–18	0 0–1	0 0
O	9.1 3.9–13.5	67 22–91	1 0–10	24* 5–71	3 0–23	0 0–1	0 0
Ref.	6–17	60–70	3–10	12–33	2–10	0–1	0–1
	BUN (mmol/l)	CRE (µmol/l)	BIL (µmol/l)	GLUK (mmol/l)	AST (IU/l,37 °C)	ALT (IU/l,37 °C)	YGT (IU/l,37 °C)
N	6.5 3.7–9.5	100 81–128	3.6 1.5–9.4	4.5 2.7–5.9	31 19–60	47 25–142	3 1–9
O	4.7* 3–12	93* 20–129	3.4 1.5–10.4	5.0 3.5–6.0	32 19–62	42 22–187	3 1–6
Ref.	3.3–8,3	44–140	1.7–8.6	3.6–6.5	–82	–88	–6

RBC red blood cells, RDW red distribution width, MCV mean cell volume, MCH mean cellular hemoglobin, MCHC mean cellular hemoglobin concentration, HB hemoglobin concentration, HTC hematocrit, WBC total leukocyte count, NEU segmented neutrophils, MO monocytes, LY lymphocytes, EO eosinophils, NS nonsegmented neutrophils, Ba basophils, BUN blood urea nitrogen, CRE creatinine, GLUC glucose, BIL total bilirubin, AST aspartate aminotransferase, ALT alanine aminotransferase, YGT gamma glutamyl transferase, N control normal weight dogs (N = 28), O total overweight and obese dogs (N = 37), median, minimum and maximum is shown, ref. reference range in our laboratory, *$p \leq 0.05$

Fibrinogen concentration, clotting factor activity, pro-thrombine time (PT) and activated partial thrombo-plastine time (aPTT) were measured in citrate plasma by a coagulometric method, using ACL 7000 analyser (Instrumentation Laboratory, Bedford, USA) based on a canine calibration curve with original reagents from the manufacturer. We used a coagulometric assay with specific factor-depleted plasma to assess the biological activity of the measured clotting factors. The clotting factors FVII, FIX and FX were measured by procoagulant activity as F VII:C, F IX:C and F X:C in a coagulation end point assay using specific factor – depleted plasma, having less than 1% activity for the specific factor being measured and close to 100% activity of all other factors. The activity of the factors was determined relative to a canine pool of samples obtained from healthy animals and expressed as %. The calibration curve was made using the citrate plasma pool obtained from healthy animals. The intraassay coefficient of variation was less than 4%, while interassay precision was less than 7%.

Prothrombin time is dependent on the functional activity of clotting factors FVII, FX, FV, FII and fibrinogen. Platelet poor plasma was mixed with tissue factor at 37 °C and an excess of calcium chloride was added to initiate coagulation. The time taken from the addition of calcium to the formation of the fibrin clot is known as the PT. The aPTT measures the activity of the intrinsic and common pathways of coagulation. Platelet poor plasma was incubated at 37 °C and phospholipid and a contact activator were added followed by calcium. The aPTT is the time taken from the addition of calcium to the formation of a fibrin clot, expressed in seconds.

The number of platelets (PLT) and their mean volumen (MPV) were evaluated using an automatic blood cell counter "Horiba ABX" (Diagnostics, Montpellier, France) and original manufacturer's reagents.

High mobility group box – 1, sICAM-1, hsCRP, IL-6, PAI-1 and suPAR were determined using ELISA kits specific for canine samples manufactured by Biotang (Biotang Source International, Camarillo, USA) following the manufacturer's instructions. All of the measurements were performed at the same time in order to avoid procedural variations. All the species specific ELISA kits used had a similar basis. Purified canine specific antibodies against the analyte to be measured were pre-coated onto a microplate. The standards, controls and samples were added into the wells. After washing away any unbound substances, a HRP-labeled antibody was added to form a complex of antibody-antigen-enzyme labeled antibody. After a second washing to remove any unbound antibody- enzyme reagent, tetramethylbenzidine substrate was added, producing a blue color when catalyze by the HRP enzyme. The reaction was terminated by addition of a stop solution that changes the solution color from blue to yellow. Optical density was measured with a microplate reader at 450 nm (BioTek Instruments, Vermont, USA). A standard curve, prepared from five standard dilutions in duplicate, was used for calculating the concentration of analyte in the canine samples, expressed in µg/ml, ng/ml or pg/ml. The intraassay coefficients of variation were less than

10%, and the interassay coefficients of variation were less than 12% for all measured analytes. The lower limit of assay detection was 6 ng/ml for HMGB-1, 1.25 µg/ml for sICAM-1, 16 pg/ml for IL-6, 0.30 µg/ml for hsCRP, 2 ng/ml for PAI-a and 20 pg/ml for suPAR.

Statistical analysis

Distribution of all variables was tested by the Kolmogorov-Smirnov test. Analytes with a normal distribution were expressed as mean and SD and analytes with non-normal distribution by median and the 25th and 75th percentile. Differences between lean and weight excess dogs were tested by either t test or Mann–Whitney U test. Multiple linear regression analysis was performed to evaluate correlations between analytes in normalweight and overweight/obese dogs. Statistical analyses were performed with computer software (Statistica for Windows, StatSoft Inc.), with the level of significance set at $p < 0.05$.

Ethical approval

The study protocol was approved by the Ethics Committee for Animal Experimentation, Faculty of Veterinary Medicine, University of Zagreb, Croatia. All dog owners gave written informed consent before entering the study. The study complied with local and international laws for the use of animals in clinical research.

Results

All lean, overweight and obese dogs had concentrations of plasma HMGB-1, sICAM-1, IL-6, hsCRP, PAI-1 and suPAR in the range of the ELISA assay detection. Overweight and obese dogs had significantly elevated IL-6 and hsCRP compared with normal weight dogs (261 pg/ml vs. 227 pg/ml, $p = 0.001$ for IL-6; 4.2 µg/ml vs. 3.7 µg/ml, $p = 0.027$ for hsCRP).

When hemostatic variables were studied, overweight and obese dogs showed significantly higher values of average PLT number, activity of factor X and factor VII (315x10^9/L vs. 234 x10^9/L, $p = 0.001$ for PLT; 115% vs. 104%, $p = 0.007$ for FX, 131% vs 109%, $p = 0.054$ for FVII) and significantly lower values of aPTT and suPAR compared with lean dogs (10 s vs. 11 s, $p = 0.022$ for aPTT, 1990 pg/ml vs. 2598 pg/ml, $p = 0.002$ for suPAR).

Statistical analysis of HMGB-1, sICAM-1, PAI-1 concentrations and MPV did not show significant differences between the total overweight and obese group and the lean dogs (Tables 2 and 3).

A significant positive correlation was found for IL-6 and HMGB-1 ($p < 0.05$, $r = 0.62$), and for FX and FIX ($p < 0.05$, $r = 0.48$), while a significant negative correlation was found for aPTT and FIX ($p < 0.05$, $r = -0.51$).

Discussion

The connection between weight excess and inflammation, haemostasis and endothelial disturbances has mostly been explored in humans, as well as in mouse and rat models, while similar investigations are in their early stages in canine medicine.

Biomarkers of inflammation, IL-6 and hsCRP were increased in overweight and obese dogs ($p = 0.001$; $p = 0.027$). Although no changes in these inflammatory biomarkers have been detected after short-term experimentally induced obesity or weight loss [30], and some authors even reported decreased CRP in obese dogs [31], our results would be more in line with those obtained by German et al. [32], for obese dogs in a clinical setting. These values could reflect a chronic low degree of inflammation or even that relatively minor changes in CRP under reference ranges could reflect genetic, demographic, behavioural or dietary factors [33]. The primary source of circulating IL-6 in obesity could be macrophages that have infiltrated white adipose tissue and accumulated during obesity due to local hypoxia. One of the main effects of IL-6 is the induction of hepatic CRP and FIB production, playing a key role in the inflammatory processes associated with obesity [34, 35]. In addition, there is evidence that CRP is produced in the adipose tissue itself [36], so in addition to increased hepatic production, proliferating adipose tissue could also represent a source of this acute-phase marker in overweight and obese dogs.

Weight excess in dogs shifts the hemostatic balance and features a hypercoagulable state, which is characterised by increased activity of FX ($p = 0.007$) and FVII ($p = 0.054$), shortened aPTT ($p = 0.022$) and increased number of PLT in circulation ($p = 0.001$). Similar results indicating increased activity of vitamin K-dependent clotting factors were found in obesity in humans [37] and mices [38]. A connection between body fat content and altered haemostasis is also found in pigs [39]. An explanation could be increased liver production of clotting factor as a consequence of a chronic inflammatory state, but Cleuren et al. [38] found that in obesity the factors activity in plasma was not paralleled by changes in transcription levels in the liver. Moreover, Takahashi et al. [40] found that obese adipose tissue itself produced FVII, and that the production and secretion of FVII by adipocytes was enhanced by proinflammatory cytokines, so the possible role of chronic inflammatory state on canine adipocytes as an alternative source of some clotting factors remains to be investigated. A significantly shorter aPTT has been found in obese rats [16], humans [41] and mices [38], which is in line with our results. The clinical significance of short aPTT in diagnostics has recently gained interest, because aPTT might be usefull as a widely available and inexpensive marker of hypercoagulability [41].

Table 3 Values of the inflammatory, hemostatic and endothelial biomarkers measured in this study in normal weight and overweight/obese dogs

Parameter/unit	Normal weight	Dogs	Overweight	And obese dogs	R and *P* -value
	Mean ± SEM	Median; CI (P 25–P 75)	Mean ± SEM	Median; CI (P 25–P 75)	
sICAM-1 µg/ml	320 ±13	321; 275–356	329 ± 8.2	326; 288–361	9.021; pd 0.536
IL–6 pg/ml	227 ± 8.9	220; 197–256	261 ± 4.9	259; 235–287	34.829; pd 0.001 **
HMGB-1 ng/ml	85 ± 4.5	83; 70–93	89 ± 2.6	89; 76–98	4.343; pd 0.384
hsCRP µg/ml	3.7 ± 0.17	3.7; 3.2–4.3	4.2 ± 0.14	3.9; 3.6–4.7	0.502; pd 0.027 *
suPAR pg/ml	2598 ± 136	2559; 2195–2923	1990 ± 126	1869; 1542–2486	−608.314; pd 0.002 *
PAI-1 ng/ml	70 ± 5.9	61; 44–94	75 ± 6.9	70; 43–86	1.145; np 0.611
FIB g/L	2.6 ± 0.16	2.6; 2.0–3.0	3.0 ± 0.20	2.6; 2.2–3.5	1.312; np 0.185
FIX %	96 ± 5.6	93; 77–106	112 ± 6.8	100; 84–140	1.385; np 0.081
FVII %	109 ± 6.2	110; 82–136	131 ± 8.7	125; 100–147	1.492; pd 0.054 *
FX %	104 ± 2.2	106; 94–112	115 ± 2.9	110; 102–128	11.557; pd 0.007 **
PT sec	6.1 ± 0.04	6.1; 6.0–6.2	6.1 ± 0.04	6.1 6.0–6.2	0.989; np 0.580
aPTT sec	11 ± 0.23	11; 10–12	10 ± 0.20	10; 9.3–11	−0.749; pd 0.022 *
MPV fl	8.3 ± 0.14	8; 8–9	8.6 ± 0.17	8; 8–9	0.318; pd 0.169
PLT x10^9/L	234 ± 13	228; 201–265	315 ± 18	298; 253–401	80.916; pd 0.001 **

HMGB-1 high mobility group box – 1 protein, *sICAM-1* soluble intercellular adhesive molecule -1, *IL-6* interleukin – 6, *hsCRP* high sensitivity C reactive protein, *PAI-1* plasminogen activator inhibitor type 1, *suPAR* soluble plasminogen activator receptor, *FIB* fibrinogen, *FX, FIX, FVII* clotting factors X, IX and VII, *PT* prothrombine time, *aPTT* activated partial thromboplastine time, *MPV* mean platelet volume, *PLT* number of platelets, *np* nonparametric distribution, *pd* parametric distribution
*$p \leq 0.05$, **$p < 0.01$,

The primary haemostasis in dogs with weight excess was affected due to increased platelet count, while the mean platelet volume remained unchanged compared with normal lean dogs. Similar findings have been found in obese dogs [19], pigs [18] and children [42]. Cytokine IL-6 was found to acts as a promotor of the maturation of megakaryocyte precursors, and this prothrombotic effect may explain the association between the increased markers of chronic inflammation and the elevated platelet count in obese humans [43], and possibly also in dogs.

In spite of the fact that obesity is characterized by decreased fibrinolysis in humans [13] where PAI-1 represents a part of the fibrinolytic system that is most disordered, in our experiments we did not find any changes in the PAI-1 concentration. In addition the soluble form of urokinase PAR, suPAR, was decreased in dogs with weight excess ($p = 0.002$). These findings disagree with other authors that investigated the effect of human obesity on the fibrinolytic system, where increased levels of suPAR was found [44, 45]. Further studies should be performed to determine the reason for these divergences in the behaviour of suPAR in canine and human obesity.

Proteins belonging to the HMGB-1 goup did not show a significant increase in dogs with weight excess. These proteins have been reported to increase in dogs with acute inflammation and neoplasms [46–49]. In our study we used species-specific canine antibodies and a highly sensitive assay for HMGB-1 that allowed us to quantify this protein in healthy control dogs, in contrast to other

studies that reported no detectable concentration using assays designed for humans [47]. Our findings suggest that overweight condition and obesity are not associated with greater impairment of endothelial function in dogs. Similarly, HMGB-1 and sICAM-1 did not show significant increases in obese dogs in our study, contrary to what has been described in humans [50, 51]. One of the risk factors for atherosclerosis is an increase of sICAM-1. Therefore, the lack of increase of this protein in obese dogs could be related to the low frequency of atherosclerosis found in this species compared with humans, where it is a leading cause of mortality and is responsible for much of the morbidity [52].

Interleukin -6 was positively correlated with HMGB-1. A similar relationship between these two proteins was found by Zeng et al. [53] in human infectious disease. Moreover, Nativel et al. [54] concluded that HMGB-1 is an adipokine, which stimulates IL-6 secretion and may contribute to chronic inflammation in fat tissue of humans. Our finding suggest that HMGB-1 may play a role in the chronic inflammatory state in dogs.

The main study limitation was that client-owned animals living in a home environment were used, which contributed to study variability, where diet, exercise and husbandry were variable. In addition, we did not have the opportunity to follow the effect of weight loss on the measured biomarkers. Despite these limitations, this study provides a comprehensive analysis of proinflammatory events, haemostasis and endothelial function associated with weight excess in dogs. Further studies should be made in the future with a larger population of dogs to confirm these findings and in addition it would be interesting to compare in obese dogs whether the existence of obesity related metabolic symdrome (ORMD) could alter these analytes.

Conclusions

In this report we showed that weight excess in dogs potentiates the prothrombotic state in apparently healthy animals. This could at least in part, be due to a chronic proinflammatory state. Altered haemostasis may be relevant as a pathological contributor to other haemostatic diseases if dog is overweight or obese. The fibrinolytic system in canine obesity and the role of decreased suPAR is not yet clear and needs to be further investigated. The positive correlation of IL-6 with HMGB-1 suggests that HMGB-1 could also have a role in the chronic inflammatory state in dogs.

Abbreviations

ALT: Alanine aminotransferase; aPTT: Activated partial thromboplastine time; AST: Aspartate aminotransferase; Ba: Basophils; BCS: Body condition scoring system; BIL: Total bilirubin; BUN: Blood urea nitrogen; CRE: Creatinine; EO: Eosinophils; F VII:C, F IX:C and F X:C: Clotting factors coagulation end point assay; FIB: Fibrinogen; FX, FIX, FVII: Clotting factors X, IX and VII; GLUC: Glucose; HB: Hemoglobin concentration; HMGB-1: High mobility group box – 1 protein; hsCRP: High sensitivity C reactive protein; HTC: Hematocrit; IL-6: Interleukin – 6; LY: Lymphocytes; MCH: Mean cellular hemoglobin; MCHC: Mean cellular hemoglobin concentration; MCV: Mean cell volume; MO: Monocytes; MPV: Mean platelet volume; NEU: Segmented neutrophils; NS: Nonsegmented neutrophils; ORMD: Obesity related metabolic symdrome; PAI-1: Plasminogen activator inhibitor type 1; PLT: Number of platelets; PT: Prothrombine time; RBC: Red blood cells; RDW: Red distribution width; sICAM-1: Soluble intercellular adhesive molecule -1; suPAR: Soluble plasminogen activator receptor; WBC: Total leukocyte count; YGT: Gamma glutamyl transferase

Acknowledgements
The authors thank the owners of the dogs for their participation in this study, the laboratory personnel at the Clinic for Internal Diseases and Branimir Rebselj, DVM, for their help with this study. This study was presented in part as an abstract at the XXXVth World Congress of the International Society of Hematology, Beijing, September 2014.

Funding
This study (experimental part) was supported through the Fond for development, University of Zagreb. Publishing was supported through FP7 project " Upgrading the research performance in molecular medicine at the Faculty of Veterinary Medicine University of Zagreb" (grant agreement No: 621394).

Authors' contributions
Conceived and designed the experiments: RBR. Sample collection, ELISA analyses, coagulation test performed by: JK, AT, and AM. Conducted data analyses: ŽM. Prepared and revised the manuscript: RBR, VM, JC. All authors read and approved the final manuscript.

Competing interests
The authors declare that they have no competing interests

Consent for publication
Not applicable.

Author details
[1]Department of Chemistry and Biochemistry, Faculty of Veterinary Medicine, University of Zagreb, Heinzelova 55, 10 000 Zagreb, Croatia. [2]ERA Chair team VetMedZg, Internal Diseases Clinic, Faculty of Veterinary Medicine, University of Zagreb, Heinzelova 55, 10 000 Zagreb, Croatia. [3]Department of Parasitology and Parasitic Diseases with Clinic, Faculty of Veterinary Medicine, University of Zagreb, Heinzelova 55, 10 000 Zagreb, Croatia. [4]Department of Animal Medicine and Surgery, Faculty of Veterinary Medicine, Regional Campus of International Excellence Campus Mare Nostrum, University of Murcia, Murcia 30100, Espinardo, Spain. [5]Veterinary Institute, Savska cesta 143, 10 000 Zagreb, Croatia. [6]Clinic for Internal Dieaases, Faculty of Veterinary Medicine, University of Zagreb, Heinzelova 55, 10 000 Zagreb, Croatia.

References
1. German AJ. The growing problem of obesity in dogs and cats. J Nutr. 2006; 136:1940–46.
2. Bland IM, Guthrie-Jones A, Taylor RD, Hill J. Dog obesity: Veterinary practices and owners opinions on cause and management. Prev Vet Med. 2010;94:310–15.
3. Zoran DL. Obesity in Dogs and Cats: A Metabolic and Endocrine Disorder. Vet Clin N Anim Small Pract. 2010;40:221–39.
4. Juhan-Vague I, Thompson SG, Jespersen J. Involvement of the hemostatic system in the insulin resistance syndrome. A study of 1500 patients with angina pectoris. The ECAT Angina Pectoris Study Group. Arterioscler Thromb. 1993;13:1865–73.
5. Hotamisligil GS. Inflammation and metabolic disorders. Nature. 2006;444: 860–67.
6. Stenlöf K, Wernstedt I, Fjällman T, Wallenius V, Wallenius K, Jansson JO. Interleukin-6 levels in the central nervous system are negatively correlated with fat mass in overweight/obese subjects. J Clin Endocrinol Metabol. 2003;88:4379–83.
7. Bartsch R, Woehrer S, Raderer M, Hejna M. Serum Interleukin-6 Levels in Patients with Gastric MALT Lymphoma Compared to Gastric and Pancreatic Cancer. Anticancer Res. 2006;26:3187–90.
8. Kishimoto T. IL-6: from its discovery to clinical applications. Int Immunol. 2010;22:347–52.
9. Gruys E, Toussaint MJM, Niewold TA, Koopmans SJ. Acute phase reaction and acute phase proteins. J Zhejiang Univ Sci B. 2005;6:1045–56.
10. Ceron JJ, Eckersall PD, Martinez-Subiela S. Acute phase proteins in dogs and cats: current nowledge and future perspectives. Vet Clin Pathol. 2005; 34:85–99.
11. Bastard JP, Maachi M, Lagathu C, Kim MJ, Caron M, Vidal H, et al. Recent advances in the relationship between obesity, inflammation, and insulin resistance. Eur Cytokine Netw. 2006;17:4–12.
12. Verhamme P, Hoylaerts MF. Haemostasis and inflammation: two of a kind? Thromb J. 2009. doi:10.1186/1477-9560-7-15.
13. Mertens I, Van Gaal LF. Obesity, haemostasis and the fibrinolytic system. Obes Rev. 2002;3:85–101.
14. Russo I. The Prothrombotic Tendency in Metabolic Syndrome: Focus on the Potential Mechanisms Involved in Impaired Haemostasis and Fibrinolytic Balance. Scientifica. 2012. doi:10.6064/2012/525374.
15. Anfossi G, Russo I, Doronzo G, Pomero A, Trovati M. Adipocytokines in Atherothrombosis: Focus on Platelets and Vascular Smooth Muscle Cells. Mediat Inflamm. 2010. doi:10.1155/2010/174341.
16. Kaji N, Nagakubo D, Hashida SI, Takahashi S, Kuratani M, Hirai N, et al. Shortened Blood Coagulation Times in Genetically Obese Rats and Diet-Induced Obese Mice. J Vet Med Sci. 2013;75(9):1245–48.
17. Bjornvad CR, Wiinberg B, Kristensen AT. Obesity increases initial rate of fibrin formation during blood coagulation in domestic shorthaired cats. J Anim Physiol Anim Nutr. 2012;96:834–41.
18. Duburcq T, Tournoys A, Gnemmi V, Hubert T, Gmyr V, Pattou F, et al. Impact of obesity on endotoxin-induced disseminated intravascular coagulation. Shock. 2015;44:341–7.

19. Pasquini A, Roberti S, Meucci V, Luchetti E, Canello S, Guidetti G, Biagi G. Association between Body Condition and Oxidative Status in Dogs. FNS. 2012;4:191–6.

20. Yamamoto K, Takeshita K, Kojima T, Takamatsu J, Saito H. Aging and plasminogen activator inhibitor-1 (PAI-1) regulation: implication in the pathogenesis of thrombotic disorders in the elderly. Cardiovasc Res. 2005; 66:276–85.

21. Thunø M, Machoa B, Eugen-Olsenb J. suPAR: The molecular crystal ball. Dis Markers. 2009;27:157–72.

22. Wang H, Yang H, Czura CJ, Sama AE, Tracey K. HMGB1 as a Late Mediator of Lethal Systemic Inflammation. AJRCCM. 2001;164:1768–73.

23. Juge-Aubry CE, Henrichot E, Meier CA. Adipose tissue: a regulator of inflammation. Best Pract Res Clin Endocrinol Metab. 2005;19:547–66.

24. Mutch NJ, Wilson HM, Booth NA. Plasminogen activator inhibitor-1 and haemostasis in obesity. Proc Nutr Soc. 2001;60:341–47.

25. Brake RDK, O'Brian Smith E, Mersmann H, Wayne Smith C, Robker RL. ICAM-1 expression in adipose tissue: effects of diet-induced obesity in mice. Am J Physiol Cell Physiol. 2006;291:1232–39.

26. Fiuza C, Bustin M, Talwar S, Tropea M, Gerstenberger E, Shelhamer JH, Suffredini AF. Inflammation-promoting activity of HMGB1 on human microvascular endothelial cells. Blood. 2003;101:2652–60.

27. Kaur H, Devaraj S, Jialal I. Circulating biomarkers of TLR activity in metabolic syndrome. Endocr Rev. 2013;34:33–4.

28. Laflamme D. Development and validation of a body condition score system for dogs. Canine Pract. 1997;22:10–5.

29. Burkholder WJ, Toll PW. Obesity. In: Hand MS, Thatcher CD, Reimillard RL, Roudebush P, Morris ML, Novotny BJ, editors. Small animal clinical nutrition. 4th ed. Topeka, KS: Mark Morris Institute; 2000. p. 401–30.

30. Tvarijonaviciute A, Tecles F, Martínez-Subiela S, Ceron JJ. Effect of weight loss on inflammatory biomarkers in obese dogs. Vet J. 2012;193:570–72.

31. Veiga APM, Price CA, de Oliveira ST, dos Santos AP, Campos R, Barbosa PR, González HDFD. Association of canine obesity with reduced serum levels of C-reactive protein. J Vet Diagn Invest. 2008;20:224–8.

32. German AJ, Hervera M, Hunter L, Holden SL, Morris PJ, Biourge V, Trayhurn P. Improvement in insulin resistance and reduction in plasma inflammatory adipokines after weight loss in obese dogs. Domest Anim Endocrinol. 2009; 37:214–26.

33. Kushner I, Rzewnicki D, Samols D. What does minor elevation of C-reactive protein signify? Am J Med. 2006;119:17–28.

34. Stapleton PA, James ME, Goodwill AG, Frisbee JC. Obesity and vascular dysfunction. Pathophysiology. 2008;15:79–89.

35. Cucuianu M, Coca M. Thrombotic Tendency in Diabetes Mellitus. Revisiting and revising a study initiated 30 years ago. Rom J Intern Med. 2012;50:107–15.

36. Calabro P, Chang DW, Willerson JT, Yeh ET. Release of C reactive protein in response to inflammatory cytokines by human adipocytes: linking obesity to vascular inflammation. J Am Coll Cardiol. 2005;46:1112–13.

37. Juhan-Vague I, Alessi MC. Abdominal obesity, insulin resistance, and alterations in hemostasis. Cardiometab Risk J. 2008;1:11–6.

38. Cleuren ACA, Blankevoort VT, van Diepen JA, Verhoef D, Voshol PJ, Reitsma1 PH, van Vlijmen BJM. Changes in Dietary Fat Content Rapidly Alters the Mouse Plasma Coagulation Profile without Affecting Relative Transcript Levels of Coagulation Factors. PLoS ONE. 2015;10(7):e0131859. doi:10.1371/journal.pone.0131859.

39. Kreutz RP, Alloosh M, Mansour K, Neeb Z, Kreutz Y, Flockhard DA, Sturek M. Morbid obesity and metabolic syndrome in Ossabaw miniature swine are associated with increased platelet reactivity. Diabetes Metab Syndrom Obes. 2011;4:99–105.

40. Montilla M, Santi MJ, Carrozas MA. Ruiz FA. Biomarkers of the prothrombotic state in abdominal obesity. Nutr Hosp. 2015;31(3):1059–66.

41. Takahashi N, Yoshizaki T, Hiranaka N, Kumano O, Suzuki T, Akanuma M, Yui T, Kanazawa K, Yoshida M, Naito S, Fujiya M, Kohgo Y, Ieko M. The production of coagulation factor VII by adipocytes is enhanced by tumor necrosis factor-α or isoproterenol. Int J Obes. 2014. doi:10.1038/ijo.2014.208.

42. Bilge YD, Alioglu B, Simşek E, Tapci AE, Ozen C. Increased coagulation in childhood obesity. Pediatr Hemat Oncol. 2012;29:721–7.

43. Samocha-Bonet D, Justo D, Rogowski O, et al. Platelet counts and platelet activation markers in obese subjects. Mediat Inflamm. 2008;2008:834153. doi:10.1155/2008/834153.

44. Heraclides A, Jensen TM, Rasmussen SS, Eugen-Olsen J, Haugaard SB, Borch-Johnsen K, et al. The pro-inflammatory biomarker soluble urokinase plasminogen activator receptor (suPAR) is associated with incident type 2 diabetes among overweight but not obese individuals with impaired glucose regulation: effect modification by smoking and body weight status. Diabetologia. 2013;56:1542–46.

45. Chen JS, Wu CZ, Chu NF, Chang LC, Pei D, Lin YF. Association among Fibrinolytic Proteins, Metabolic Syndrome Components, Insulin Secretion, and Resistance in Schoolchildren. Int J Endocrinol. 2015;doi:10.1155/2015/170987.

46. Escobar HM, Meyer B, Richter A, Becker K, Flohr AM, Bullerdiek J, Nolte I. Molecular characterization of the canine HMGB1. Cytogenet Genome Res. 2003;101:33–8.

47. Yu DH, Kim SH, Lee MJ, Nemzek JA, Nho DH, Park J, Song RH. High-mobility group box 1 as a surrogate prognostic marker in dogs with systemic inflammatory response syndrome. J Vet Emerg Crit Care. 2010;20:298–302.

48. Meyer A, Eberle N, Bullerdiek J, Nolte I, Simon D. High-mobility group B1 proteins in canine lymphoma: prognostic value of initial and sequential serum levels in treatment outcome following combination chemotherapy. Vet Comp Oncol. 2010;8:127–37.

49. Sterenczak KA, Joetzke AE, Willenbrock S, Eberle N, Lange S, Junghanss C, et al. High-mobility group B1 (HMGB1) and receptor for advanced glycation end-products (RAGE) expression in canine lymphoma. Anticancer Res. 2010; 30:5043–48.

50. Shankar SS, Steinberg HO. Obesity and endothelial dysfunction. Sem Vasc Med. 2005;5:56–64.

51. Weil BR, Stauffer BL, Mestek ML, deSouza CA. Influence of abdominal obesity on vascular endothelial function in overweight/obese adult men. Obesity. 2011;19:1742–6.

52. Robinson JG, Gidding SS. Curing Atherosclerosis should be the next major cardiovascular prevention goal. J Am Coll Cardiol. 2014;63:2779–85.

53. Zeng JC, Xiang WY, Lin DZ, Zhang JA, Liu GB, Kong B, et al. Elevated HMGB1-related interleukin-6 is associated with dynamic responses of monocytes in patients with active pulmonary tuberculosis. Int J Clin Exp Pathol. 2015;8:1341–53.

54. Nativel B, Marimoutou M, Thon-Hon VG, Gunasekaran MK, Andries J, Stanislas G, et al. Soluble HMGB1 Is a Novel Adipokine Stimulating IL-6 Secretion through RAGE Receptor in SW872 Preadipocyte Cell Line: Contribution to Chronic Inflammation in Fat Tissue. PLoS One 2013; doi:10.1371/journal.pone.0076039.

6

Treatment of 5 dogs with immune-mediated thrombocytopenia using Romiplostim

Barbara Kohn[1], Gürkan Bal[2], Aleksandra Chirek[1], Sina Rehbein[1] and Abdulgabar Salama[2*]

Abstract

Background: Immune thrombocytopenia (ITP) in dogs is analogous to that in humans. Romiplostim, a novel thrombopoietin receptor (TPO-R) agonist, is currently used for the treatment of refractory ITP in humans, but not in dogs. Here, we describe the response to romiplostim in five dogs with refractory ITP. Five dogs with severe and refractory ITP (three primary and two secondary) received romiplostim subcutaneously. Four dogs were administered 3–5 µg/kg and one dog received 10–13 µg/kg body weight once weekly.

Results: Romiplostim was well-tolerated and administration was associated with an increase in platelet counts in all five dogs. Four of the five dogs entered remission and relapses were not observed over a follow-up period of 3–10 months.

Conclusions: Romiplostim is effective in the treatment of ITP in dogs at least as well as in humans. This finding may help to develop and use new therapeutics for ITP in dogs and humans.

Keywords: Immune thrombocytopenia, ITP, Dog, Romiplostim, Thrombopoietin, mpl

Background

Immune thrombocytopenia (ITP) is a well-characterized autoimmune bleeding disease in humans that is accompanied by the immune-mediated destruction of platelets and impaired thrombopoiesis [1–4]. Comparable to humans, dogs develop ITP spontaneously [5] or secondary following infectious or neoplastic diseases [6–8]. Differential diagnosis of ITP in both species is based on the exclusion of known causes or underlying diseases [5, 9].

The current treatment options for ITP in humans and dogs are largely identical. Corticosteroid administration is generally accepted as the first-line treatment option in affected human patients and dogs [10, 11]. However, the effect of steroids is not predictable in a single patient [12]. Approximately two-thirds of human patients achieve a complete or partial response with corticosteroids, although a high proportion of patients relapse and require alternative therapy [13]. Similarly, steroid treatment may remain ineffective and may result in severe adverse reactions in dogs [8, 10, 14–16].

A second line therapy in dogs is not well-defined and may include platelet transfusions and high dose intravenous immunoglobulins (IVIgG) for acute management, or vincristine, azathioprine, mycophenolate mofetil, cyclophosphamide, cyclosporine, danazol, leflunomide, and ultimately splenectomy for long-term management and in cases of relapse or refractory ITP [8, 10, 16–19]. These treatment options are not performed analogously and there are no generally accepted guidelines on when they should be used [16]. The rates of relapse and mortality in dogs range between 9% and 43% [8, 10, 15, 18, 20–22].

During the last decade, significant new aspects regarding the pathogenesis and treatment of ITP in humans have been highlighted. Patients with ITP have been found to have increased platelet destruction due to autoantibodies and an impaired thrombopoiesis in the bone marrow [3, 23]. Consequently, two thrombopoietin receptor (TPO-R) agonists, romiplostim and eltrombopag, have been shown to be effective in the treatment of human ITP [24]. Romiplostim is a 59 kDa peptibody that

---

* Correspondence: abdulgabar.salama@charite.de
[2]Institut für Transfusionsmedizin, Charité – Universitätsklinikum, Augustenburger Platz 1, 13353 Berlin, Germany
Full list of author information is available at the end of the article

binds to the extracellular domain of TPO-R on megakaryocytes and platelets, activates the receptor, and increases platelet counts [25]. In contrast, eltrombopag is a small molecule with a molecular weight of 442 Da, and is a non-peptide TPO-R agonist that selectively binds to the transmembrane domain of the TPO-R and increases platelet counts [26]. The safety and efficiency of TPO agonists in the treatment of ITP has been previously studied in well-designed controlled and randomized clinical trials. Eltrombopag is administered orally at a dosage ranging between 25 and 75 mg/d, and 1–10 µg/kg romiplostim is administered subcutaneously once weekly [22, 27–29]. Treatment with TPO agonists is usually indicated in patients with refractory ITP and in patients who do not adequately respond to standard therapy [22, 27].

Dogs with therapy refractory ITP are at a high risk of life-threatening bleeding. In such cases, there are no alternative therapeutic options, and affected dogs either die or are euthanized due to thrombocytopenia [5]. As ITP in dogs is largely analogous to ITP in humans, we questioned whether human TPO agents such as the Food and Drug Administration (FDA) approved human TPO-R agonists can be used as a new therapeutic measure in dogs with ITP that cannot be controlled by standard therapy.

Methods

Five dogs with primary or secondary ITP were admitted to the Small Animal Clinic at the Freie Universität Berlin between 10/2014 and 6/2015 and were treated with romiplostim. Inclusion criteria were diagnosed primary or secondary ITP based on complete medical records, platelet counts < 150,000/µl and a positive platelet-bound antibody test. Primary ITP was only diagnosed, if there was no evidence of any other underlying disease or cause which might have triggered platelet destruction. In presence of an additionally positive direct Coombs' test, Evans' syndrome was diagnosed. Discrimination of primary and secondary forms of ITP was based on the complete diagnostic work-up that comprised of a complete blood count, blood smear evaluation, testing for erythrocyte agglutination, clinical chemistry, coagulation panel, diagnostic imaging including thoracic and abdominal radiography and ultrasonography, direct and indirect tests for infectious diseases, and immunological testing [7, 8]. The dogs had been pre-treated with prednisolone and adjunctive immunosuppressive drugs and were either non-responders or were readmitted due to a relapse. A response to therapy (complete remission) was defined as an increase of the platelet count to ≥ 150,000/µl. A relapse was defined as a decrease of the platelet count below 150,000/µl after the value had already been within reference range. A dog was classified as non-responder when, the platelet counts did not increase or did not reach values above 150.000/µl.(references) The

dosage for each dog was extrapolated from human data, and was dependent on the clinical responses [30]. Consent from the owners was obtained. Romiplostim is licensed in human medicine and a comparable product is not available in veterinary medicine. Therefore this drug can be used in veterinary medicine without approval of an ethics committee. Moreover all the dogs were treated using standard therapy (best practice of veterinary care) first before using this novel agent.

Results

Depending on the availability of romiplostim and the severity of ITP in affected dogs, treatment was initially commenced with a dosage of 3–5 µg/kg per week. Prior to treatment with romiplostim, all dogs had underwent conventional treatment (Tables 1 and 2) and had experienced one or more relapses. Treatment was either ineffective or was discontinued to avoid the development of severe side effects (e.g. in the case of ehrlichiosis). Administration of romiplostim resulted in an increase of platelet counts within 3–6 days following the commencement of treatment in 4 of the 5 treated dogs (Table 2). The remaining dog suffered from ehrlichiosis and hepatopathy, and did not respond to the administration of 5.3 µg/kg of romiplostim. Bone marrow examination revealed the presence of numerous megakaryocytes. A dose escalation was attempted after the following 2 months and the dog received first 13 µg/kg and then 10 µg/kg after one week. Simultaneously, prednisolone was re-administered due to the deterioration of hepatopathy. One week after the second injection, an increase in platelet counts was observed (Table 2). We report here a mean length of treatment of 13.8 (min. 3, max. 35 and median 11 weeks) weeks, which were varying for each individual dog. None of the treated dogs developed any side effects. Concomitant therapy with other drugs was gradually reduced and halted in three of the dogs when the platelet count was stabilized. Interestingly, none of the five dogs relapsed during observation. Moreover, the initially given dose of romiplostim could be reduced in four cases (Table 2).

Discussion

ITP is the most common cause of severe thrombocytopenia in dogs [31]. Corticosteroids are considered as the cornerstone of treatment. However, in cases where these drugs remain ineffective, contraindicated, or may cause severe side effects, other treatment options are desirable [8, 16, 32]. Furthermore, dogs are, unlike humans, unable to verbally express themselves. Therefore, the true incidence of intolerability to immunosuppressive drugs remains obscure in the treated animals.

Romiplostim is produced by covalently linking two tandem dimers to the C-terminus of endogenous TPO. Thus, exposure of cells expressing TPO-R (BaF3-mpl) to

Table 1 Signalment and history of five dogs with primary and secondary immune thrombocytopenia treated with romiplostim

Dog	Signalment	ITP – diagnoses month/year	Recurrences	Previous immunosuppressive therapy	Therapy (in addition to immunosuppressive medication)
1	Bearded Collie 7-year-old, female 22 kg	7/2012: primary ITP	1) 10/2012 2) 3/2013 3) 9/2014 4) 10/2014	pred 1 mg/kg twice daily + MMF 8 mg/kg twice daily Recurrence 1) Pred, cyclosporine 2) only pred 3) pred, MMF, then dexamethasone 4) pred, MMF	omeprazole, sucralfate (to prevent gastrointestinal ulcers) ursodeoxycholic acid (due to increase in liver enzymes)
2	Border Collie 10-year-old, female-spayed 25 kg (obese)	2014: primary AIHA 5/2015: Evans' syndrome (primary ITP and AIHA)	after 3 weeks	short-acting methyl-pred 10 mg/kg once, pred 0.8 mg/kg twice daily	doxycycline omeprazole, sucralfate
3	Poodle 3-year-old, male-neutered 25 kg	12/2014: Evans' syndrome (primary ITP and AIHA)	after 3 weeks	pred 1.5 mg/kg twice daily, MMF 5 mg/kg twice daily	omeprazole, sucralfate
4	Mixed-breed 3-year-old, female-spayed, 22 kg	ITP associated with monocytic ehrlichiosis	after 4 weeks	pred 1 mg/kg twice daily	doxycycline omeprazole, sucralfate
5	Mixed-breed 2.5-year-old, female 14 kg	ITP associated with monocytic ehrlichiosis	2 weeks	pred 0.4 mg/kg once daily	chloramphenicole/ imidocarb amoxicillin-clavulanic acid omeprazole, sucralfate ursodeoxycholic acid S-adenosyl-methionine

Pred prednisolone, *MMF* mycofenolate mofetil, *ITP* immune thrombocytopenia, *AIHA* autoimmune hemolytic anemia

romiplostim results in rapid tyrosine phosphorylation of mpl, JAK2, and STAT5, and stimulation of megakaryopoiesis and platelet production. Pharmacodynamic studies in animals including mice, rats, rabbits, monkeys, and dogs have shown well-tolerability, and dose-dependent increases in platelet counts [24, 27, 33]. Subsequently, well-designed human studies have been conducted in patients with chronic ITP. The drug was well-tolerated in all studies and most events were mild to moderate. Furthermore, there was no evidence of an increased risk of thromboembolic complications or development of antibodies against natural TPO. In 2008, romiplostim was licensed for the treatment of ITP in humans and long-term treatment appears to be well-tolerable [34–36].

Depending on the phylogenetic differences of TPO-R in canines and humans, dual usage of TPO-R agonists in

Table 2 Romiplostim therapy in five dogs with primary and secondary immune thrombocytopenia: Dosage, response and outcome

Dog	Current therapy at the commencement of romiplostim	Platelets count x10^3/µl	Romiplostim µg/kg (initial dose)	Response Day	Response Platelets count x10^3/µl	Maintenance therapy	Outcome
1	pred 0.5 mg/kg twice daily MMF 5 mg/kg twice daily	19	5	6 / 73	13 / 226	2.3 µg romi	CR > 10 mon
2	pred 0.6 mg/kg twice daily	57	3	3 / 83 5 / 131	8 / 222 15 / 332	now 2 µg/kg romi 0.1 mg/kg pred every other day[a]	CR > 3 mon
3	pred 0.6 mg/kg twice daily MMF 5 mg/kg twice daily	25	5	4 7 10	58 189 217	2.5 µg	ITP CR but euthanized due to AIHA after 2.5 mon
4	pred 0.5 mg/kg twice daily	123	4.5	3 / 178	5 / 213	3.4	CR > 5 mon
5	a) pred 0.4 mg/kg once daily, doxycycline b) 2 months later: pred 0.5 mg/kg, amoxicillin	a) 4 b) 1	a) 5.3 b) 13	a) No response b) 4 11 15	7 3 115		b) Lost for follow-up

Romi romiplostim, *pred* prednisolone, *MMF* mycofenolate mofetil, *CR* complete remission (platelet counts > 200 × 10^3/µl), *ITP* immune thrombocytopenia, *AIHA* autoimmune hemolytic anemia, *mon* months
[a]due to autoimmune hemolysis

both species may be evolutionally encouraging or discouraging. As shown in Fig. 1, TPO-R protein sequences of canines and humans are very highly conserved at the C-terminus and the possible binding site for TPO (EpoR-lig-bind domains) is localised in this highly conserved area. As romiplostim interacts with an extracellularly located part of TPO-R and canine and human protein sequences are highly conserved, this may be the molecular basis of this therapeutic effect in canine ITP. Consistently, the safety and haematological efficiency of recombinant human TPO peptide has been demonstrated in chemotherapy-induced thrombocytopenia in dogs [37]. To date, two TPO-R agonists, romiplostim and eltrombopag, have been approved by the FDA for the treatment of ITP in humans. Although both of these drugs activate TPO-R and are used for the same indications, their binding properties and their mode of action in activating TPO-R is rather different. In contrast to romiplostim, eltrombopag interacts with the transmembrane domain of TPO-R, where the protein sequences are not phylogenetically highly conserved. Therefore, we preferred to use romiplostim as a potential candidate drug for the treatment of ITP in dogs.

In this observational study, we treated five dogs with ITP with romiplostim. All five dogs appeared not only to tolerate the drug quite well, but four of the five dogs also responded relatively quickly with a significant increase of platelet counts. One dog with secondary ITP that had not responded to prednisolone and romiplostim at a dosage of 5 μg/kg responded to a higher dosage of romiplostim. Based on the dogs' medical history, the increase of platelet counts did not appear to be related to concomitant treatment with prednisolone.

One limitation of this pilot study is the low sample size and the inclusion of primary and secondary ITP forms. In some cases, contaminant immunosuppressive drugs was also necessary, at least, at the beginning of romiplostim therapy. Because of these limitations, dogs were treated with individual therapy protocol, inside of a clinical trial set-up. Depend on the duration of response, length of treatments were also varying for each individual dog. We report here a mean length of treatment of 13.8 weeks, whereas a mean treatment duration in human has been recently reported as 60 weeks and a maximum duration of 96 weeks [38]. Romiplostim dosage was reduced in 4 dogs (information is given in Table 2,

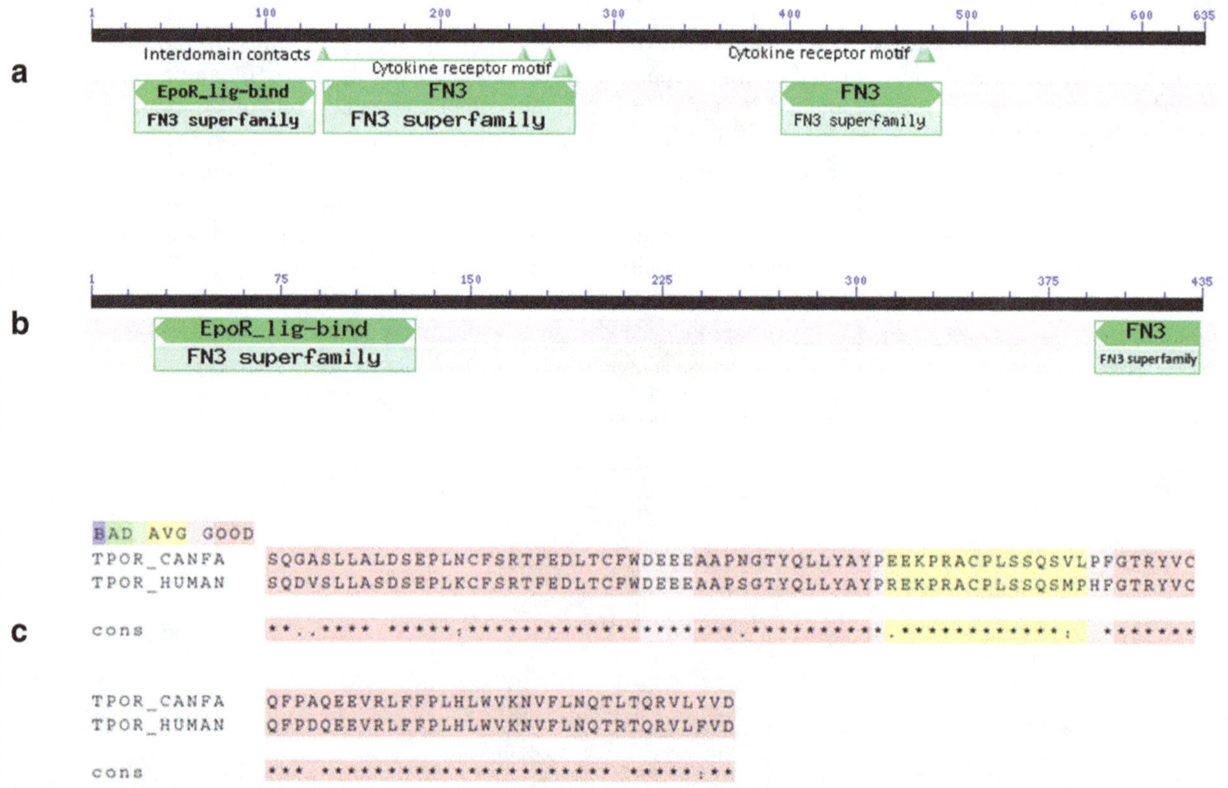

Fig. 1 Multiple sequence analysis of thrombopoietin receptor protein sequences in canines and humans. **a** Conserved domains on the human thrombopoietin receptor gi|730980|sp|P40238.1|TPOR_HUMAN; **b** Conserved domains on the canine thrombopoietin receptor gi|73978050|ref|XP_853442.1|Canis lupus familiaris; **c** Protein sequence alignments of conserved Erythropoietin receptor, ligand binding (EpoR-lig-bind) domains in extracellular part of canines and human thrombopoietin receptor (MPL)

initial dose – maintenance dose). In 3 cases romiplostim was given until the end of the observation period, one case (no. 3) was euthanized, case no. 5 was lost for follow-up.

Interestingly, the start of the increase in platelets in treated dogs appears to occur within two days after the first administration. The question whether this effect would be faster via the administration of higher doses, i.e. initially 10 μg/kg, remains to be answered in future studies. If this assumption would be true, romiplostim would be indicated as a first-line therapy in dogs requiring emergency treatment, i.e. dogs with life-threatening bleeding. The question why romiplostim appears to increase platelet counts in dogs faster than in humans remains obscure.

Romiplostim and other TPOs such as eltrombopag represent a new therapeutic measure for ITP in dogs that cannot be treated with conventional drugs or where these drugs are ineffective. Interestingly, the rapid effect is comparable with that observed in dogs treated with vincristine or IVIgG [18, 19].

Availability of romiplostim for usage in veterinary medicine may be limited by its high cost. We would therefore like to highlight one possible solution. The required amount of romiplostim for each human patient is dependent on the patient's response and is extremely variable. Some patients may require less than 100 μg, while others may require > 500 μg. Since the drug is only available in 250 μg and 500 μg vials, it cannot be avoided that the rest of the drug will be discarded. Based on our experience, the rest of the dissolved romiplostim can be stored for several weeks (6–8 weeks) under sterile conditions at 4 ° C without a dramatic loss in biological activity. On the other hand, dogs need in total less amounts of the drug than humans. Thus, the available vials might be used in parallel for treatment of three or more dogs at the same time.

We presented here the results of a pilot study and showed that the approved human drug romiplostim may represent a novel therapeutic option in refractory dog ITP.

Conclusions
Romiplostim is effective in the treatment of ITP in dogs at least as well as in humans. This finding may help to develop and use new therapeutics for ITP in dogs and humans.

Acknowledgements
Not applicable.

Funding
This study was funded by the German Research Foundation (DFG) (Project number SA 405/3-1).

Authors' contributions
GB, BK and AS conceived the study, analysed the data and wrote the paper; BK, AC, SR diagnosed and treated the dogs, and provided all relevant data. All authors critically revised the manuscript. All authors read and approved the final manuscript.

Authors' information
Not applicable.

Competing interests
The authors declare that they have no competing interests.

Consent for publication
Consent from the owners was obtained.

Author details
[1]FB Veterinärmedizin, Klinik für Kleine Haustiere, Freie Universität Berlin, Oertzenweg 19 b, 14163 Berlin, Germany. [2]Institut für Transfusionsmedizin, Charité – Universitätsklinikum, Augustenburger Platz 1, 13353 Berlin, Germany.

References
1. Harrington WJ, Minnich V, Hollingsworth JW, Moore CV. Demonstration of a thrombocytopenic factor in the blood of patients with thrombocytopenic purpura. J Lab Clin Med. 1951;38(1):1–10.
2. Cines DB, Schreiber AD. Immune thrombocytopenia. Use of a Coombs antiglobulin test to detect IgG and C3 on platelets. N Engl J Med. 1979; 300(3):106–11.
3. Ballem PJ, Segal GM, Stratton JR, Gernsheimer T, Adamson JW, Slichter SJ. Mechanisms of thrombocytopenia in chronic autoimmune thrombocytopenic purpura. Evidence of both impaired platelet production and increased platelet clearance. J Clin Invest. 1987;80(1):33–40.
4. Cines DB, Bussel JB, Liebman HA, Luning Prak ET. The ITP syndrome: pathogenic and clinical diversity. Blood. 2009;113(26):6511–21.
5. Lewis DC, Meyers KM. Canine idiopathic thrombocytopenic purpura. J Vet Intern Med. 1996;10(4):207–18.
6. Lewis DC, Meyers KM, Callan MB, Bucheler J, Giger U. Detection of platelet-bound and serum platelet-bindable antibodies for diagnosis of idiopathic thrombocytopenic purpura in dogs. J Am Vet Med Assoc. 1995;206(1):47–52.
7. Kohn B, Engelbrecht R, Leibold W, Giger U. Clinical findings, diagnostics and treatment results in primary and secondary immune-mediated thrombocytopenia in the dog. Kleintierpraxis. 2000;45(12):893–907.
8. Putsche JC, Kohn B. Primary immune-mediated thrombocytopenia in 30 dogs (1997–2003). J Am Anim Hosp Assoc. 2008;44(5):250–7.
9. Bussel JB, Cines D. Immune thrombocytopenic purpura, neonatal alloimmune thrombocytopenia and post-transfusion purpura. In: Hoffman EJB R, Shattil S, Furie B, Cohen HJ, Silberstein LE, editors. Hematology: Basic Principles and Practice. 3rd ed. 1999. p. 2096–114.
10. O'Marra SK, Delaforcade AM, Shaw SP. Treatment and predictors of outcome in dogs with immune-mediated thrombocytopenia. J Am Vet Med Assoc. 2011;238(3):346–52.
11. Provan D, Stasi R, Newland AC, Blanchette VS, Bolton-Maggs P, Bussel JB, Chong BH, Cines DB, Gernsheimer TB, Godeau B, et al. International consensus report on the investigation and management of primary immune thrombocytopenia. Blood. 2010;115(2):168–86.
12. Salama A. Current treatment options for primary immune thrombocytopenia. Expert Rev Hematol. 2011;4(1):107–18.
13. Force BCfSiHGHT. Guidelines for the investigation and management of idiopathic thrombocytopenic purpura in adults, children and in pregnancy. Br J Haematol. 2003;120(4):574–96.

14. Carr AP, Panciera DL, Kidd L. Prognostic factors for mortality and thromboembolism in canine immune-mediated hemolytic anemia: a retrospective study of 72 dogs. J Vet Intern Med. 2002;16(5):504–9.

15. Williams DA, Maggio-Price L. Canine idiopathic thrombocytopenia: clinical observations and long-term follow-up in 54 cases. J Am Vet Med Assoc. 1984;185(6):660–3.

16. Nakamura RK, Tompkins E, Bianco D. Therapeutic options for immune-mediated thrombocytopenia. J Vet Emerg Crit Care (San Antonio). 2012;22(1):59–72.

17. Rozanski EA, Callan MB, Hughes D, Sanders N, Giger U. Comparison of platelet count recovery with use of vincristine and prednisone or prednisone alone for treatment for severe immune-mediated thrombocytopenia in dogs. J Am Vet Med Assoc. 2002;220(4):477–81.

18. Balog K, Huang AA, Sum SO, Moore GE, Thompson C, Scott-Moncrieff JC. A prospective randomized clinical trial of vincristine versus human intravenous immunoglobulin for acute adjunctive management of presumptive primary immune-mediated thrombocytopenia in dogs. J Vet Intern Med. 2013;27(3):536–41.

19. Bianco D, Armstrong PJ, Washabau RJ. A prospective, randomized, double-blinded, placebo-controlled study of human intravenous immunoglobulin for the acute management of presumptive primary immune-mediated thrombocytopenia in dogs. J Vet Intern Med. 2009;23(5):1071–8.

20. Jackson ML, Kruth SA. Immune-mediated Hemolytic Anemia and Thrombocytopenia in the Dog: A retrospective study of 55 cases diagnosed from 1979 through 1983 at the Western College of Veterinary Medicine. Can Vet J. 1985;26(8):245–50.

21. Jans HE, Armstrong PJ, Price GS. Therapy of immune mediated thrombocytopenia. A retrospective study of 15 dogs. J Vet Intern Med. 1990;4(1):4–7.

22. Cines DB, Gernsheimer T, Wasser J, Godeau B, Provan D, Lyons R, et al. Integrated analysis of long-term safety in patients with chronic immune thrombocytopaenia (ITP) treated with the thrombopoietin (TPO) receptor agonist romiplostim. Int J Hematol. 2015;102(3):259–70.

23. Lev PR, Grodzielski M, Goette NP, Glembotsky AC, Espasandin YR, Pierdominici MS, Contrufo G, Montero VS, Ferrari L, Molinas FC, et al. Impaired proplatelet formation in immune thrombocytopenia: a novel mechanism contributing to decreased platelet count. Br J Haematol. 2014;165(6):854–64.

24. Kuter DJ. Thrombopoietin and thrombopoietin mimetics in the treatment of thrombocytopenia. Annu Rev Med. 2009;60:193–206.

25. Frederickson S, Renshaw MW, Lin B, Smith LM, Calveley P, Springhorn JP, Johnson K, Wang Y, Su X, Shen Y, et al. A rationally designed agonist antibody fragment that functionally mimics thrombopoietin. Proc Natl Acad Sci U S A. 2006;103(39):14307–12.

26. Jenkins JM, Williams D, Deng Y, Uhl J, Kitchen V, Collins D, Erickson-Miller CL. Phase 1 clinical study of eltrombopag, an oral, nonpeptide thrombopoietin receptor agonist. Blood. 2007;109(11):4739–41.

27. Wang B, Nichol JL, Sullivan JT. Pharmacodynamics and pharmacokinetics of AMG 531, a novel thrombopoietin receptor ligand. Clin Pharmacol Ther. 2004;76(6):628–38.

28. Kuter DJ, Rummel M, Boccia R, Macik BG, Pabinger I, Selleslag D, Rodeghiero F, Chong BH, Wang X, Berger DP. Romiplostim or standard of care in patients with immune thrombocytopenia. N Engl J Med. 2010;363(20):1889–99.

29. Gonzalez-Porras JR, Mingot-Castellano ME, Andrade MM, Alonso R, Caparros I, Arratibel MC, Fernandez-Fuertes F, Cortti MJ, Pascual C, Sanchez-Gonzalez B, et al. Use of eltrombopag after romiplostim in primary immune thrombocytopenia. Br J Haematol. 2015;169(1):111–6.

30. Bussel JB, Kuter DJ, Pullarkat V, Lyons RM, Guo M, Nichol JL. Safety and efficacy of long-term treatment with romiplostim in thrombocytopenic patients with chronic ITP. Blood. 2009;113(10):2161–71.

31. Grindem CB, Breitschwerdt EB, Corbett WT, Jans HE. Epidemiologic survey of thrombocytopenia in dogs: a report on 987 cases. Vet Clin Pathol. 1991;20(2):38–43.

32. Yau VK, Bianco D. Treatment of five haemodynamically stable dogs with immune-mediated thrombocytopenia using mycophenolate mofetil as single agent. J Small Anim Pract. 2014;55(6):330–3.

33. Molineux G, Newland A. Development of romiplostim for the treatment of patients with chronic immune thrombocytopenia: from bench to bedside. Br J Haematol. 2010;150(1):9–20.

34. Newland A, Caulier MT, Kappers-Klunne M, Schipperus MR, Lefrere F, Zwaginga JJ, Christal J, Chen CF, Nichol JL. An open-label, unit dose-finding study of AMG 531, a novel thrombopoiesis-stimulating peptibody, in patients with immune thrombocytopenic purpura. Br J Haematol. 2006;135(4):547–53.

35. Kuter DJ, Bussel JB, Lyons RM, Pullarkat V, Gernsheimer TB, Senecal FM, Aledort LM, George JN, Kessler CM, Sanz MA, et al. Efficacy of romiplostim in patients with chronic immune thrombocytopenic purpura: a double-blind randomised controlled trial. Lancet. 2008;371(9610):395–403.

36. Chalmers S, Tarantino MD. Romiplostim as a treatment for immune thrombocytopenia: a review. J Blood Med. 2015;6:37–44.

37. Case BC, Hauck ML, Yeager RL, Simkins AH, de Serres M, Schmith VD, Dillberger JE, Page RL. The pharmacokinetics and pharmacodynamics of GW395058, a peptide agonist of the thrombopoietin receptor, in the dog, a large-animal model of chemotherapy-induced thrombocytopenia. Stem Cells. 2000;18(5):360–5.

38. Bussel JB, Hsieh L, Buchanan GR, Stine K, Kalpatthi R, Gnarra DJ, et al. Long-term use of the thrombopoietin-mimetic romiplostim in children with severe chronic immune thrombocytopenia (ITP). Pediatr Blood Cancer. 2014.

7

Is CCNU (lomustine) valuable for treatment of cutaneous epitheliotropic lymphoma in dogs? A critically appraised topic

Aurore Laprais[1] and Thierry Olivry[1,2]* iD

Abstract

Background: CCNU and other treatment protocols are commonly offered to owners for the treatment of dogs diagnosed with cutaneous (epitheliotropic) T-cell lymphoma (CTCL). Chemotherapy protocols provide variable benefits; they have different side-effects, and they typically require monitoring to detect drug toxicity at a non-negligible cost to the owner. At this time, even though CCNU is most often recommended to treat dogs with CTCL, there is no clear consensus on the benefit of this drug. Knowing which chemotherapy protocol yields the highest rate of complete remission and longest survival times would help veterinarians and pet owners select treatment options based on the best evidence available. Our objective was to review the literature to compare the complete remission rates and survival times of CCNU-based protocols to those of other interventions. We critically assessed the data included in articles reporting treatment outcome in at least five dogs with CTCL. Single case reports and case series with less than five patients were not reviewed to avoid anecdotal evidence of lower quality.

Results: The search for, and review and analysis of, the best evidence available as of February 8, 2017, suggests that CCNU and pegylated liposomal doxorubicin appear to yield the highest rate of complete remission in approximately one-third of dogs with CTCL. Other treatment protocols did not report usable information on remission rates. Without any treatment, the mean/median survival time in dogs with CTCL varied between 3 and 5 months. With CCNU protocols, the median survival time was 6 months and the one with retinoids (isotretinoin and/or etretinate), PEG L-asparaginase or prednisolone monotherapy was 11, 9 and 4 months, respectively; all these durations were obtained from small numbers of dogs, however.

Conclusions: CCNU leads to a complete remission of signs in approximately one-third of dogs with CTCL, but such remissions are of short duration. The median survival time after CCNU appears longer than that without treatment, but other drugs appear to provide a better long-term prognosis. Further studies are required to investigate the effect of CCNU, alone or in combination, on remission rates, survival times and impact on quality of life.

Keywords: Canine, Chemotherapy, Dog, Epitheliotropic, Lomustine, Lymphosarcoma, Mycosis fungoides, Neoplasia

Background

Lomustine (CCNU) or other chemotherapy protocols are commonly offered to owners for the treatment of their dogs diagnosed with cutaneous (epitheliotropic) T-cell lymphoma (CTCL). Although these regimens are expected to lead to a temporary partial or complete remission (CR) of skin lesions, monitoring for the detection of common severe adverse events requires regular laboratory monitoring that might represent a significant financial burden to the clients [1]. At this time, there is no clear consensus on the benefit of the various treatment regimens for dogs with CTCL.

Knowing which chemotherapy protocol has the strongest evidence for yielding the best complete remission rates and longest survival times would help veterinarians and pet owners select treatment options based on the best evidence available. Our objective was to review the literature to compare the complete remission rates and survival times of CCNU-based protocols to those of other interventions.

* Correspondence: tolivry@ncsu.edu
[1]Department of Clinical Sciences, College of Veterinary Medicine, North Carolina State University, Raleigh, NC, USA
[2]Comparative Medicine Institute, College of Veterinary Medicine, North Carolina State University, Raleigh, NC, USA

Clinical scenarios

You have two patients: The first one is a 5-year-old female Labrador retriever crossbred dog. The owners report that the lesions started 2.5 months beforehand and that they consisted, at first, of generalized scaling and pruritus. They evolved into multifocal areas of truncal alopecia and erythema along with an ulcer on the caudal abdomen. The dog was placed on a tapering course of prednisone that led to a reduction in clinical signs. After discontinuing the steroids, the dog developed alopecic erythematous macules, patches and plaques, and she became more pruritic than before.

Your second patient is a 12-year-old male golden retriever presenting with multifocal large patchy areas of hypopigmentation and depigmentation along with multifocal erythematous plaques and nodules. The owner reports that the dog may have had depigmented muzzle lesions for the past 2 years.

In both cases, skin biopsies confirmed your suspicion of CTCL. You wonder which chemotherapeutic option would be most beneficial for these two dogs.

Structured question

In a dog with CTCL, which chemotherapeutic treatment protocol would be most effective to induce the CR of clinical signs and to lead to the longest survival?

Methods

Search strategy

The CAB Abstracts and Web of Science (WoS) Science Citation Index Expanded databases were searched on April 26, 2016 for relevant articles using the following string: (dog or dogs or canine) and (cutaneous or epitheliotropic or epidermotropic) and (lymphoma or lymphosarcoma) and (CCNU or lomustine or vincristine or cyclophosphamide or chlorambucil or predniso* or chemotherap*). The search was limited to the period 1980–2016. We then screened the bibliographies of identified articles for additional relevant reports. At the time of revision of this manuscript (Febuary 08, 2017), a second broad literature search was done to identify papers published since the first search.

Results and discussion

Identified evidence

Our literature search found 63 and 65 articles in the CAB Abstract and Web of Science (WoS) databases, respectively. Citations were initially examined for the identification of articles reporting the outcome of treatment in dogs with CTCL diagnosed via histopathology. We then evaluated abstracts, and articles with potentially relevant information were read in full. The bibliography of these papers was analyzed further for additional pertinent reports.

We only selected articles that provided definite information on the rate of CR /or survival times after diagnosis or treatment of at least five dogs with CTCL; articles and information on partial remission were not reviewed further.

Two retrospective [2, 3] and one prospective studies [4] providing clear information on CR rates in dogs with CTCL were found in both CAB and WoS databases. One preclinical trial [5] and one pilot study [6] were subsequently added following the review of the bibliographies of articles identified in the electronic searches. Finally, we added one last article that had been published after the performance of our initial literature search [7].

For survival times after diagnosis or treatment, one retrospective study [8] and one prospective study [9] were identified in the CAB abstracts, one of which was also found in the WoS [8]. A prospective [10] and a retrospective study [11] were added following the review of bibliographies of articles found in the electronic search.

Evaluation of evidence

Complete remission rates

The rates of CR in studies involving five or more dogs were given for protocols using CCNU, pegylated liposomal doxorubicin, the prodrug VDC-1101 (a guanine analog) and masitinib (Table 1).

Altogether, CCNU, alone or in conjunction with other concurrent medications, yielded a combined rate of CR of 30% of the 87 dogs reported [2, 3, 6]. The median duration of CR, estimated from only 15 dogs in one article [2], was 132 days (range: 26–258 days). The time to achieve CR was not identified in any article. In one report of 46 dogs [2], the overall median number of treatments needed to observe a response (type not specified) was one (range: one to six cycles).

A similar rate of CR occurred with pegylated liposomal doxorubicin, but the number of dogs treated (nine) was low [5]. The median duration of CR was shorter (90 days, range: 21–340) than with CCNU; the time to CR was not reported either.

The prednisone and VDC-1101 combination did not lead to CR in any of the ten dogs to which it was administered [4].

Finally, masitinib induced a CR of signs of CTCL in 2/10 treated dogs (20%); this remission lasted for 126 days in one dog and over 3 years in the other [7].

Survival times after diagnosis or treatment initiation

The survival times were only available for a few dogs treated with each intervention (Table 2). Without any treatment, the median survival time in dogs with CTCL varied between 3 [11] and 5 months [8].

Table 1 Rates of complete remission in dogs with CTCL

References	CCNU		Pegylated liposomal doxorubicin		VDC-1101 and prednisone		Masitinib	
	N	CR (N, %)	N	CR (N, %)	N	CR (N, %)	N	CR (N, %)
Morges, 2014 [4]					10	0 (0%)		
Risbon, 2006 [2]	46[a]	15 (33%)						
Williams, 2006 [3]	36	6[b] (33%)						
Graham, 1999 [6]	5	5[c] (100%)						
Vail, 1997 [5]			9	3 (33%)				
Holtermann, 2016 [7]							10[d]	2 (20%)
TOTAL	87	26 (30%)	9	3 (33%)	10	0 (0%)	1-	2 (20%)

Abbreviations: *CR* complete remission, *N* number of dogs
[a]14 dogs received CCNU monotherapy, 27 also received glucocorticoids that were later either tapered, discontinued or maintained. The co-administration of prednisone was reported not to be significantly associated with the response or its duration. Other concurrent medications included PEG L-asparaginase (6 dogs), essential fatty acids (8), nonsteroidal anti-inflammatory drugs (3), retinoids (2), and interferon (1)
[b]67% of the dogs experiencing a CR also received concurrent glucocorticoids
[c]2 dogs may have received concurrent surgery
[d]the response was assessed on the three most dominant "target" lesions

The median/mean survival times were, in order of decreasing durations, 11 months after treatment with the retinoids isotretinoin and/or etretinate [9], 9 months after PEG L-asparaginase [10], 6 months after CCNU protocols [8] and 4 months after prednisolone alone [8].

Limitations

The main limitation of this compilation is that any confounding effect of the dog's age, CTCL severity, CTCL stage or time before the diagnosis was made or treatment initiated were not evaluated for their possible impact on CR or survival times in any of these studies. Another limitation is that CCNU was used alone in only one-third of dogs in the largest case series [2, 3], and the rates of CR were not compared between dogs receiving CCNU monotherapy and those treated with combination regimens. Furthermore, the survival times provided were likely to have been influenced by euthanasia decisions by the owner, thereby not reflecting disease-induced death. Finally, many of the estimates provided herein were only assembled from a small number of patients.

Conclusions
Implications for practitioners

In spite of the limitations raised above, and taking into consideration the best evidence available, CCNU protocols, when used alone or in combination with other drugs, appear to lead to CR rates of 30%, but the median duration of such CRs remains unclear. The median survival time of CTCL after CCNU protocols is 6 months following diagnosis. Retinoids or PEG L-asparaginase appear to offer longer median survival times, but these drugs are not routinely available.

At the time of this writing, CCNU—alone or in combination with other drugs—appears to be a valuable option to treat dogs with CTCL; unfortunately, the common occurrence of myelopoietic and/or gastrointestinal side effects requires frequent blood test monitoring that increases the cost of treatment.

Implication for research

Additional studies are needed to compare the rates of CR and survival times using glucocorticoids, CCNU or retinoids (e.g. bexarotene), either alone or in various

Table 2 Survival times in dogs with CTCL (in months)

References	CCNU		Prednisolone		Retinoids[a]		PEG L-asparaginase[b]		No treatment	
	N	S	N	S	N	S	N	S	N	S
Fontaine, 2010 [8][c]	7	6	6	4					3	5
White, 1993 [9][c]					5	11				
Moriello, 1993 [10][d]							7	9		
Beale, 1993 [11][e]									8	3

Abbreviations: *N* number, *S* median or mean survival times (in months) after diagnosis or treatment
[a]the concurrent use of glucocorticoids was allowed
[b]three patients also received glucocorticoids, one patient was also treated with vincristine/cyclophosphamide and doxorubicin
[c]Most dogs were euthanized; the specific number of dogs was not specified
[d]All dogs were euthanized
[e]the number of dogs euthanized was not specified

combinations thereof. Because of the potential toxicity and side effects of CCNU, the quality of life in dogs receiving CCNU protocols should be compared to that without any treatment or with other medications. Future studies should also attempt to compare CR rates and survival times in dogs of various age groups as well as in those with variable duration of clinical signs, stages or severities of CTCL.

Abbreviations
CCNU: 1-(2-chloroethyl)-3-cyclohexyl-1-nitrosourea (i.e. lomustine); CR: complete remission; CTCL: cutaneous T-cell lymphoma; PEG: polyethylene glycol

Acknowledgement
None needed.

Funding
None.

Authors' contributions
The two authors selected the topic of this CAT; AFL performed the literature search, extracted and summarized the evidence; TO verified the evidence and both authors contributed to the writing of this article.

Competing interests
The authors declare that they have no competing interests.

Consent for publication
Not needed or relevant.

References

1. Heading KL, Brockley LK, Bennett PF. CCNU (lomustine) toxicity in dogs: a retrospective study (2002-07). Aust Vet J. 2011;89:109–16.
2. Risbon RE, de Lorimier LP, Skorupski K, Burgess KE, Bergman PJ, Carreras J, Hahn K, Leblanc A, Turek M, Impellizeri J, Fred 3rd R, Wojcieszyn JW, Drobatz K, Clifford CA. Response of canine cutaneous epitheliotropic lymphoma to lomustine (CCNU): a retrospective study of 46 cases (1999-2004). J Vet Intern Med. 2006;20:1389–97.
3. Williams LE, Rassnick KM, Power HT, Lana SE, Morrison-Collister KE, Hansen K, Johnson JL. CCNU in the treatment of canine epitheliotropic lymphoma. J Vet Intern Med. 2006;20:136–43.
4. Morges MA, Burton JH, Saba CF, Vail DM, Burgess KE, Thamm DH. Phase II evaluation of VDC-1101 in canine cutaneous T-cell lymphoma. J Vet Intern Med. 2014;28:1569–74.
5. Vail DM, Kravis LD, Cooley AJ, Chun R, MacEwen EG. Preclinical trial of doxorubicin entrapped in sterically stabilized liposomes in dogs with spontaneously arising malignant tumors. Cancer Chemother Pharmacol. 1997;39:410–6.
6. Graham JC, Myers RK. Pilot study on the use of lomustine (CCNU) for the treatment of cutaneous lymphoma in dogs [abstract 125]. Proceedings of the Proceedings of the 17th Annual Forum of the College of Veterinary Internal Medicine. Chicago: American College of Veterinary Internal Medicine; 1999.
7. Holtermann N, Kiupel M, Kessler M, Teske E, Betz D, Hirschberger J. Masitinib monotherapy in canine epitheliotropic lymphoma. Vet Comp Oncol. 2016;14 Suppl 1:127–35.
8. Fontaine J, Heimann M, Day MJ. Canine cutaneous epitheliotropic T-cell lymphoma: a review of 30 cases. Vet Dermatol. 2010;21:267–75.
9. White SD, Rosychuk RA, Scott KV, Trettien AL, Jonas L, Denerolle P. Use of isotretinoin and etretinate for the treatment of benign cutaneous neoplasia and cutaneous lymphoma in dogs. J Am Vet Med Assoc. 1993;202:387–91.
10. Moriello KA, Macewen G, Schultz KT. Peg L-asparaginase in the treatment of canine epitheliotropic lymphoma and histiocytic proliferative dermatitis. In: Ihrke PJ, Mason IS, White SD, editors. Advances in veterinary dermatology, vol. 2. 1993. p. 293–9.
11. Beale KM, Bolon B. Canine cutaneous lymphosarcoma: epitheliotropic and non-epitheliotropic, a retrospective study. In: Ihrke PJ, Mason IS, White SD, editors. Advances in veterinary dermatology, vol. 2. New York: Pergamon Press; 1993. p. 273–84.

8

Localization of neonatal Fc receptor for IgG in aggregated lymphoid nodules area in abomasum of Bactrian camels (*Camelus bactrianus*) of different ages

Wang-Dong Zhang, Wen-Hui Wang[*], Shu-Xian Li, Shuai Jia, Xue-Feng Zhang and Ting-Ting Cao

Abstract

Background: The neonatal Fc receptor (FcRn) plays a crucial role in transporting IgG and associated antigens across polarized epithelial barriers in mucosal immunity. However, it was not clear that FcRn expression in aggregated lymphoid nodules area (ALNA) in abomasum, a unique and important mucosal immune structure discovered only in Bactrian camels. In the present study, 27 Alashan Bactrian camels were divided into the following five age groups: fetus (10–13 months of gestation), young (1–2 years), pubertal (3–5 years), middle-aged (6–16 years) and old (17–20 years). The FcRn expressions were observed and analyzed in detail with histology, immunohistochemistry, micro-image analysis and statistical methods.

Results: The results showed that the FcRn was expressed in mucosal epithelial cells of ALNA from the fetus to the old group, although the expression level rapidly declined in old group; moreover, after the ALNA matured, the FcRn expression level in the non-follicle-associated epithelium (non-FAE) was significantly higher than that in FAE ($P < 0.05$). In addition, the FcRn was also expressed in the vessel endothelium, smooth muscle tissue, and macrophages and dendritic cells (DCs) of secondary lymphoid follicles (sLFs).

Conclusions: It was demonstrated that FcRn was mainly expressed in non-FAE, the effector sites, although which was expressed in FAE, the inductive sites for mucosal immunity. And it was also expressed in DCs and macrophages in sLFs of all ages of Bactrian camels. The results provided a powerful evidence that IgG (including HCAb) could participate in mucosal immune response and tolerance in ALNA of Bactrian camels through FcRn transmembrane transport.

Keywords: Neonatal Fc receptor (FcRn), Expression, Aggregated lymphoid nodules area (ALNA), Bactrian camels, Epithelium, Mucosal immunity

Background

In mucosal immunity, polymeric immunoglobulin receptor (pIgR) is an important receptor, which helps to maintain mucosal barrier integrity and gastroenteric homeostasis by transporting secretory immunoglobulin A (SIgA) antibodies across intestinal epithelial cells (IECs) into gut secretions [1–5]. As well, the neonatal Fc receptor (FcRn) also plays a crucial role in transporting IgG and associated antigens across polarized barriers [6–11]. It is another important receptor regulating mucosal immune response.

FcRn, originally discovered in the intestinal epithelium of newborn rat [12], is also referred to as the major histocompatibility complex (MHC) class I-related receptor due to their structural similarities [13]. The heterodimer composed of a soluble light chain β2-microglobulin (β2m) and a membrane-bound heavy chain that consists of three soluble domains (α1, α2 and α3), a single transmembrane helix, and a small cytoplasmic domain [14]. Although FcRn was originally named according to its expression

* Correspondence: wwh777@126.com
College of Veterinary Medicine, Gansu Agricultural University, Lanzhou, Gansu 730070, China

pattern in rodent IECs where it was first identified, FcRn is now known to be expressed throughout life in many different cell types across the body [15–25]. However, the FcRn expression characteristics markedly differ with different species. For instance, in human intestinal epithelial cells, FcRn is expressed in both fetus and adult [15, 26]. By contrast, it is only highly in newborns and the level rapidly declines after weaning in mouse [27, 28]. In addition, the range of animals in which FcRn orthologs have also been identified includes rabbit [29], pig [30], sheep [31], bovine [32], Egyptian water buffalo [33], and dromedary [34].

Bactrian camel is an important livestock of economic characteristics in northwest of China and has some special immunological features. First, compared with the structure of conventional IgG, the Camelidae IgG2 and IgG3 are special heavy chain antibodies (HCAbs) [35], which are naturally devoid of light chain and their antigen binding site only consists of a single domain [36]. Second, compared with other livestock [37], Chinese Alashan Bactrian camels have a unique aggregated lymphoid nodule area (ALNA) in the abomasum [38]. This species-specific anatomical structure could be divided into the reticular mucosal folds region (RMFR) and longitudinal mucosal folds region (LMFR) [38–40]. They belonged to the organized mucosa-associated lymphoid tissue (MALT). However, the FcRn expression in this region has not been reported at present. Based on our previous researches on the morphology and histology of ALNA [38–40], the characteristics of FcRn expression with age in this area were studied in this paper. We hope that it will provide the necessary immunomorphology support for further studying whether FcRn could participate in mucosal immunity in this area or not.

Methods
Experimental animals
Twenty-seven Alashan Bactrian camels of different ages (half male and half female, except fetus group) were divided into five age groups: fetus (10–13 months' gestation, $n = 3$, two males and one female), young (1–2 years, $n = 6$), pubertal (3–5 years, $n = 6$), middle-aged (6–16 years, $n = 6$) and old (17–20 years, $n = 6$). Fetus tissues were collected from animal carcasses submitted to the necropsy service in College of Veterinary Medicine, Gansu Agricultural University. Other animals were from the slaughterhouse (Xining, Qinghai province of China) and were not starved before slaughter, which were anaesthetised intravenously with sodium pentobarbital (20 mg/kg) and then exsanguinated to death.

Microsection
The whole abomasum from the isthmus to the pyloric ostium was incised along the greater curvature. The gastric contents were cleaned with saline. Samples from RMFR and LMFR of ANLNA were rapidly taken after death and fixed in 10 % neutral formalin. The paraffin sections were made and stained with haematoxylin and eosin (H&E) by a routine method [41] as well as SABC-immunohistochemistry (IHC) by the method as follows: the samples were sectioned (4 μm) and placed on the polylysine-coated slides (molecular weight: 150, 000–300,000; working concentration: 0.10 % (w/v) solution in water, Sigma, USA). After deparaffination, we used 1.0 mg/ml trypsin 1: 250 (250.N.F.U/mg, Sigma, USA) for enzyme-induced epitope retrieval, which was followed by endogenous peroxidase blocking (3 % H_2O_2). For blocking, 5 % bovine serum albumin (BSA, from easy-to-use immunohistochemical kit, Lot No.07H3OCJ, Boster, Wuhan, Hubei, China) was used. All samples with the primary antibody were incubated at 4 °C overnight. After being rinsed with PBS 2 min × 3 times; HRP conjugated goat anti-rabbit IgG (from easy-to-use immunohistochemical kit, Lot No.07H3OCJ, Boster, Wuhan, Hubei, China) as secondary antibody was applied for 1 h in humidified box at 37 °C. After being rinsed with PBS 5 min × 4 times. The SABC was applied for 30 min in humidified box at 37 °C. After being rinsed with PBS 5 min × 4 times. For detection, DAB Kit (ZSGB-BIO, Beijing, China) was used at room temperature. Slides were counterstained with Hematoxylin (Solarbio, Beijing, China) and mounted with Neutral Balsam (Solarbio, Beijing, China). Sections were examined with an Olympus microscope (Olympus, Hamburg, Germany) [42].

Primary antibodies selection and analysis
Rabbit polyclonal antibodies against human FcRn, diluted with the buffer at 3.33 μg/ml before use, was supported by BIOSS (Lot No. 140226, BIOSS, Beijing, China).

Some studies reported that the drFcRn/ Fc contact residues were highly conserved, and the structures of FcRn in different species were similar [14, 34, 43]. Hence, the epitopes of FcRn are similar among different species. Moreover, in immune responses, MHCII presents antigens to $CD4^+$ T cells, and the antigen peptide should be composed of more than 12 amino acid residues. The molecular weight of human FcRn is about 50 kDa. Moreover, the similarity of FcRn between dromedary and human was 78.6 % by analyzing the genes of phylogenetic relatedness of the extracellular domains (α1–α2–α3) [34]. Therefore, this primary antibody well met the sequent experiment request.

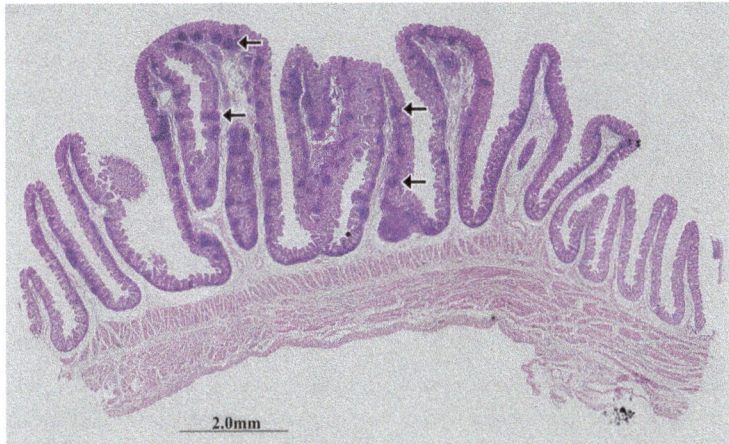

Fig. 1 Histological characteristics of the RMFR in fetus group. A plenty of primary lymphatic follicles (pLFs) (*arrow*) were seen in this area and they were mainly distributed in the lamina propria (LP). Original magnification: 40×

Second antibodies

SABC goat anti-rabbit IgG polyclonal antibodies immunohistochemical kit (Lot No.07H3OCJ, Boster, Wuhan, Hubei, China). The kit contained 1.5% BSA:12 ml. Second antibodies: Biotin goat anti rabbit IgG: 12 ml. SABC: 12 ml. It is an easy-to-use kit, which can be used directly and is unnecessary to be diluted with the buffer.

Light microscopy

In each group, the expression sites and characteristics of FcRn were observed in detail under microscope and photomicrographed using Olympus DP-71 microscopy system.

Statistical analysis

Five sections were randomly selected for each sample. Ten microscopic fields were randomly selected, observed and photomicrographed for FAE, non-FAE, vascular, smooth muscle and lymphoid follicle in each section. The mean optical density (MOD) of each site was calculated (Image-Pro Plus 6.0), respectively. The main steps contain: 1. the background correction of the IHC photos (this can make the light intensity in the central and around the IHC photos become consistent); 2. the correction of the optical density of the IHC photos (this can change the image intensity to the optical density); 3. the parameter setting (select the integrated optical density (IOD) as the measurement value of the ICH image); 4. selection the measurement region through the software tools; 5. color settings; 6. measurement of the IOD and the area of the selected region; 7. the calculation of the MOD through IOD/selected areas. The MOD differences among groups were analyzed by one-way ANOVA followed by Duncan's new multiple range test using IBM SPSS v. 23.0 (SPSS Inc., Chicago, USA). The significant difference was considered at $P < 0.05$.

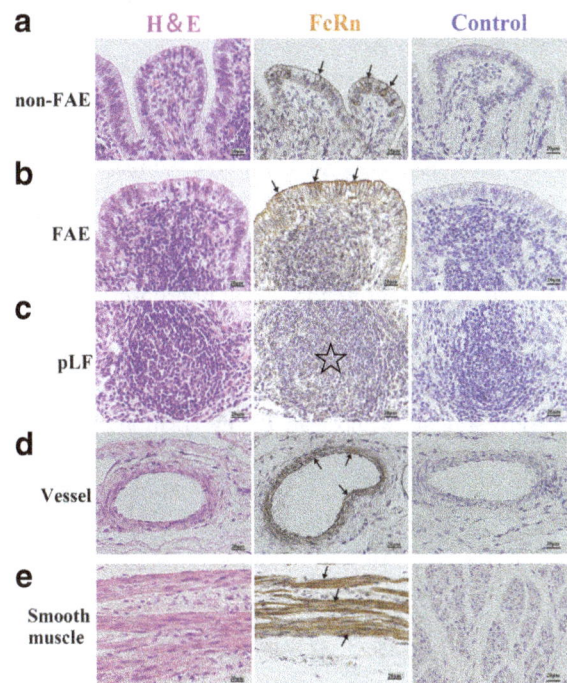

Fig. 2 Localization of FcRn in RMFR of fetus' abomasum ALNA. From left to right column, the paraffin sections were stained with hematoxylin and eosin (H&E), immunohistochemistry for FcRn, hematoxylin counterstain (as negative control), respectively. **a** non-FAE represents non-follicle-associated epithelium in the top panel, and FcRn positive expression was mainly distributed in membrane of the epithelial cells (*arrow*); **b** FAE represents follicle-associated epithelium in the second panel from top to bottom, and FcRn positive expression was mainly distributed in membrane of the epithelial cells (*arrow*); **c** pLF represents primary lymphatic follicles in the third panel (*star*), and typical macrophages and dendritic cells (DCs) with high FcRn expression were not observed; **d** Vessel, FcRn was highly expressed both in vascular endothelial cells and smooth muscle cells (*arrow*); **e** Smooth muscle, FcRn was also highly expressed in basement membrane of smooth muscle (*arrow*). Original magnification: 400×

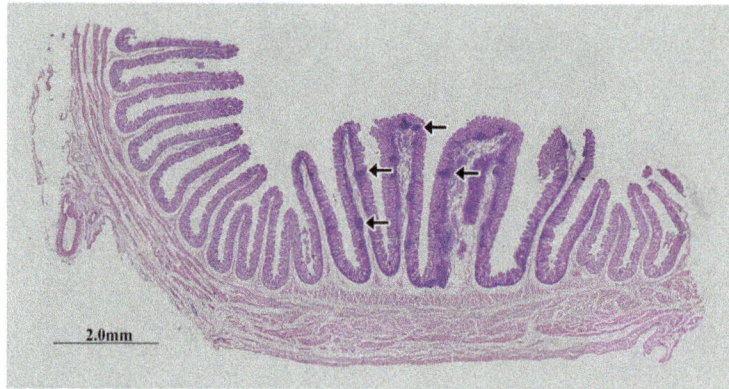

Fig. 3 Histological characteristics of the LMFR in fetus group. A certain amount of primary lymphatic follicles (pLFs) (*arrow*) were seen in this area. The distribution characteristics of pLFs were similar to those in RMFR, i.e., they were mainly distributed in the lamina propria (LP). Original magnification: 40×

Results

Localization of FcRn in abomasum ALNA in Bactrian camels of different ages

Fetus group

(1') In RMFR, a plenty of primary lymphatic follicles (pLFs) were primary densely-distributed in the lamina propria (LP) (Fig. 1). And FcRn was expressed in both non-follicle-associated epithelium (non-FAE) (Fig. 2a) and FAE (Fig. 2b), and mainly at the apical membrane. However, typical macrophages and dendritic cells (DCs) with high FcRn expression were not observed in the pLFs (Fig. 2c). In addition, the FcRn was also expressed in vessel endothelium (Fig. 2d) and smooth muscle tissue (Fig. 2e). (2') In LMFR, the histological characteristics were similar to those in RMFR. Lymphatic follicles were also pLFs. But the distribution density was lower than that in RMFR (Fig. 3). The localization of FcRn was similar to that in RMFR (Fig. 4a–e).

Young group

(1') In RMFR, a plenty of secondary lymphatic follicles (sLFs) were concentrated in the LP and submucosa (Fig. 5a). FcRn was highly expressed in typical macrophages and DCs in sLFs (Fig. 5b, c and d). Meanwhile, the FcRn was also expressed in non-FAE (Fig. 6a), FAE (Fig. 6b), vessel endothelium (Fig. 6c) and smooth muscle tissue (Fig. 6d). (2') In LMFR, the localization of FcRn was similar to that in RMFR (Figs. 7 and 8).

Pubertal and middle-aged groups

The localization of FcRn was in the two groups were both similar to those in young group.

Old group

The localization of FcRn was in RMFR and LMFR were similar. It was highly expressed in macrophages and

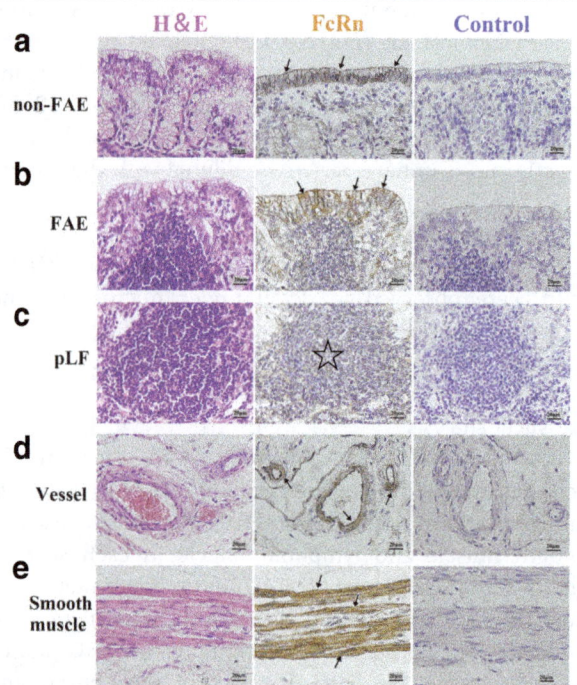

Fig. 4 Localization of FcRn in LMFR of fetus' abomasum ALNA. From left to right column, the paraffin sections were stained with hematoxylin and eosin (H&E), immunohistochemistry for FcRn, hematoxylin counterstain (as negative control), respectively. **a** non-FAE represents non-follicle-associated epithelium in the top panel, and FcRn positive expression was mainly distributed in membrane of the epithelial cells (*arrow*); **b** FAE represents follicle-associated epithelium in the second panel from top to bottom, and FcRn positive expression was mainly distributed in membrane of the epithelial cells (*arrow*); **c** pLF represents primary lymphatic follicles in the third panel (*star*), and typical macrophages and dendritic cells (DCs) with high FcRn expression were not observed; **d** Vessel, FcRn was highly expressed both in vascular endothelial cells and smooth muscle cells (*arrow*); **e** Smooth muscle, FcRn was also highly expressed in basement membrane of smooth muscle (*arrow*). Original magnification: 400×

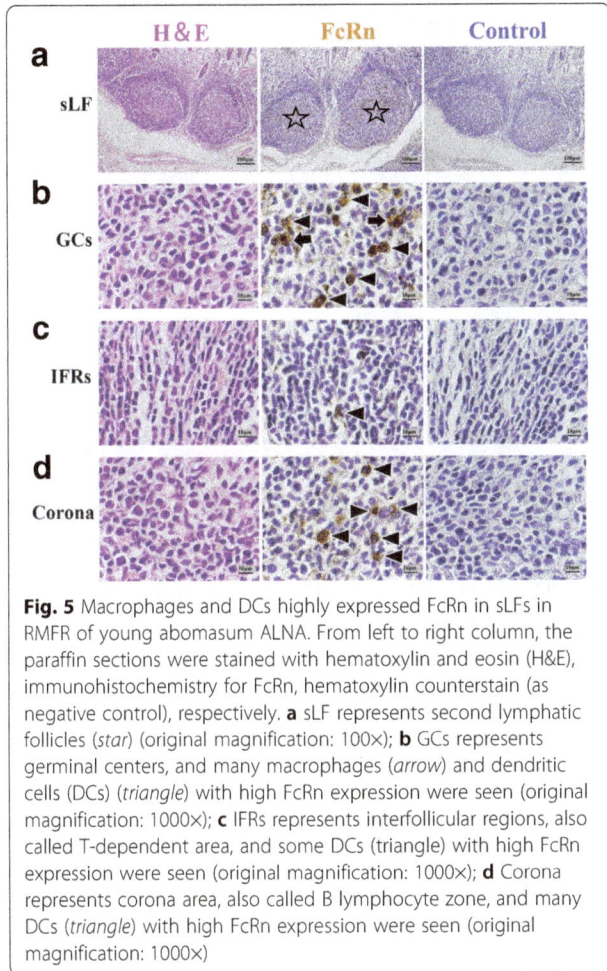

Fig. 5 Macrophages and DCs highly expressed FcRn in sLFs in RMFR of young abomasum ALNA. From left to right column, the paraffin sections were stained with hematoxylin and eosin (H&E), immunohistochemistry for FcRn, hematoxylin counterstain (as negative control), respectively. **a** sLF represents second lymphatic follicles (*star*) (original magnification: 100×); **b** GCs represents germinal centers, and many macrophages (*arrow*) and dendritic cells (DCs) (*triangle*) with high FcRn expression were seen (original magnification: 1000×); **c** IFRs represents interfollicular regions, also called T-dependent area, and some DCs (triangle) with high FcRn expression were seen (original magnification: 1000×); **d** Corona represents corona area, also called B lymphocyte zone, and many DCs (*triangle*) with high FcRn expression were seen (original magnification: 1000×)

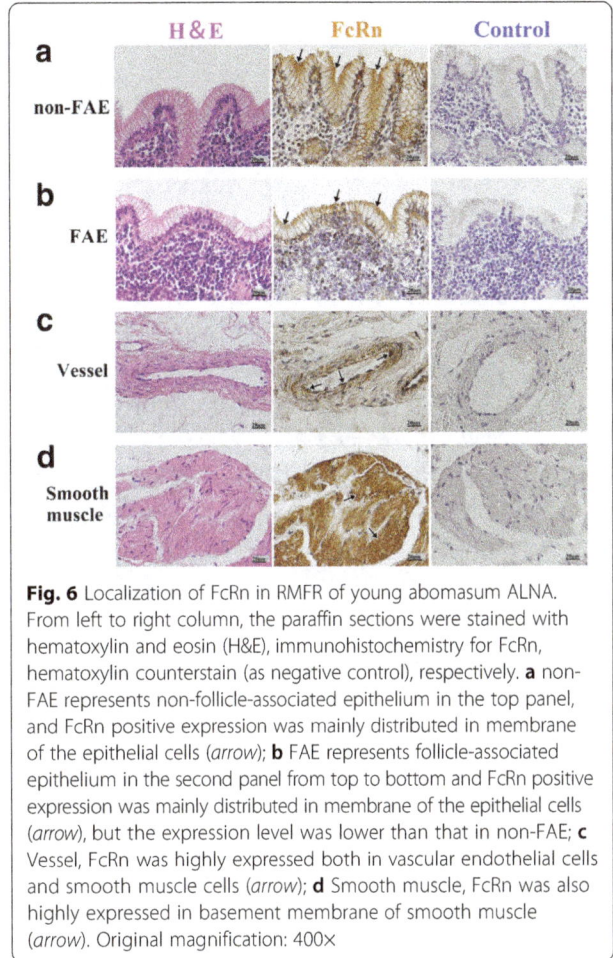

Fig. 6 Localization of FcRn in RMFR of young abomasum ALNA. From left to right column, the paraffin sections were stained with hematoxylin and eosin (H&E), immunohistochemistry for FcRn, hematoxylin counterstain (as negative control), respectively. **a** non-FAE represents non-follicle-associated epithelium in the top panel, and FcRn positive expression was mainly distributed in membrane of the epithelial cells (*arrow*); **b** FAE represents follicle-associated epithelium in the second panel from top to bottom and FcRn positive expression was mainly distributed in membrane of the epithelial cells (*arrow*), but the expression level was lower than that in non-FAE; **c** Vessel, FcRn was highly expressed both in vascular endothelial cells and smooth muscle cells (*arrow*); **d** Smooth muscle, FcRn was also highly expressed in basement membrane of smooth muscle (*arrow*). Original magnification: 400×

DCs in sLFs, however, the expression levels were very low in other tissues.

FcRn expression levels in mucosal epithelium of abomasum ALNA with age
FcRn expression levels

The MOD value detection results showed: (**1'**) In RMFR, the FcRn expression level in non-FAE was significantly higher than that in FAE in young, pubertal and middle-aged groups, respectively ($P < 0.05$) (Fig. 9b, c and d), but it had no significant difference in fetus and old groups ($P > 0.05$) (Fig. 9a and e); (**2'**) In LMFR, the FcRn expression level in non-FAE was significantly higher than that in FAE in pubertal and middle-aged groups, respectively ($P < 0.05$) (Fig. 9c and d), and it had no significant difference in other groups ($P > 0.05$) (Fig. 9a, b and e).

Changes in the FcRn expression with age
(**1'**) In RMFR, the FcRn expression level in FEA and non-FAE both gradually increased from fetus to pubertal groups with increasing age, peaked in pubertal group, and subsequently gradually declined (Fig. 10a and b). (**2'**) In LMFR, the FcRn expression level in FAE peaked in young and kept the high level to pubertal period, then subsequently significantly declined, but that in non-FAE gradually increased with increasing age, peaked in the middle-aged group (Fig. 10c and d). In addition, the FcRn expression level significantly decreased in the mucosa epithelium in old group ($P < 0.05$) (Fig. 10e).

Discussion
Organized MALT is a critical part of the mucosal immune system [44]. Wang et al. reported that there were developed ALNA in abomasum of Bactrian camel [38–40], which belonged to the organized MALT. Our result showed that FcRn was expressed in non-FAE of ALNA at different levels in all groups, which was compatible with the expression of FcRn in human enterocytes (FcRn was expressed in adult human enterocyte) [15]. However, this was very different from the FcRn expression in the intestinal mucosal epithelium of rat [8], which was only

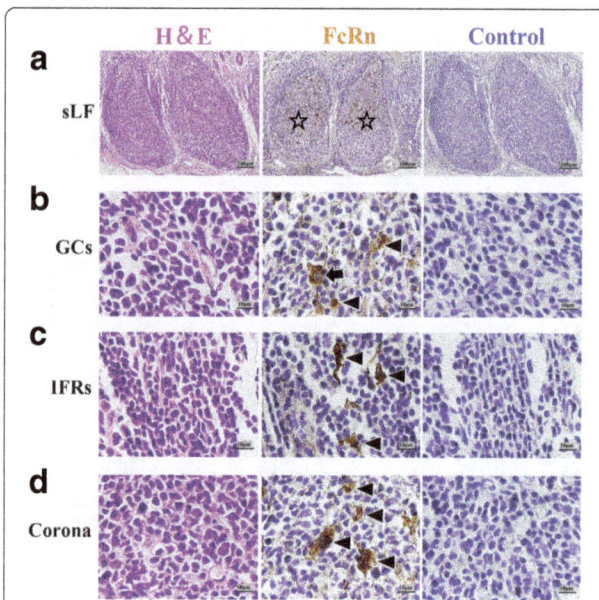

Fig. 7 Macrophages and DCs highly expressed FcRn in sLFs in LMFR of young abomasum ALNA. From left to right column, the paraffin sections were stained with hematoxylin and eosin (H&E), immunohistochemistry for FcRn, hematoxylin counterstain (as negative control), respectively. **a** sLF represents second lymphatic follicles (*star*) (original magnification: 100×); **b** GCs represents germinal centers, and many macrophages (*arrow*) and dendritic cells (DCs) (*triangle*) with high FcRn expression were seen (original magnification: 1000×); **c** IFRs represents interfollicular regions, also called B lymphocyte zone, and some DCs (*triangle*) with high FcRn expression were seen (original magnification: 1000×); **d** Corona represents corona area, also called B lymphocyte zone, and many DCs (*triangle*) with high FcRn expression were seen (original magnification: 1000×)

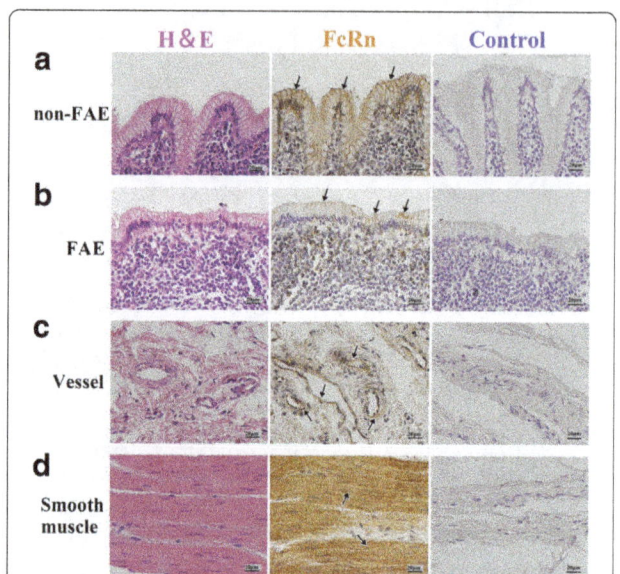

Fig. 8 Localization of FcRn in LMFR of young abomasum ALNA. From left to right column, the paraffin sections were stained with hematoxylin and eosin (H&E), immunohistochemistry for FcRn, hematoxylin counterstain (as negative control), respectively. **a** non-FAE represents non-follicle-associated epithelium in the top panel, and FcRn positive expression was mainly distributed in membrane of the epithelial cells (*arrow*); **b** FAE represents follicle-associated epithelium in the second panel from top to bottom and FcRn positive expression was mainly distributed in membrane of the epithelial cells (*arrow*), but the expression level was lower than that in non-FAE; **c** Vessel, FcRn was highly expressed both in vascular endothelial cells and smooth muscle cells (*arrow*); **d** Smooth muscle, FcRn was also highly expressed in basement membrane of smooth muscle (*arrow*). Original magnification: 400×

expressed in newborns enterocyte and rapidly declined after weaning in mouse. Researches have demonstrated that FcRn was pH-dependent binding to IgG, with relatively strong binding at acidic pH (pH ≤ 6.5) and negligible binding at physiological pH (7.3–7.4) [43]. Some studies reported that the pH was 5.55 in the camel abomasum [45], which was just within the range of optimal pH value for FcRn binding to IgG. Thus, FcRn expression in the mucosal epithelial cells of ALNA in abomasum of Bactrian camels of different ages could provide a powerful evidence for FcRn participating in the transmembrane transport of IgG and associated antigens (especially the transportation of HCAb).

Compared with non-FAE, the FAE is a kind of specialized epithelium, on which the unique microfolds cell (M cell) could efficiently uptake and transport macromolecules and microorganisms in gut lumen to the underlying lymphoid tissue [46]. The MOD measuring results of FcRn expression in epithelial cell of this area found

that the FcRn expression level in FAE and non-FAE had no difference in the fetus and young groups, respectively ($P > 0.05$), while that in FAE was significantly lower than that in non-FAE in pubertal and middle-aged groups, respectively ($P < 0.05$). The expression characteristics were similar to those of pIgR, transport receptor of SIgA, in this area [46]. In ALNA of the fetus to middle-aged Bactrian camels, although the FcRn was expressed in mucosal immune inductive sites FAE, in ALNA of the fetus to old Bactrian camels, mainly in effector sites non-FAE. As for whether FcRn participated in M cells uptaking and transporting associated antigens in FAE of ALNA in abomasum of Bactrian camels remains a further study.

In addition, our results showed that FcRn was expressed in the vessel endothelium and smooth muscle in this area, which was similar to the FcRn expression characteristics in the vessel and smooth of mice and humans [47]. It suggested that the FcRn expression in these sites was mainly related to regulating the half-life of IgG and albumin and homeostasis in this local region.

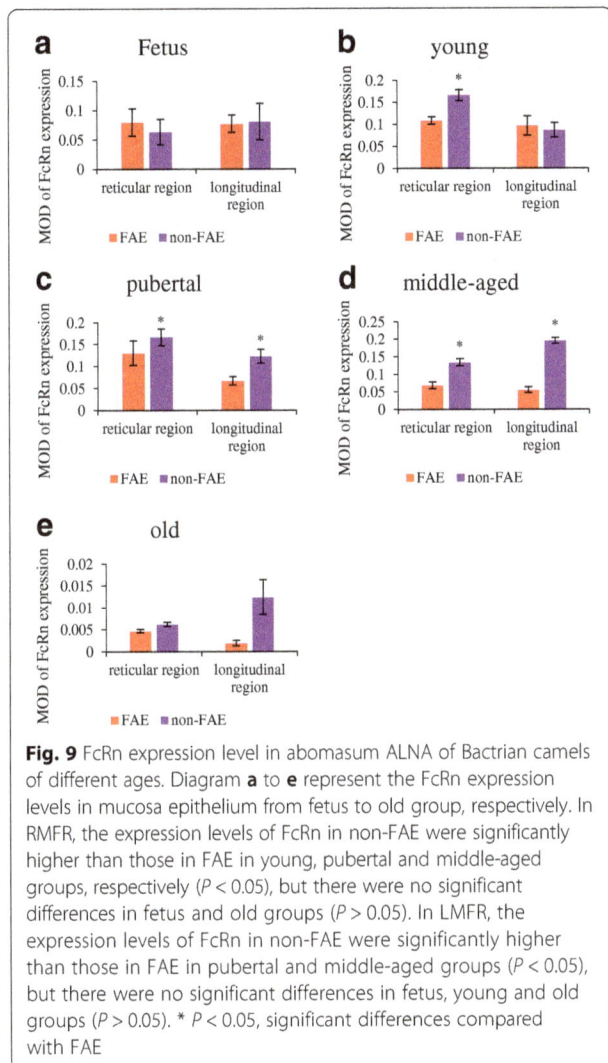

Fig. 9 FcRn expression level in abomasum ALNA of Bactrian camels of different ages. Diagram **a** to **e** represent the FcRn expression levels in mucosa epithelium from fetus to old group, respectively. In RMFR, the expression levels of FcRn in non-FAE were significantly higher than those in FAE in young, pubertal and middle-aged groups, respectively ($P < 0.05$), but there were no significant differences in fetus and old groups ($P > 0.05$). In LMFR, the expression levels of FcRn in non-FAE were significantly higher than those in FAE in pubertal and middle-aged groups ($P < 0.05$), but there were no significant differences in fetus, young and old groups ($P > 0.05$). * $P < 0.05$, significant differences compared with FAE

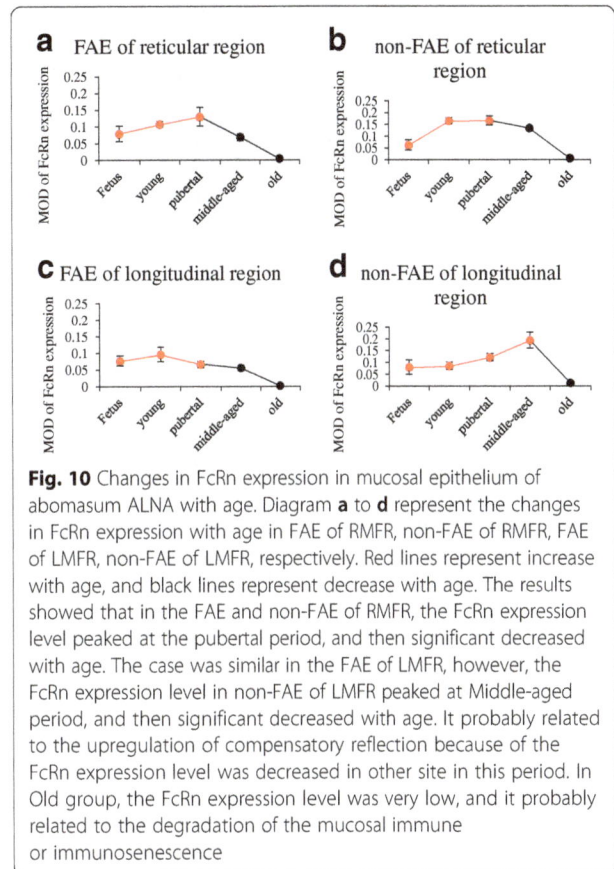

Fig. 10 Changes in FcRn expression in mucosal epithelium of abomasum ALNA with age. Diagram **a** to **d** represent the changes in FcRn expression with age in FAE of RMFR, non-FAE of RMFR, FAE of LMFR, non-FAE of LMFR, respectively. Red lines represent increase with age, and black lines represent decrease with age. The results showed that in the FAE and non-FAE of RMFR, the FcRn expression level peaked at the pubertal period, and then significant decreased with age. The case was similar in the FAE of LMFR, however, the FcRn expression level in non-FAE of LMFR peaked at Middle-aged period, and then significant decreased with age. It probably related to the upregulation of compensatory reflection because of the FcRn expression level was decreased in other site in this period. In Old group, the FcRn expression level was very low, and it probably related to the degradation of the mucosal immune or immunosenescence

In the present study, both macrophages and DCs in sLFs of ALNA in abomasum of Bactrian camels highly expressed FcRn, respectively. Researches have shown that there was mononuclear phagocyte system composed of monocytes, DCs and macrophages in sLFs. And in this system, different types of cells had different subtypes, respectively, and were distributed in special regions [48–53]. They played an important role in antigen capture, processing and presentation, secreting cytokines and regulating immune tolerance [54, 55]. These results provided an evidence that FcRn could participate in regulating the immune response and tolerance in the sLFs of ALNA in abomasum of Bactrian camels.

Conclusions
Our results showed that FcRn was mainly expressed in non-FAE, the effector sites, although which was expressed in FAE, the inductive sites for mucosal immunity. And it was also expressed in DCs and macrophages in sLFs of all ages of Bactrian camels. This provided a powerful evidence that IgG could participate in mucosal immune and immune response and tolerance in this area.

Abbreviations
FcRn: Neonatal Fc receptor; ALNA: Aggregated lymphoid nodules area; RMFR: Reticular mucosal folds region; LMFR: Longitudinal mucosal folds region; MALT: Mucosa-associated lymphoid tissue; MECs: Mucosal epithelial cells; non-FAE: Non-follicle-associated epithelium; DCs: Dendritic cells; pLFs: Primary lymphoid follicles; sLFs: Secondary lymphoid follicles; HCAb: Heavy chain antibody; IHC: Immunohistochemistry; MOD: Mean optical density; SED: Subepithelial dome; IFRs: Interfollicular regions; M cell: Microfolds cell

Acknowledgements
We would like to thank Dr. Wanling Yao. (Institute of Traditional Chinese Veterinary Medicine, College of Veterinary Medicine, Gansu Agricultural University) for her assistance with English.

Funding
This study was supported by Grant sponsor: National Natural Science Foundation of China; Grant number: 31260595. Grant sponsor: National Natural Science Foundation of China; Grant number: 30671549. The Fostering Foundation for the Excellent Ph. D. Dissertation of Gansu Agricultural University; Grant number: 2013001.

Authors' contributions

Conceived and designed the experiments: WHW, WDZ. Performed the experiments: WDZ. Analyzed the data: WDZ. Contributed reagents/materials/analysis tools: WDZ, SXL, SJ, XFZ and TTC. Contributed to the writing of the manuscript: WDZ. All authors read and approved the final manuscript.

Competing interests

The authors declare no financial or commercial conflict of interest.

Consent for publication

Not applicable.

References

1. Fagarasan S, Honjo T. Intestinal IgA synthesis: regulation of front-line body defences. Nat Rev Immunol. 2003;3(1):63–72.
2. Mostov KE. Transepithelial transport of immunoglobulins. Annu Rev Immunol. 1994;12(1):63–84.
3. Macpherson AJ, McCoy KD, Johansen FE, Brandtzaeg P. The immune geography of IgA induction and function. Mucosal Immunol. 2008;1(1):11–22.
4. Norderhaug I, Johansen F, Schjerven H, Brandtzaeg P. Regulation of the formation and external transport of secretory immunoglobulins. Crit Rev Immunol. 1999;19(5–6):481–508.
5. Kaetzel CS, Bruno ME. Epithelial transport of IgA by the polymeric immunoglobulin receptor. US: Springer; 2007:43–89.
6. Dickinson BL, Badizadegan K, Wu Z, Ahouse JC, Zhu X, Simister NE, et al. Bidirectional FcRn-dependent IgG transport in a polarized human intestinal epithelial cell line. J Clin Invest. 1999;104(7):903–11.
7. Yoshida M, Claypool SM, Wagner JS, Mizoguchi E, Mizoguchi A, Roopenian DC, et al. Human neonatal Fc receptor mediates transport of IgG into luminal secretions for delivery of antigens to mucosal dendritic cells. Immunity. 2004;20(6):769–83.
8. Yoshida M, Kobayashi K, Kuo TT, Bry L, Glickman JN, Claypool SM, et al. Neonatal Fc receptor for IgG regulates mucosal immune responses to luminal bacteria. J Clin Invest. 2006;116(8):2142–51.
9. Jones EA, Waldmann TA. The mechanism of intestinal uptake and transcellular transport of IgG in the neonatal rat. J Clin Invest. 1972;51(11):2916–27.
10. Rodewald R. pH-dependent binding of immunoglobulins to intestinal cells of the neonatal rat. J Cell Biol. 1976;71(2):666–9.
11. Rodewald R, Kraehenbuhl JP. Receptor-mediated transport of IgG. J Cell Biol. 1984;99(1 Pt 2):159s–64s.
12. Borthistle BK, Kubo RT, Brown WR, Grey HM. Studies on receptors for IgG on epithelial cells of the rat intestine. J Immunol. 1977;119(2):471–6.
13. Simister NE, Mostov KE. An Fc receptor structurally related to MHC class I antigens. Nature. 1989;337(6203):184–7.
14. Burmeister WP, Gastinel LN, Simister NE, Blum ML, Bjorkman PJ. Crystal structure at 2.2 A resolution of the MHC-related neonatal Fc receptor. Nature. 1994;372(6504):336–43.
15. Israel E, Taylor S, Wu Z, Mizoguchi E, Blumberg R, Bhan A, et al. Expression of the neonatal Fc receptor, FcRn, on human intestinal epithelial cells. Immunology. 1997;92(1):69–74.
16. Haymann JP, Levraud JP, Bouet S, Kappes V, Hagege J, Nguyen G, et al. Characterization and localization of the neonatal Fc receptor in adult human kidney. J Am Soc Nephrol. 2000;11(4):632–9.
17. Kobayashi N, Suzuki Y, Tsuge T, Okumura K, Ra C, Tomino Y. FcRn-mediated transcytosis of immunoglobulin G in human renal proximal tubular epithelial cells. Am J Physiol Renal Physiol. 2002;282(2):F358–65.
18. Spiekermann GM, Finn PW, Ward ES, Dumont J, Dickinson BL, Blumberg RS, et al. Receptor-mediated Immunoglobulin G Transport Across Mucosal Barriers in Adult Life: Functional Expression of FcRn in the Mammalian Lung. J Exp Med. 2002;196(3):303–10.
19. Cianga P, Cianga C, Cozma L, Ward ES, Carasevici E. MHC class I related Fc receptor, FcRn, is expressed in the epithelial cells of the human mammary gland. Human Immunology. 2003;64(12):1152–59.
20. Korthagen NM, van Bilsen K, Dik WA, Bastiaans J, Kolijn M, Kuijpers RW, et al. FcRn mediated IgG transport by retinal pigment epithelium cells. J Transl Med. 2012;10 Suppl 3:2.
21. Li Z, Palaniyandi S, Zeng R, Tuo W, Roopenian DC, Zhu X. Transfer of IgG in the female genital tract by MHC class I-related neonatal Fc receptor (FcRn) confers protective immunity to vaginal infection. Proc Natl Acad Sci. 2011;108(11):4388–93.
22. Ober RJ, Martinez C, Vaccaro C, Zhou J, Ward ES. Visualizing the Site and Dynamics of IgG Salvage by the MHC Class I-Related Receptor, FcRn. J Immunol. 2004;172(4):2021–9.
23. Antohe F, Rădulescu L, Gafencu A, Gheţie V, Simionescu M. Expression of functionally active FcRn and the differentiated bidirectional transport of IgG in human placental endothelial cells. Hum Immunol. 2001;62(2):93–105.
24. Baker K, Qiao SW, Kuo TT, Aveson VG, Platzer B, Andersen JT, et al. Neonatal Fc receptor for IgG (FcRn) regulates cross-presentation of IgG immune complexes by CD8-CD11b + dendritic cells. Proc Natl Acad Sci U S A. 2011;108(24):9927–32.
25. Zhu X, Meng G, Dickinson BL, Li X, Mizoguchi E, Miao L, et al. MHC Class I-Related Neonatal Fc Receptor for IgG Is Functionally Expressed in Monocytes, Intestinal Macrophages, and Dendritic Cells. J Immunol. 2001;166(5):3266–76.
26. Shah U, Dickinson BL, Blumberg RS, Simister NE, Lencer WI, Walker WA. Distribution of the IgG Fc receptor, FcRn, in the human fetal intestine. Pediatr Res. 2003;53(2):295–301.
27. Yoshida M, Masuda A, Kuo TT, Kobayashi K, Claypool SM, Takagawa T, et al. IgG transport across mucosal barriers by neonatal Fc receptor for IgG and mucosal immunity. Springer Semin Immunopathol. 2006;28(4):397–403.
28. Ghetie V, Hubbard JG, Kim JK, Tsen MF, Lee Y, Ward ES. Abnormally short serum half-lives of IgG in β2-microglobulin-deficient mice. Eur J Immunol. 1996;26(3):690–6.
29. Catunda Lemos AP, Cervenak J, Bender B, Hoffmann OI, Baranyi M, Kerekes A, et al. Characterization of the rabbit neonatal Fc receptor (FcRn) and analyzing the immunophenotype of the transgenic rabbits that overexpresses FcRn. PLoS One. 2012;7(1):e28869.
30. Ye L, Tuo W, Liu X, Simister NE, Zhu X. Identification and characterization of an alternatively spliced variant of the MHC class I-related porcine neonatal Fc receptor for IgG. Dev Comp Immunol. 2008;32(8):966–79.
31. Mayer B, Zolnai A, Frenyó LV, Jancsik V, Szentirmay Z, Hammarström L, et al. Redistribution of the sheep neonatal Fc receptor in the mammary gland around the time of parturition in ewes and its localization in the small intestine of neonatal lambs. Immunology. 2002;107(3):288–96.
32. Kacskovics I, Wu Z, Simister NE, Frenyó LV, Hammarström L. Cloning and characterization of the bovine MHC class I-like Fc receptor. J Immunol. 2000;164(4):1889–97.
33. Sayed-Ahmed A, Kassab M, Abd-Elmaksoud A, Elnasharty M, El-Kirdasy A. Expression and immunohistochemical localization of the neonatal Fc receptor (FcRn) in the mammary glands of the Egyptian water buffalo. Acta Histochem. 2010;112(4):383–91.
34. Kacskovics I, Mayer B, Kis Z, Frenyo LV, Zhao Y, Muyldermans S, et al. Cloning and characterization of the dromedary (Camelus dromedarius) neonatal Fc receptor (drFcRn). Dev Comp Immunol. 2006;30(12):1203–15.
35. Hamers-Casterman C, Atarhouch T, Muyldermans S, Robinson G, Hamers C, Songa EB, et al. Naturally occurring antibodies devoid of light chains. Nature. 1993;363(6428):446–8.
36. Deschacht N, De Groeve K, Vincke C, Raes G, De Baetselier P, Muyldermans S. A novel promiscuous class of camelid single-domain antibody contributes to the antigen-binding repertoire. J Immunol. 2010;184(10):5696–704.
37. Liebler-Tenorio EM, Pabst R. MALT structure and function in farm animals. Vet Res. 2006;37(3):257–80.
38. Wang W-H. Observations on aggregated lymphoid nodules in the cardiac glandular areas of the Bactrian camel (Camelus bactrianus). Vet J. 2003;166(2):205–9.
39. Xu XH, Wang WH, Gao Q, Qi SS, He WH, Tai LF, et al. The anatomical characteristics of the aggregated lymphoid nodule area in the stomach of Bactrian camels (Camelus bactrianus) of different ages. Vet J. 2010;184(3):362–5.
40. Zhang WD, Wang WH, Xu XH, Zhaxi YP, Zhang LJ, Qi SS, et al. The histological characteristics of the aggregated lymphoid nodules area in abomasum of Bactrian camels (Camelus bactrianus) of different ages. Vet Immunol Immunopathol. 2012;147(3–4):147–53.
41. Liu S: Practical bio-histological techniques. Beijing: Beijing Science Press; 2006.
42. Wang-dong Z: Study on the purification, preparation of polyclonal antibody of Ig Gs of the Bactrian Camels and the characteristics of distribution of the secrete Ig Gs plasma cells in small intestine. Master's Degree. Lanzhou: Gansu Agricultural University; 2012.

43. Martin WL, West Jr AP, Gan L, Bjorkman PJ. Crystal structure at 2.8 A of an FcRn/heterodimeric Fc complex: mechanism of pH-dependent binding. Mol Cell. 2001;7(4):867–77.

44. Brandtzaeg P, Kiyono H, Pabst R, Russell MW. Terminology: nomenclature of mucosa-associated lymphoid tissue. Mucosal Immunol. 2008;1(1):31–7.

45. Maloiy GM, Clemens ET. Gastrointestinal osmolality electrolyte and organic acid composition in five species of East African herbivorous mammals. J Anim Sci. 1980;51(4):917–24.

46. Kraehenbuhl J-P, Neutra MR. Epithelial M cells: differentiation and function. Annu Rev Cell Dev Biol. 2000;16(1):301–32.

47. Borvak J, Richardson J, Medesan C, Antohe F, Radu C, Simionescu M, et al. Functional expression of the MHC class I-related receptor, FcRn, in endothelial cells of mice. Int Immunol. 1998;10(9):1289–98.

48. Bonnardel J, Da Silva C, Henri S, Tamoutounour S, Chasson L, Montanana-Sanchis F, et al. Innate and adaptive immune functions of peyer's patch monocyte-derived cells. Cell Rep. 2015;11(5):770–84.

49. Contractor N, Louten J, Kim L, Biron CA, Kelsall BL. Cutting Edge: Peyer's Patch Plasmacytoid Dendritic Cells (pDCs) Produce Low Levels of Type I Interferons: Possible Role for IL-10, TGF, and Prostaglandin E2 in Conditioning a Unique Mucosal pDC Phenotype. J Immunol. 2007;179(5):2690–4.

50. Grouard G, Durand I, Filgueira L, Banchereau J, Liu Y-J. Dendritic cells capable of stimulating T cells in germinal centres. Nature. 1996;384(6607):364–7.

51. Iwasaki A, Kelsall BL. Unique Functions of CD11b+, CD8 +, and Double-Negative Peyer's Patch Dendritic Cells. J Immunol. 2001;166(8):4884–90.

52. Lelouard H, Henri S, De Bovis B, Mugnier B, Chollat-Namy A, Malissen B, Meresse S, Gorvel JP: Pathogenic bacteria and dead cells are internalized by a unique subset of Peyer's patch dendritic cells that express lysozyme. Gastroenterology 2010, 138(1):173–184 e171–173.

53. Lindquist RL, Shakhar G, Dudziak D, Wardemann H, Eisenreich T, Dustin ML, et al. Visualizing dendritic cell networks in vivo. Nat Immunol. 2004;5(12):1243–50.

54. Lelouard H, Fallet M, de Bovis B, Meresse S, Gorvel JP. Peyer's patch dendritic cells sample antigens by extending dendrites through M cell-specific transcellular pores. Gastroenterology. 2012;142(3):592–601. e593.

55. Baker K, Rath T, Flak MB, Arthur JC, Chen Z, Glickman JN, et al. Neonatal Fc receptor expression in dendritic cells mediates protective immunity against colorectal cancer. Immunity. 2013;39(6):1095–107.

9

In situ detection of GM1 and GM2 gangliosides using immunohistochemical and immunofluorescent techniques for auxiliary diagnosis of canine and feline gangliosidoses

Moeko Kohyama[1], Akira Yabuki[1], Kenji Ochiai[2], Yuya Nakamoto[3], Kazuyuki Uchida[4], Daisuke Hasegawa[5], Kimimasa Takahashi[6], Hiroaki Kawaguchi[7], Masaya Tsuboi[4] and Osamu Yamato[1*]

Abstract

Background: GM1 and GM2 gangliosidoses are progressive neurodegenerative lysosomal storage diseases resulting from the excessive accumulation of GM1 and GM2 gangliosides in the lysosomes, respectively. The diagnosis of gangliosidosis is carried out based on comprehensive findings using various types of specimens for histological, ultrastructural, biochemical and genetic analyses. Therefore, the partial absence or lack of specimens might have resulted in many undiagnosed cases. The aim of the present study was to establish immunohistochemical and immunofluorescent techniques for the auxiliary diagnosis of canine and feline gangliosidoses, using paraffin-embedded brain specimens stored for a long period.

Results: Using hematoxylin and eosin staining, cytoplasmic accumulation of pale to eosinophilic granular materials in swollen neurons was observed in animals previously diagnosed with GM1 or GM2 gangliosidosis. The immunohistochemical and immunofluorescent techniques developed in this study clearly demonstrated the accumulated material to be either GM1 or GM2 ganglioside.

Conclusions: Immunohistochemical and immunofluorescent techniques using stored paraffin-embedded brain specimens are useful for the retrospective diagnosis of GM1 and GM2 gangliosidoses in dogs and cats.

Keywords: Gangliosidosis, Dog, Cat, Lysosomal Storage Disease, Immunohistochemistry, Immunofluorescence

Background

GM1 and GM2 gangliosidoses are progressive neurodegenerative lysosomal storage diseases resulting mainly from the excessive accumulation of GM1 and GM2 gangliosides in the lysosomes, respectively [1]. These diseases are inherited in an autosomal recessive manner and result in the premature death of affected individuals due to brain damage with progressive neurological signs. In GM1 gangliosidosis, the accumulation of GM1 ganglioside is caused by an inherited deficiency of the lysosomal acid β-galactosidase [2]. In GM2 gangliosidosis, the accumulation of GM2 ganglioside is caused by an inherited deficiency of the lysosomal acid β-hexosaminidase A or GM2 activator protein in GM2 gangliosidosis, and the disease is accordingly categorized into three variants: Tay-Sachs disease (B variant), Sandhoff disease (0 variant), and GM2 activator protein deficiency (AB variant) [3].

Gangliosidosis is more likely to occur in many animal species and breeds compared to other lysosomal diseases. Naturally occurring GM1 gangliosidosis has been reported in dogs, including mixed Beagles [4], English Springer Spaniels [5], Portuguese Water dogs [6], Alaskan Huskies [7], Shiba Inus [8], and a mixed-

* Correspondence: osam@vet.kagoshima-u.ac.jp
[1]Laboratory of Clinical Pathology, Department of Veterinary Medicine, Joint Faculty of Veterinary Medicine, Kagoshima University, 1-21-24 Kohrimoto, Kagoshima-shi, Kagoshima 890-0065, Japan

breed dog [9], and in cats, including Siamese [10, 11], Korat [12], and several families of domestic cats [13–17]. In addition, GM1 gangliosidosis has been reported in ruminants such as Friesian calves [17, 18], Suffolk sheep [19], Coopworth Romny-cross sheep [20], and Romny sheep [21], and in wild species such as American black bears [22] and emus [23]. Naturally occurring GM2 gangliosidosis has been reported in dogs, including German Shorthair Pointers [24], Japanese Spaniels (Chins) [25, 26], a Golden Retriever [27], Toy Poodles [28], and mixed-breed dogs [29, 30], and in cats, including Korat [31], European Burmese [32], and several families of domestic cats [33–35]. In addition, GM2 gangliosidosis has been reported in Yorkshire pigs [36], Jacob sheep [37], a rabbit [38], Muntjak deer [39], and American flamingos [40].

The diagnosis of GM1 and GM2 gangliosidoses is carried out based on comprehensive findings, which include clinical, biochemical, histopathological, and genetic findings using various types of specimens [2, 3]. The clinical findings are progressive neurological, motor, and visual dysfunctions, but they are not specific to these diseases [41]. The biochemical findings include the cerebral accumulation of specific glycoconjugates and deficiency of specific enzyme activities, which are determined by specialized techniques such as thin-layer chromatography (TLC) and fluorometric enzymatic assays, respectively, using fresh or frozen tissues [42, 43]. The histopathological and ultrastructural findings demonstrate swollen neurons filled with periodic acid-Schiff stain-positive storage materials and osmiophilic membranous cytoplasmic bodies in the lysosomes of neurons, respectively, but these characteristics are not completely specific to these diseases [8, 28, 30, 34]. Genetic tests can be used to directly diagnose the diseases, but they are limited to diseases for which specific mutations have been identified [44–46]. Therefore, it is possible that a correct diagnosis has not been established in many animal cases, as a result of the partial absence or lack of specimens for biochemical, histological, ultrastructural, or genetic examination.

The aim of the present study was to establish immunohistochemical and immunofluorescent techniques for the auxiliary diagnosis of canine and feline gangliosidoses using paraffin-embedded brain specimens, which are often stored for a long time in veterinary diagnostic laboratories worldwide.

Methods

Specimens

Stored paraffin-embedded cerebral cortex samples of dogs and cats with GM1 or GM2 gangliosidosis were used in this study. These cases occurred in different parts of Japan and the original diagnosis was made using specific genetic tests and biochemical analyses at the Laboratory of Clinical Pathology, Joint Faculty of Veterinary Medicine, Kagoshima University, which has been exclusively supporting the diagnosis of inherited metabolic diseases in animals in Japan. These animals included a 14-month-old Shiba Inu with GM1 gangliosidosis diagnosed in 2009, an 11-month-old domestic shorthair cat with GM1 gangliosidosis diagnosed in 2004, a 20-month-old Toy Poodle with GM2 gangliosidosis diagnosed in 2006, and a 20-month-old domestic shorthair cat with GM2 gangliosidosis diagnosed in 2010. The diagnosis of these animals was established using genetic and/or biochemical tests reported previously [11, 43–45]. Stored paraffin-embedded cerebral cortex samples of a dog and a cat without any brain disease were also used as controls. Thin sections at 4 μm were prepared from these paraffin-embedded tissue blocks by standard method. These sections were stained with hematoxylin and eosin (HE) and subjected to the immunohistochemical and immunofluorescent techniques described below. All experimental procedures and ethical issues involving animals and their samples were approved by the the Animal Research Committee at Kagoshima University with the approval number VM15041.

Immunohistochemical study

Each section was deparaffinized with xylene and rehydrated through a graded ethanol series. Antigen retrieval was conducted by heating the sample in a 10 mM citrate buffer (pH 6.0) in a microwave oven. Thereafter, the samples were washed in deionized water, treated with 3 % hydrogen peroxide, and washed in 0.01 M phosphate-buffered saline (PBS; pH 7.4). Blocking was performed with 0.25 % casein in 0.01 M PBS and incubated overnight at 4°C with the respective reagents.

For the detection of GM1 ganglioside, biotinylated cholera toxin B subunit (1:1000; List Biological Laboratories, Inc., Campbell, CA, USA) was used. For the detection of GM2 ganglioside, mouse anti-GM2 ganglioside monoclonal IgM antibody (1:1000; Tokyo Chemical Industry, Co., Ltd., Tokyo, Japan) was used as a primary antibody, and biotinylated goat anti-mouse IgM antibody (1:200; Vector Laboratories, Inc., Burlingame, CA, USA) was used as a secondary antibody. Subsequently, these sections were incubated with peroxidase-labeled streptavidin (KPL, Kirkegaard & Perry Laboratories, Inc., Gaithersburg, MD, USA). The immunoreactivity was detected by a 3,3′-diaminobenzidine (DAB) system using DAB Tablet (Merck KGaA, Darmstadt, Germany) as a peroxidase substrate. The sections were counterstained with hematoxylin.

Immunofluorescent study

Each section was pretreated in the same way as described above for immunohistochemistry. For the detection of GM1 ganglioside, biotinylated cholera toxin B subunit (1:500; List Biological Laboratories, Inc.) and Alexa Fluor 488-conjugated streptavidin (1:1000; Life Technologies, Inc., Gaithersburg, MD, USA) were used. For the detection of GM2 ganglioside, mouse anti-GM2 monoclonal IgM antibody (1:500; Vector Laboratories, Inc.) was used as a primary antibody, and Alexa Fluor 488-conjugated goat anti-mouse IgM antibody (1:1000; Life Technologies, Inc.) was used as a secondary antibody. Subsequently, these sections were incubated with a 4′,6-diamidino-2-phenylindole dihydrochloride (DAPI) solution (1:1000; Dojindo Laboratories, Inc., Kumamoto, Japan) for nuclear staining. The fluorescence was observed using a fluorescence microscopy (BX53-33-FL2, Olympus, Corp., Tokyo, Japan).

Results

Using the HE stain, cytoplasmic accumulation of pale to eosinophilic granular materials in balloon-swollen neurons was observed in the cerebral cortex samples of dogs and cats previously diagnosed with GM1 or GM2 gangliosidosis (Fig. 1a–d), whereas there was no such abnormal change observed in the samples of the control animals (Fig. 1e and f).

Using the immunohistochemical technique for the detection of GM1 ganglioside, the accumulated cytoplasmic materials were positively stained and mainly identified as GM1 ganglioside in cells of animals with confirmed GM1 gangliosidosis (Fig. 2a and b). In animals with GM2 gangliosidosis, the accumulated cytoplasmic materials were very weakly positively stained in a portion of the cells of the affected cat (Fig. 2c and d).

In the control animals, the cytoplasm in some normal-shaped cells was also positively stained to indicate the presence of GM1 ganglioside (Fig. 2e and f). The nuclei of several cells were positively stained in a portion of the samples such as in the case of feline GM2 gangliosidosis and in both control animals (Fig. 2d–f).

Using the immunohistochemical technique for the detection of GM2 ganglioside, the accumulated cytoplasmic materials were positively stained and mainly identified as GM2 ganglioside in the cells of animals with GM2 gangliosidosis (Fig. 3c and d), whereas these materials were not strongly stained in animals with GM1 gangliosidosis (Fig. 3a and b). In the control animals, the cytoplasm in some normal-shaped cells was also weakly stained using this method (Fig. 3e and f). The nuclei of several cells were weakly positively stained in a portion of the samples such as in the case of canine GM1 gangliosidosis and in both control animals (Fig. 3a, e and f).

The results of the immunofluorescent technique were almost identical to those of the immunohistochemical technique. The accumulated materials in the swollen neurons of animals with gangliosidoses were positively stained and clearly identified as either GM1 or GM2 ganglioside by using the respective detection techniques for each ganglioside (Figs. 4 and 5). The accumulated materials in the neurons of animals with GM2 gangliosidosis were very weakly stained using the technique for GM1 ganglioside (Fig. 4c and d), and vice versa (Fig. 5a and b). In the control animals, some cells showed

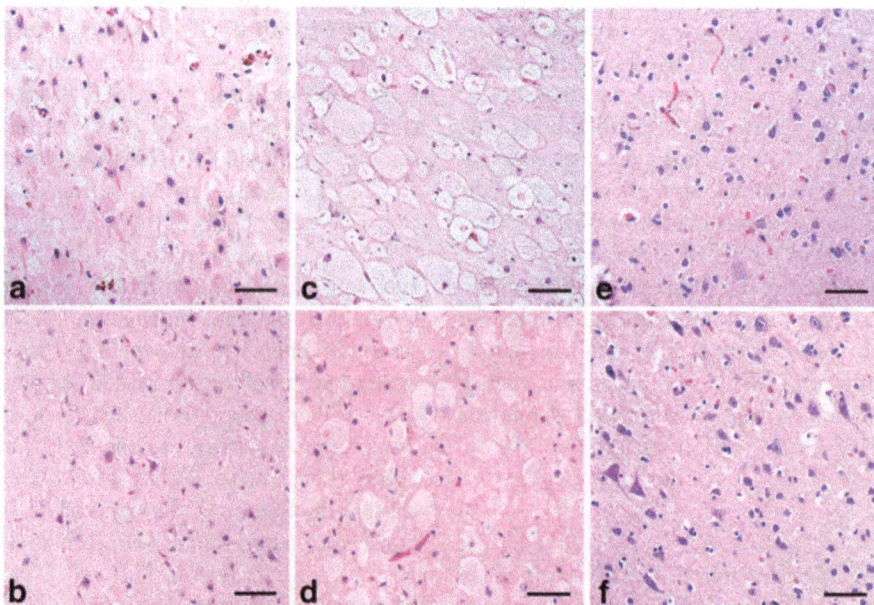

Fig. 1 Histopathological findings in animals affected and unaffected with gangliosidoses. Hematoxylin and eosin staining was performed on paraffin-embedded sections of the cerebral cortex from the following animals: a dog (a) and a cat (b) affected with GM1 gangliosidosis; a dog (c) and a cat (d) affected with GM2 gangliosidosis; an unaffected control dog (e) and cat (f). Bar = 50 μm

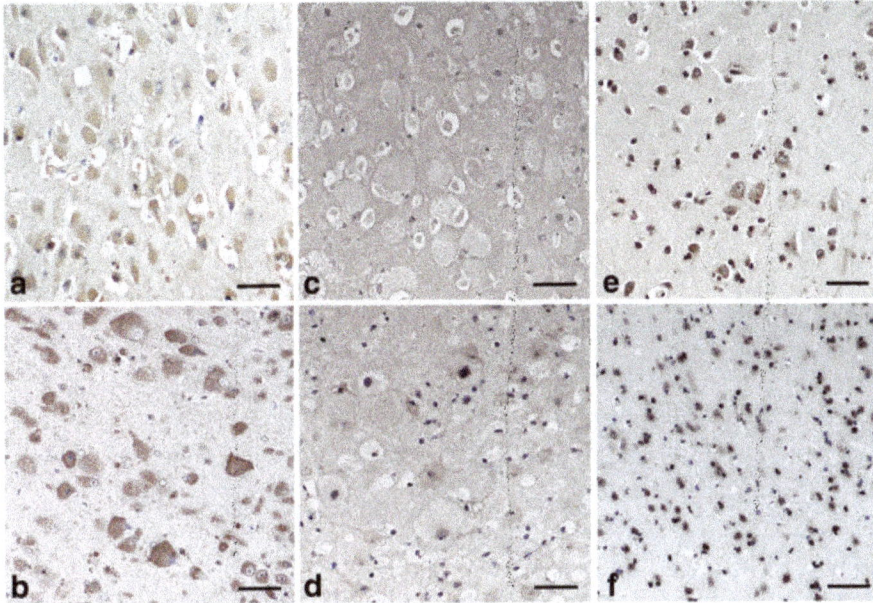

Fig. 2 Immunohistochemical findings for the detection of GM1 ganglioside in animals affected and unaffected with gangliosidoses. The immunohistochemical technique for the detection of GM1 ganglioside was performed on paraffin-embedded sections of the cerebral cortex from the following animals: a dog (**a**) and a cat (**b**) affected with GM1 gangliosidosis; a dog (**c**) and a cat (**d**) affected with GM2 gangliosidosis; an unaffected control dog (**e**) and cat (**f**). For the detection of GM1 ganglioside, biotinylated cholera toxin B subunit and peroxidase-labeled streptavidin were used. The immunoreactivity was detected by 3,3′-diaminobenzidine as a peroxidase substrate. The sections were counterstained with hematoxylin. Bar = 50 μm

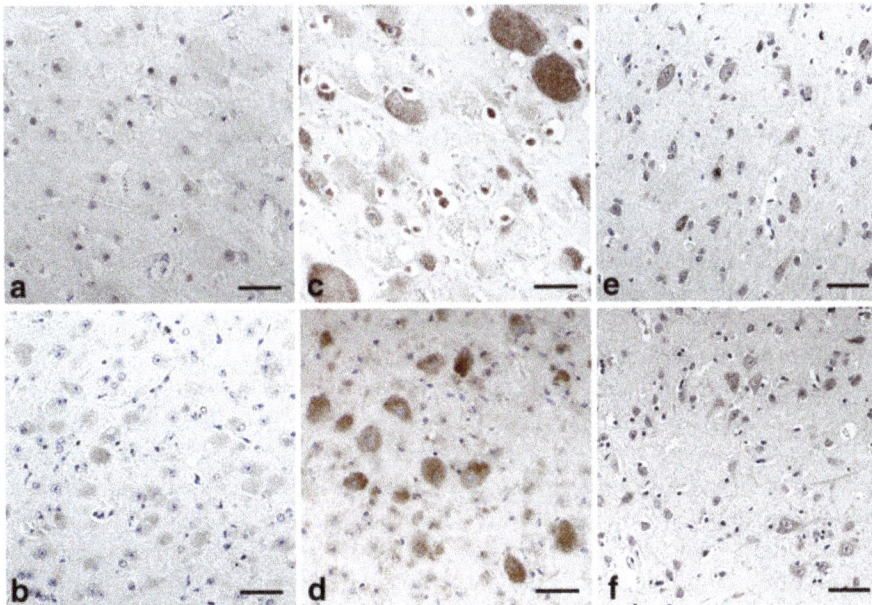

Fig. 3 Immunohistochemical findings for the detection of GM2 ganglioside in animals affected and unaffected with gangliosidoses. The immunohistochemical technique for the detection of GM2 ganglioside was performed on paraffin-embedded sections of the cerebral cortex from the following animals: a dog (**a**) and a cat (**b**) affected with GM1 gangliosidosis; a dog (**c**) and a cat (**d**) affected with GM2 gangliosidosis; an unaffected control dog (**e**) and cat (**f**). For the detection of GM2 ganglioside, mouse anti-GM2 ganglioside monocloncal IgM antibody was used as a primary antibody, and biotinylated goat anti-mouse IgM antibody was used as a secondary antibody. Subsequently, these sections were incubated with peroxidase-labeled streptavidin. The immunoreactivity was detected by 3,3′-diaminobenzidine as a peroxidase substrate. The sections were counterstained with hematoxylin. Bar = 50 μm

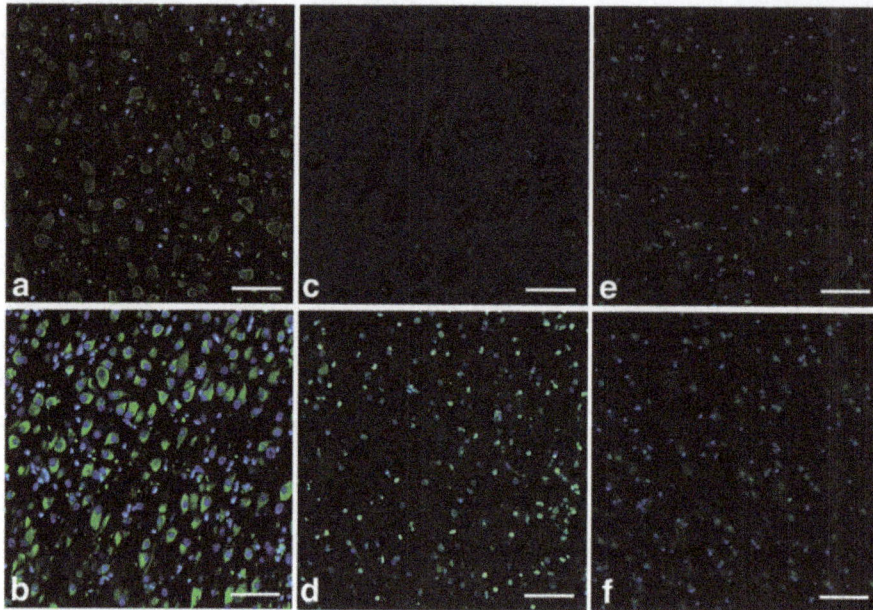

Fig. 4 Immunofluorescent findings for the detection of GM1 ganglioside in animals affected and unaffected with gangliosidoses. The immunofluorescent technique for the detection of GM1 ganglioside was performed on paraffin-embedded sections of the cerebral cortex from the following animals: a dog (**a**) and a cat (**b**) affected with GM1 gangliosidosis; a dog (**c**) and a cat (**d**) affected with GM2 gangliosidosis; an unaffected control dog (**e**) and cat (**f**). For the detection of GM1 ganglioside, biotinylated cholera toxin B subunit and Alexa Fluor 488-conjugated streptavidin were used. Subsequently, these sections were incubated with 4',6-diamidino-2-phenylindole dihydrochloride for nuclear staining. Bar = 30 μm

cytoplasm that was positively stained for GM1 and GM2 gangliosides (Figs. 4 and 5e and f). In addition, some of the cells of a cat with GM2 gangliosidosis and both control animals showed positive staining of nuclei using the technique for the detection of GM1 ganglioside (Fig. 4d–f). Some of the cells of a control cat showed weakly positive staining of nuclei using the technique for the detection of GM2 ganglioside (Fig. 5f).

Discussion

Gangliosides are glycosphingolipids consisting of a hydrophobic ceramide (*N*-acylsphingosine) and a hydrophilic oligosaccharide chain bearing one or more *N*-acetylneuraminic acid (silalic acid) residues, and are typical components of the outer leaflet of the plasma membranes of animal cells [2, 3]. GM1 and GM2 gangliosides are present as the main glycolipids in neurons and are likely to be involved in cell differentiation and cell–cell interactions, but their specific physiological functions remain obscure. Therefore, developing techniques for the detection of GM1 and GM2 gangliosides is important not only for advancement in brain science but also for the correct diagnosis of gangliosidoses, because the intralysosomal accumulation of each ganglioside in neurons is characteristic to either GM1 or GM2 gangliosidosis. Therefore, in the past few decades, various determination methods for the profiling, quantification, or evaluation of gangliosides, including GM1 and GM2

gangliosides, in tissues, cultured cells, or extracellular fluids have been reported. These methods include TLC coupled with densitometric or immunochemical detection [43, 47], high-performance liquid chromatography coupled with tandem mass spectrometric detection [48], enzyme-linked immunosorbent assay [49], and matrix-assisted laser desorption ionization time-of-flight mass spectrometry [50].

The *in situ* detection of gangliosides in tissue sections is also very important not only for diagnosis of the diseases but also to obtain reliable information on their tissue, cellular, and subcellular distributions [51]. Furthermore, confirming that the histological detection of GM1 and GM2 gangliosides is applicable to paraffin-embedded specimens stored for a long period would also be useful for the retrospective diagnosis of the diseases, but very few studies have evaluated such *in situ* detection methods using long-term stored paraffin-embedded specimens from canine and feline gangliosidoses. In the present study, immunohistochemical and immunofluorescent techniques for the detection of GM1 and GM2 gangliosides were developed, and their application was evaluated using canine and feline paraffin-embedded specimens stored for 5 to 11 years. As a result, these two techniques could clearly detect the presence of both GM1 and GM2 gangliosides in neurons of the control animals (Figs. 2, 3, 4 and 5e and f) as well as the accumulation of either GM1 or GM2 ganglioside in neurons

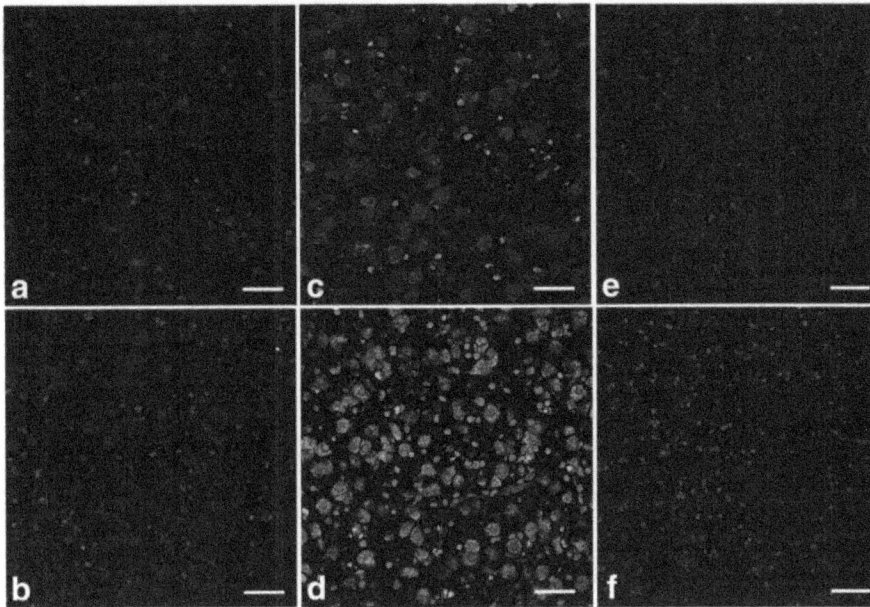

Fig. 5 Immunofluorescent findings for the detection of GM2 ganglioside in animals affected and unaffected with gangliosidoses. The immunofluorescent technique for the detection of GM2 ganglioside was performed on paraffin-embedded sections of the cerebral cortex from the following animals: a dog (**a**) and a cat (**b**) affected with GM1 gangliosidosis; a dog (**c**) and a cat (**d**) affected with GM2 gangliosidosis; an unaffected control dog (**e**) and cat (**f**). For the detection of GM2 ganglioside, mouse anti-GM2 monoclonal IgM antibody was used as a primary antibody, and Alexa Fluor 488-conjugated goat anti-mouse IgM antibody was used as a secondary antibody. Subsequently, these sections were incubated with 4′,6-diamidino-2-phenylindole dihydrochloride for nuclear staining. Bar = 30 μm

of animals with diagnosed GM1 (Figs. 2, 3, 4 and 5a and b) and GM2 gangliosidoses (Figs. 2, 3, 4 and 5c and d). These data demonstrate that the two techniques are applicable to the retrospective *in situ* detection of GM1 and GM2 gangliosides, and consequently to the auxiliary diagnosis of gangliosidoses in dogs and cats. However, gangliosides can be accumulated as the secondary products without direct link to the primary protein defect in some lysosomal and a few non-lysosomal diseases [2, 52]. Therefore, in cases in which the abnormal accumulation of each ganglioside is found in swollen neurons, a definitive diagnosis should ultimately be made using DNA extracted from the same paraffin-embedded specimen via the identification of pathogenic mutation(s) in the responsible genes: the *GLB1* gene for GM1 gangliosidosis and the *HEXA*, *HEXB*, and *GM2A* genes for GM2 gangliosidosis.

Comparing the two techniques developed in the present study, the immunofluorescent technique provided relatively less histopathological information than the immunohistochemical technique, due to the dark background when using immunofluorescence. Therefore, the tissue, cellular, and subcellular distributions of stained materials could not be easily determined in the immunofluorescent technique; however, this technique does have the advantage of requiring a lower amount of reagents (nearly half) because of its

higher detection sensitivity compared to the immunohistochemical technique.

In addition, in the experiments conducted to detect GM1 and GM2 gangliosides, the nuclei were stained in some specimens using both techniques. The positive staining of the nuclei in some cells from affected and control animals may result from the natural components of GM1 and GM2 gangliosides because the nuclei of neuronal cells in rat brain contain these gangliosides [53]. However, this stain of the nucleus was easily differentiated from the specific stain of cytoplasmic GM1 and GM2 gangliosides when using the immunohistochemical technique but not when using the immunofluorescent technique, owing to the reduced morphological visibility. Therefore, the simultaneous observation of HE-stained cerebral tissues (Fig. 1) is necessary for accurate judgment of the results, especially when using an immunofluorescent technique.

Conclusions

The immunohistochemical and immunofluorescent techniques for the detection of GM1 and GM2 gangliosides established in this study are useful for the auxiliary diagnosis of GM1 and GM2 gangliosidoses in dogs and cats before a definitive diagnosis can be made using molecular analysis for identification of causative mutations.

These techniques may also be useful for the retrospective diagnosis of suspected cases of all animal species for which paraffin-embedded cerebral tissues are stored.

Abbreviations

DAB: 3,3′-diaminobenzidine; DAPI: 4′,6-diamidino-2-phenylindole dihydrochloride; HE: hematoxylin and eosin; PBS: phosphate-buffered saline; TLC: thin-layer chromatography.

Competing interests

The authors declare that they have no competing interests.

Authors' contributions

MK carried out the histopathological, immunohistochemical, and immunofluorescent studies and drafted the manuscript. AY participated in the design of the study. KO, YN, KU, DH, KT, HK, and MT prepared the paraffin-embedded tissues samples for the original diagnosis of animals used in this study. OY supervised the project, designed the study, and reviewed the results and manuscript. All authors read and approved the final version of the manuscript.

Acknowledgements

This study was supported financially by grants (25292181 and 26660242 OY) from the Ministry of Education, Culture, Sports, Science and Technology of Japan.

Author details

[1]Laboratory of Clinical Pathology, Department of Veterinary Medicine, Joint Faculty of Veterinary Medicine, Kagoshima University, 1-21-24 Kohrimoto, Kagoshima-shi, Kagoshima 890-0065, Japan. [2]Laboratory of Veterinary Pathology, Department of Veterinary Medicine, Faculty of Agriculture, Iwate University, 3-18-8 Ueda, Morioka-shi, Iwate 020-8550, Japan. [3]Kyoto Animal Referral Medical Center, 208-4 Shin-arami, Tai, Kumiyama-cho, Kuse-gun, Kyoto 613-0036, Japan. [4]Laboratory of Veterinary Pathology, Graduate School of Agricultural and Life Sciences, The University of Tokyo, 1-1-1 Yayoi, Bunkyou-ku, Tokyo 113-8657, Japan. [5]Department of Veterinary Radiology, Nippon Veterinary and Life Science University, 1-7-1 Kyouman-chou, Musashino-shi, Tokyo 180-8602, Japan. [6]Department of Veterinary Pathology, Nippon Veterinary and Life Science University, 1-7-1 Kyouman-chou, Musashino-shi, Tokyo, 180-8602, Japan. [7]Laboratory of Veterinary Histopathology, Department of Veterinary Medicine, Joint Faculty of Veterinary Medicine, Kagoshima University, 1-21-24 Kohrimoto, Kagoshima-shi, Kagoshima 890-0065, Japan.

References

1. Haskins M, Giger U. Lysosomal storage diseases. In: Kaneko JJ, Harvey JW, Bruss ML, editors. Clinical biochemistry of domestic animals. 6th ed. Burlington: Academic; 2008. p. 731–50.
2. Suzuki Y, Oshima A, Nanba E. β-Galactosidase deficiency (β-galactosidosis): GM1 gangliosidosis and Morquio B disease. In: Scriver CR, Beaudet AL, Sly WS, Valle D, editors. The metabolic and molecular bases of inherited disease. 8th ed. New York: McGraw-Hill; 2001. p. 3775–809.
3. Gravel RA, Kaback MM, Proia RL, Sandhoff K, Suzuki K. The GM2 gangliosidosis. In: Scriver CR, Beaudet AL, Sly WS, Valle D, editors. The metabolic and molecular bases of inherited disease. 8th ed. McGraw-Hill: New York; 2001. p. 3824–76.
4. Read DH, Harrington DD, Keenana TW, Hinsman EJ. Neuronal-visceral GM1 gangliosidosis in a dog with beta-galactosidase deficiency. Science. 1976;194:442–5.
5. Alroy J, Orgad U, Ucci AA, Schelling SH, Schunk KL, Warren CD, et al. Neurovisceral and skeletal GM1-gangliosidosis in dogs with beta-galactosidase deficiency. Science. 1985;229:470–2.
6. Saunders GK, Wood PA, Myers RK, Shell LG, Carithers R. GM1 gangliosidosis in Portuguese water dogs: pathologic and biochemical findings. Vet Pathol. 1988;25:265–9.
7. Müller G, Baumgärtner W, Moritz A, Sewell A, Kustermann-Kuhn B. Biochemical findings in a breeding colony of Alaskan huskies suffering from GM1-gangliosidosis. J Inherit Metab Dis. 1998;21:430–1.
8. Yamato O, Ochiai K, Masuoka Y, Hayashida E, Tajima M, Omae S, et al. GM1 gangliosidosis in shiba dogs. Vet Rec. 2000;146:493–6.
9. Whitfield P, Johnson AW, Dunn KA, Delauche AJN, Winchester BG, Franklin RJM. GM1-gangliosidosis in a cross-bred dog confirmed by detection of GM1-ganglioside using electrospray ionisation-tandem mass spectrometry. Acta Neuropathol. 2000;100:409–14.
10. Baker Jr HJ, Lindsey JR, McKhann GM, Farrell DF. Neuronal GM1 gangliosidosis in a Siamese cat with β-galactosidase deficiency. Science. 1971;174:838–9.
11. Uddin MM, Tanimoto T, Yabuki A, Kotani T, Kuwamura M, Chang HS, et al. Mutation analysis of GM1 gangliosidosis in a Siamese cat from Japan in the 1960s. J Feline Med Surg. 2012;14:900–2.
12. De Maria R, Divari S, Bo S, Sonnio S, Lotti D, Capucchio MT, et al. β-Galactosidase deficiency in a Korat cat: a new form of feline GM1 gangliosidosis. Acta Neuropathol. 1998;96:307–14.
13. Blakemore WF. GM1 gangliosidosis in a cat. J Comp Pathol. 1972;82:179–85.
14. Barnes IC, Kelly DF, Pennock CA, Randell DJ. Hepatic beta galactosidase and feline GM1 gangliosidosis. Neuropathol Appl Neurobiol. 1981;7:463–76.
15. Baker CG, Blakemore WF, Dell A, Palmer AC, Tiller PR, Winchester BG. GM1 gangliosidosis (type 1) in a cat. Biochem J. 1986;235:151–8.
16. Uddin MM, Hossain MA, Rahman MM, Chowdhury MA, Tanimoto T, Yabuki A, et al. Identification of Bangladesh domestic cats with GM1 gangliosidosis caused by the c.1448G>C mutation of the feline *GLB1* gene: case study. J Vet Med Sci. 2013;75:395–7.
17. Ueno H, Yamato O, Sugiura T, Kohyama M, Yabuki A, Miyoshi K, et al. GM1 gangliosidosis in a Japanese domestic cat: a new variant identified in Hokkaido, Japan. J Vet Med Sci. 2016;78:91–5.
18. Donnelly WJ, Sheahan BJ, Kelly M. Beta-galactosidase deficiency in GM1 gangliosidosis of Friesian calves. Res Vet Sci. 1973;15:139–41.
19. Ahern-Rindell AJ, Prieur DJ, Murname RD, Raghavan SS, Daniel PF, McCluer RH, et al. Inherited lysosomal storage disease associated with deficiencies of beta-galactosidase and alfa-neuraminidase in sheep. Am J Med Genet. 1988;31:39–56.
20. Skelly BJ, Jeffrey M, Franklin RJM, Winchester BG. A new form of ovine GM1-gangliosidosis. Acta Neuropathol. 1995;89:374–9.
21. Ryder SJ, Simmons MM. A lysosomal storage disease of Romney sheep that resembles human type 3 GM1 gangliosidosis. Acta Neuropathol. 2001;101: 225–8.
22. Muthupalani S, Torres PA, Wang BC, Zeng BJ, Eaton S, Erdelyi I, et al. GM1-gangliosidosis in American black bears: clinical, pathological, biochemical and molecular genetic characterization. Mol Genet Metab. 2014;111:513–21.
23. Bermudez AJ, Johnson GC, Vanier MT, Schröder M, Suzuki K, Stogsdill PL, et al. Gangliosidosis in emus (*Dromaius novaehollandiae*). Avian Dis. 1995;39: 292–303.
24. Karbe E. Animal model: canine GM2-gangliosidosis. Am J Pathol. 1973; 71:151–4.
25. Cummings JF, Wood PA, Walkley SU, de Lahunta A, DeForest ME. GM2 gangliosidosis in a Japanese spaniel. Acta Neuropathol. 1985;67:247–53.
26. Sanders DN, Zeng R, Wenger DA, Johnson GS, Johnson GC, Decker JE, et al. GM2 gangliosidosis associated with a *HEXA* missense mutation in Japanese Chin dogs: a potential model for Tay Sachs disease. Mol Genet Metab. 2013;108:70–5.
27. Yamato O, Matsuki N, Satoh H, Inaba M, Ono K, Yamasaki M, et al. Sandhoff disease in a golden retriever dog. J Inherit Metab Dis. 2002;25:319–20.
28. Tamura S, Tamura Y, Uchida K, Nibe K, Nakaichi M, Hossain MA, et al. GM2 gangliosidosis variant 0 (Sandhoff-like disease) in a family of toy poodles. J Vet Intern Med. 2010;24:1013–9.
29. Rotmistrovsky RA, Alcaraz A, Cummings JC, de Lahunta A, Farmer SF. GM2 gangliosidosis in a mix-breed dog. Prog Vet Neurol. 1991;2:203–8.
30. Kohyama M, Yabuki A, Kawasaki Y, Miura N, Kitano Y, Onitsuka T, et al. GM2 gangliosidosis variant 0 (Sandhoff disease) in a mixed-breed dog. J Am Anim Hosp Assoc. 2015;51:396–400.
31. Neuwelt EA, Johnson WG, Blank NK, Pagel MA, Masien-McClure C, McClure MJ, et al. Characterization of a new model of GM2-gangliosidosis (Sandhoff's disease) in Korat cats. J Clin Invest. 1985;76:482–90.
32. Bradbury AM, Morrison NE, Hwang M, Cox NR, Baker HJ, Martin DR. Neurodegenerative lysosomal storage disease in European Burmese cats with hexosaminidase β-subunit deficiency. Mol Genet Metab. 2009;97:53–9.
33. Cork LC, Munnell JF, Lorenz MD, Murphy JV, Baker HJ, Rattazzi MC. GM2 ganglioside lysosomal storage disease in cats with β-hexosaminidase deficiency. Science. 1977;196:1014–7.

34. Yamato O, Matsunaga S, Takata K, Uetsuka K, Satoh H, Shoda T, et al. GM2-gangliosidosis variant 0 (Sandhoff-like disease) in a family of Japanese domestic cats. Vet Rec. 2004;155:739–44.
35. Martin DR, Cox NR, Morrison NE, Kennamer DM, Peck SL, Dodson AN, et al. Mutation of the GM2 activator protein in a feline model of GM2 gangliosidosis. Acta Neuropathol. 2005;110:443–50.
36. Kosanke SD, Pierce KR, Bay WW. Clinical and biochemical abnormalities in porcine GM2 gangliosidosis. Vet Pathol. 1978;15:685–99.
37. Torres PA, Zeng BJ, Porter BF, Alroy J, Horak F, Horak J, et al. Tay-Sachs disease in Jacob sheep. Mol Genet Metab. 2010;101:357–63.
38. Rickmeyer T, Schöniger S, Petermann A, Harzer K, Kustermann-Kuhn B, Fuhrmann H, et al. GM2 gangliosidosis in an adult pet rabbit. J Comp Pathol. 2013;148:243–7.
39. Fox J, Li YT, Dawson G, Alleman A, Johnsrude J, Schumacher J, et al. Naturally occurring GM2 gangliosidosis in two Muntjak deer with pathological and biochemical features of human classical Tay-Sachs disease (type B GM2 gangliosidosis). Acta Neuropathol. 1999;97:57–62.
40. Zeng BJ, Torres PA, Viner TC, Wang ZH, Raghavan SS, Alroy J, et al. Spontaneous appearance of Tay-Sachs disease in an animal model. Mol Genet Metab. 2008;95:59–65.
41. Hasegawa D, Tamura S, Nakamoto Y, Matsuki N, Takahashi K, Fujita M, et al. Magnetic resonance findings of the corpus callosum in canine and feline lysosomal storage diseases. PLoS One. 2013;8(12):e0083455.
42. Yamato O, Kobayashi A, Satoh H, Endoh D, Shoda T, Masuoka Y, et al. Comparison of polymerase chain reaction-restriction fragment length polymorphism assay and enzyme assay for diagnosis of GM1-gangliosidosis in Shiba dogs. J Vet Diagn Invest. 2004;16:299–304.
43. Yamato O, Satoh H, Matsuki N, Ono K, Yamasaki M, Maede Y. Laboratory diagnosis of canine GM2-gangliosidosis using blood and cerebrospinal fluid. J Vet Diagn Invest. 2004;16:39–44.
44. Chang HS, Arai T, Yabuki A, Hossain MA, Rahman MM, Mizukami K, et al. Rapid and reliable genotyping technique for GM1 gangliosidosis in Shiba dogs by real-time polymerase chain reaction with TaqMan minor groove binder probes. J Vet Diagn Invest. 2010;22:234–7.
45. Rahman MM, Yabuki A, Kohyama M, Mitani S, Mizukami K, Uddin MM, et al. Real-time PCR genotyping assay for GM2 gangliosidosis variant 0 in Toy Poodles and the mutant allele frequency in Japan. J Vet Med Sci. 2014;76:295–9.
46. Rahman MM, Shoubudani T, Mizukami K, Chang HS, Hossain MA, Yabuki A, et al. Rapid and simple polymerase chain reaction-based diagnostic assays for GM2 gangliosidosis variant 0 (Sandhoff-like disease) in Japanese domestic cats. J Vet Diagn Invest. 2011;23:338–42.
47. Satoh H, Yamato O, Asano T, Yamasaki M, Maede Y. Increased concentration of GM1-ganglioside in cerebrospinal fluid in dogs with GM1- and GM2-gangliosidoses and its clinical application for diagnosis. J Vet Diagn Invest. 2004;16:223–6.
48. Huang Q, Zhou X, Liu D, Xin B, Cechner K, Wang H, Zhou A. A new liquid chromatography/tandem mass spectrometry method for quantification of gangliosides in human plasma. Anal Biochem. 2014;455:26–34.
49. Dawson RM. Characterization of the binding of cholera toxin to ganglioside GM1 immobilized onto microtitre plates. J Appl Toxicol. 2005;25:30–8.
50. Satoh H, Yamauchi T, Yamasaki M, Maede Y, Yabuki A, Chang HS, et al. Rapid detection of GM1 ganglioside in cerebrospinal fluid in dogs with GM1 gangliosidosis using matrix-assisted laser desorption ionization time-of-flight mass spectrometry. J Vet Diagn Invest. 2011;23:1202–7.
51. Petr T, Šmíd V, Šmídová J, Hůlková H, Jirkovská M, Elleder M, et al. Histochemical detection of GM1 ganglioside using cholera toxin-B subunit. Evaluation of critical factors optimal for in situ detection with special emphasis to acetone pre-extraction. Eur J Histochem. 2010;54:e23.
52. Walkley SU, Vanier MT. Secondary lipid accumulation in lysosomal disease. Biochim Biophys Acta. 2009;1793:726–36.
53. Saito M, Sugiyama K. Characterization of nuclear gangliosides in rat brain: concentration, composition, and developmental changes. Arch Biochem Biophys. 2002;398:153–9.

10

Evaluation of antigen-induced synovitis in a porcine model: Immunological, arthroscopic and kinetic studies

Francisco-Javier Vela[1†], Francisco-Miguel Sánchez-Margallo[1,5†], Rebeca Blázquez[1,5*], Verónica Álvarez[1], Raquel Tarazona[2], M. Teresa Mangas-Ballester[3], Alejandro Cristo[4] and Javier G. Casado[1,2,5]

Abstract

Background: Synovitis is an inflammation-related disease linked to rheumatoid arthritis, osteoarthritis, infections and trauma. This inflammation is accompanied by immune cells infiltration which initiates an inflammatory response causing pain, discomfort and affecting the normal joint function. The treatment of synovitis is based on the administration of anti-inflammatory drugs or biological agents such as platelet rich plasma and mesenchymal stem cells. However, the evaluation and validation of more effective therapies of synovitis requires the establishment of clinically relevant animal models.

Results: In this study, Large White pigs were pre-immunized to evaluate an antigen-induced synovitis. The immune monitoring of synovial fluids in this model allowed us the identification of IL-12p40 and T cell subsets as immune biomarkers. Moreover, the evolution of synovitis was performed by arthroscopic procedures and kinetic analysis. In summary, this paper describes an animal model of antigen-induced synovitis to be used in the evaluation of anti-inflammatory therapies.

Conclusions: The novelty of this paper lies in the development of a clinically relevant model of synovitis which permits the simultaneous evaluation of synovitis from an immunological, surgical and kinetic point of view.

Keywords: Synovitis, Animal model, Inflammation

Background

The synovial fluid (SF) is a transudate of plasma that provides low-friction for a normal joint function [1]. The homeostasis of SF depends on the continuous renewal from the lymphatic capillaries to the articular cavity and the transynovial filtration towards the lymphatic capillaries. This renewal is also facilitated by physical exercise and joint flexion [2]. The synovitis is an inflammation-related disease usually linked to rheumatoid arthritis [3], osteo-arthritis [4, 5] and viral infections [6]. The inflammation of synovial tissue is accompanied to immune cells infiltration (mainly composed by macrophages and T and B lympho-cytes) which initiates an inflammatory response causing

pain and discomfort [7] and affecting the normal joint function [8].

At the present, some of the most common treatments for synovitis are based on the administration of non-steroidal anti-inflammatory drugs [9] as well as biological agents such as platelet rich plasma [10], autologous condi-tioned medium [11] and mesenchymal stem cells isolated from different sources [12] that have become a promising therapeutic option in regenerative medicine due to their self-renewal capacity, multipotentiality and immunomo-dulatory properties [13, 14].

Similarly to other diseases, the development of more effective therapies for the treatment of synovitis requires the establishment of clinically relevant animal models. Ideally, a valuable animal model for this inflammatory-related disease should be suitable for the evaluation of immune biomarkers and kinematic parameters. At the present, several animal models of synovitis have been

* Correspondence: rblazquez@ccmijesususon.com
†Equal contributors
[1]Stem Cell Therapy Unit, Minimally Invasive Surgery Centre, 10071, Caceres, Spain
[5]CIBER de Enfermedades Cardiovasculares, Caceres, Spain
Full list of author information is available at the end of the article

described including dogs [15], rats [16] and rabbits [17]. However, due to their translational applicability, other large animal models such as pigs or sheep have been considered as the more appropriate models for this kind of studies [18]. Concretely, the morphological and physiological similarities of pigs and humans in terms of cartilage thickness, biomechanical features and joint dimensions become this animal model particularly attractive for further clinical translation.

Based on that, the aim of this work was to develop and characterize a clinically relevant large animal model of synovitis. The novelty of this manuscript lies in the development of an animal model which permits to researchers the evaluation, monitoring and follow up of synovitis from different perspectives: firstly, from an immunological point of view through the evaluation of immunological biomarkers (synovial fluid lymphocytes and IL-12p40), and secondly, from a biomechanical and surgical point of view by arthroscopic and kinetic gait analysis.

Methods
Animals and experimental design
Eight Large White pigs were housed in the animal facility at the Minimally Invasive Surgery Centre and used for all experimental procedures. Animals aged 3 months and weighed 25–35 kg at the beginning of the study were used. All experimental protocols were approved by the Committee on the Ethics of Animal Experiments of Minimally Invasive Surgery Centre and fully complied with recommendations outlined by the local government (Junta de Extremadura) and by the Directive 2010/63/EU of the European Parliament on the protection of animals used for scientific purposes.

All the animals were pre-immunized by subcutaneous injections of bovine serum albumin (BSA). Local immunizations for synovitis induction were performed by intra-articular injection of BSA on the right carpal joint of each animal. The left carpal joints received an intra-articular injection of phosphate buffer saline (PBS) to be used as negative control.

As an additional control group, three Large White pigs without BSA pre-immunization were included in this study. Intra-articular injections of PBS and BSA were performed in the left and the right carpal joints respectively.

Anesthetics procedures
Every procedure was done under anesthesia. For blood sampling and subcutaneous BSA injections, anesthesia was induced by intramuscular injection of 10 mg/kg ketamine hydrochloride and 0.02 mg/kg dexmedetomidine hydrochloride. The animals were recovered with 0.02 mg/kg atipamezole hydrochloride. For SF sampling

and arthroscopies, anesthesia was induced by the same procedure together with 2 mg/kg propofol on intravenous bolus injection, and the analgesia was performed with 3 mg/kg of tramadol. According to ethical and animal welfare concerns, all the animals received analgesic treatment with buprenorphine hydrochloride. The buprenorphine at 0.3 mg/ml was regularly administered at 0.03 ml/kg for 7 days after intra-articular injection.

Immunization protocol
For animal immunizations, a solution with 20 mg/ml of BSA (Sigma-Aldrich, St. Louis, MO, USA) was prepared and passed through a 0.2 μm sterilized microfilter. An equal volume of Freund Complete Adjuvant (FCA) (Sigma-Aldrich, St. Louis, MO, USA) was mixed with the BSA solution and emulsified. The immunization was performed by subcutaneous injection of this emulsion. A total of 0.4 ml/kg was injected on days 0, 14 and 21 (see Fig. 1). On day 28, a total of 0.5 ml of SF was aspirated from both joints (SF basal sample) and intra-articular immunizations of BSA were performed in the forelimbs. A total of 0.5 ml of BSA at 20 mg/ml was injected on the right carpal joint to induce the synovitis and 0.5 ml PBS on the left carpal joint (used as negative control).

Isolation and phenotypic characterization of synovial fluid and peripheral blood lymphocytes
Synovial fluid leukocytes (SFLs) were obtained from carpal joints. A total of 0.5–1 ml of SF was aspirated and weekly sampled for 5 weeks (see Fig. 1). Leukocytes were counted in an automatic hematology analyzer (Mindray BC-5300 Vet, Hamburg, Germany) and SFLs were isolated by centrifugation at 900×g and used for flow cytometric analysis. Supernatants were also collected and stored at –20 °C for cytokines determination.

Peripheral blood lymphocytes (PBLs) were obtained from jugular vein blood samples. Blood sampling was performed weekly from the beginning of the study. PBLs were isolated by centrifugation over Histopaque-1077 (Sigma-Aldrich) and washed twice with PBS for cytometric analysis.

For flow cytometric analysis, PBLs and SFLs were suspended in PBS containing 2% FBS. The cells were then stained with PerCP-conjugated monoclonal antibody against porcine CD4 (Mouse Anti-Pig CD4a, clone: 74–12-4, BD Pharmingen, San Jose, CA, USA) and APC-conjugated monoclonal antibody against porcine CD8 (Mouse Anti-Pig CD8a, clone: 76–2-11, BD Pharmingen). The cytometric analysis was performed as follows: 2×10^5 cells were incubated for 30 min at 4 °C with appropriate concentrations of monoclonal antibodies. The cells were washed and resuspended in PBS. The flow cytometric analysis was performed in a FACScalibur cytometer (BD Biosciences) after acquisition of

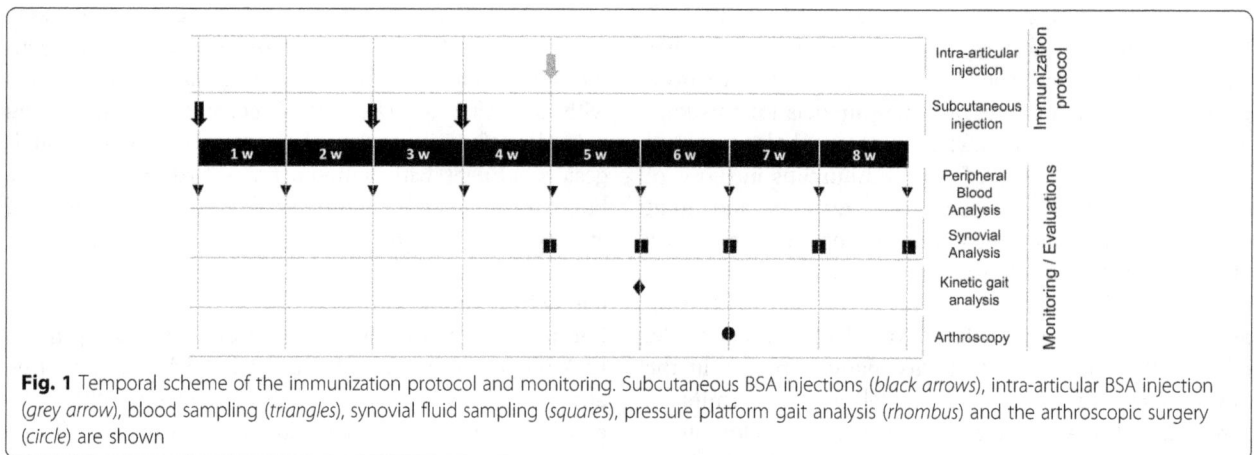

Fig. 1 Temporal scheme of the immunization protocol and monitoring. Subcutaneous BSA injections (*black arrows*), intra-articular BSA injection (*grey arrow*), blood sampling (*triangles*), synovial fluid sampling (*squares*), pressure platform gait analysis (*rhombus*) and the arthroscopic surgery (*circle*) are shown

10^5 events. Cells were primarily selected using forward and side scatter characteristics and fluorescence was analyzed using CellQuest software (BD Biosciences, San Jose, CA, USA). Isotype-matched negative control antibodies were used in all the experiments.

Quantification of anti-BSA antibodies by ELISA
In order to quantify the anti-BSA IgG titers on immunized animals, an ELISA test was performed on plasma samples. Microplate coating was performed by an overnight incubation with BSA at 20 µg/ml. The next day, coating solution was removed and wells were washed twice with 200 µl of PBS/Tween-20 (0.05%, 7.4 pH). In order to prevent the nonspecific binding of the antibodies, the remaining protein-binding sites were blocked by adding 200 µl of BSA and the plate was incubated for 2 h at 4 °C. The plate was washed four times with 200 µl PBS/Tween-20. Plasma samples were diluted on PBS at 1/200 and 100 µl of this dilution was added to each well. The plate was incubated for 2 h at 4 °C. After washing four times with PBS/Tween-20, 100 µl of 1/5000 diluted horseradish peroxidase (HRP) -conjugated secondary antibody (Rabbit Anti-Pig IgG, Thermo Fisher Scientific, Waltham, MA, USA) were added to each well and the plate was incubated for 2 h at 4 °C. Again, the plate was washed four times and 100 µl of the enzyme substrate (3,3′, 5,5′-Tetramethylbenzidineor TMB, Sigma-Aldrich) were added to each well. Two minutes later, 100 µl of 1 N HCl were added *per* well in order to stop the reaction. Plate absorbance was measured at 450 nm on a Synergy Mx spectrophotometer (BioTech Industries, Newton, NC, USA).

Cytokine detection and measurement with multiplex technology
The supernatants of SF were diluted 1:4 in PBS and stored at −20 °C. These supernatants were thawed and IFNα, IFNγ, IL-1b, IL-4, IL-6, IL-8, IL-10, IL-12p40 and

TNFα were analyzed using a multiplexed immunoassay. The measurements were performed according to the manufacturer's instructions by Luminex xMAP technology using the ProcartaPlex Porcine Cytokine & Chemokine Panel 1 (eBioscience, San Diego, CA, USA; catalog number EPX090–60829-901). The concentrations of the different cytokines were expressed as pg/ml, and calculated according to a standard curve.

Arthroscopies
In order to evaluate the potential changes on the joint status, arthroscopies were performed in the carpal joints of pre-immunized animals at two weeks after intra-articular PBS or BSA injection. The arthroscope used on surgical procedures was a HOPKINS® wide angle forward-oblique telescope 30°, 2.4 mm diameter, 10 cm length (Karl Storz, Tuttlingen, Germany).

A needle was used as a guide for the correct placement of the arthroscope through a small incision. A saline flux through the joint was maintained during all the procedure to provide a better visualization of the tissues. A careful and detailed evaluation of the joint was performed and photo recorded. Finally, the 3 mm incision was closed with a 2–0 absorbable suture and every animal received antibiotic treatment (clavulanic acid + amoxicillin) during 7 days after arthroscopy.

Pressure platform gait analysis functional evaluation by biomechanical analysis
A 174.5 cm × 36.9 cm pressure platform (PP) (Walkway™; Tekscan, South Boston, MA, USA), composed by individual sensors with a density of 1.4 sensor/cm^2 and 9152 sensors in total, was used for the biomechanical evaluation. The sensors of the PP walkway were calibrated according to the manufacturer's specifications. Seven days after intra-articular injection, animals were guided to walk along the PP and after at least 5 complete passes *per* animal, data were analyzed. Impulse (kg x sec) and vertical

maximum force (kg) were determined. Measurements were normalized to animal weights.

Statistical analysis

Data were statistically analyzed using the non-parametric Man Whitney U-test for paired comparisons and Kruskal-Wallis test for multiple comparisons. The p-values ≤ 0.05 were considered statistically significant. All the statistical determinations were made using SPSS-21 software (SPSS, Chicago, IL, USA).

Results

The BSA-immunization protocol elicits an antibody and T cell response on porcine model

The animals were subcutaneously immunized with an emulsion of BSA and FCA on days 0, 14 and 21. During the immunization protocol, peripheral blood was weekly collected from vein and analyzed by flow cytometry to evaluate the percentage of CD4 + T cells, CD8+ T cells and their ratio. It is important to note that anti-CD4 and anti-CD8 antibodies were simultaneously used for the quantification of CD4+/CD8- and CD4–/CD8+ subsets. The presence of anti-BSA antibodies in plasma samples was also quantified by ELISA test.

The analysis of peripheral blood lymphocytes from BSA-immunized animals demonstrated that the CD8 + T cell subset showed a trend to increase (non-statistically significant) whereas both CD4 + T cell subset and CD4/CD8 ratio showed a trend to decrease (Fig. 2).

Regarding the evaluation of antibodies in plasma samples, our results demonstrated that anti-BSA IgG antibody titers were detected in all of the four animals. The antibody concentrations significantly increased when compared 7 and 14 days and remained stable from days 14 to 35 showing a maximum level at 4 weeks (Fig. 3).

Based on these immunoassays, here we demonstrate that BSA-immunization protocol triggered the pre-sensitization of this animal model, which is prerequisite to generate an antigen-induced synovitis.

Intra-articular administration of BSA on pre-immunized animals modifies the leukocyte counts and synovial lymphocytes distribution

The pre-sensitized animals (subcutaneously immunized with BSA at day 0, 14 and 21) received an intra-articular injection of PBS or BSA in left or right carpal joints, respectively, at day 28. Basal samples were aspirated at day 28 prior to PBS or BSA injections. Synovial fluids were aspirated at days 35, 42, 49 and 56 (Fig. 1). The synovial fluids were centrifuged and synovial leukocytes were processed for flow cytometry analysis. Non-cellular fraction of synovial fluid was frozen for subsequent cytokine analyses.

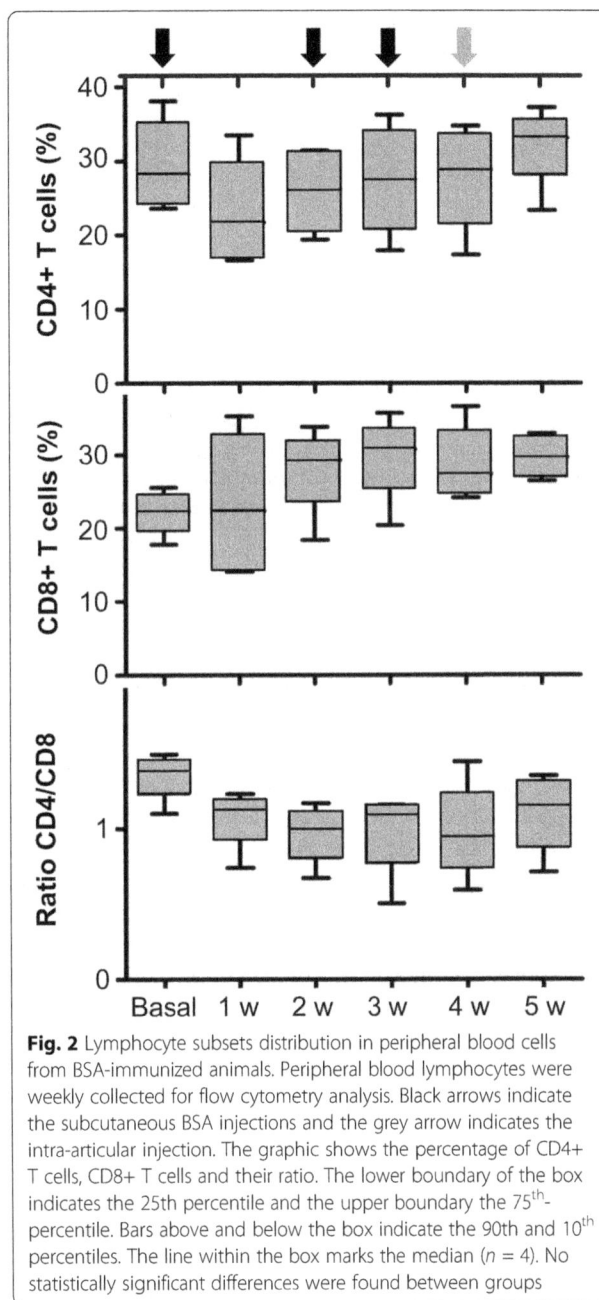

Fig. 2 Lymphocyte subsets distribution in peripheral blood cells from BSA-immunized animals. Peripheral blood lymphocytes were weekly collected for flow cytometry analysis. Black arrows indicate the subcutaneous BSA injections and the grey arrow indicates the intra-articular injection. The graphic shows the percentage of CD4+ T cells, CD8+ T cells and their ratio. The lower boundary of the box indicates the 25th percentile and the upper boundary the 75th-percentile. Bars above and below the box indicate the 90th and 10th percentiles. The line within the box marks the median (n = 4). No statistically significant differences were found between groups

The counting of leukocytes from synovial fluid samples demonstrated that, at day 35 (7 days post intra-articular BSA), the leukocyte counts were significantly increased (p = 0.04) in those carpal joints where BSA was intra-articularly injected: $0.75 \pm 1.12 \times 10^6$ /ml in control samples vs $2.40 \pm 1.19 \times 10^6$/ml in BSA-injected.

Moreover, the lymphoid and myeloid synovial cells were quantified in an automatic hematology analyzer. The distribution of lymphoid/myeloid cells in control samples was: 67.95 ± 6.57 (% of lymphoid cells) and 32.05 ± 8.11 (% of myeloid cells). On the other hand, the distribution of lymphoid/myeloid cells after intra-

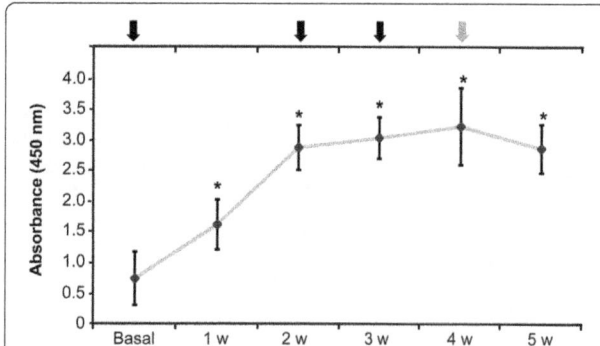

Fig. 3 Humoral response to bovine serum albumin in immunized animals. Plasma samples were weekly collected and anti-BSA IgG levels were quantified by ELISA immunoassay. In the graphic, *black* arrows indicate the subcutaneous BSA injections and the *grey* arrow indicates the intra-articular injection. Values show the mean ± SD (*n* = 4). *Statistically significant difference (*p* ≤ 0.05) compared to basal level

articular BSA injections was: 40.9 ± 19.93 (% of lymphoid cells) and 59.1 ± 20.79 (% of myeloid cells).

Once demonstrated that leukocyte counts were significantly increased, the analysis of synovial lymphocytes CD4 + T cells, CD8 + T cells and their ratio was performed at day 7, 14 and 21 after intra-articular BSA or PBS injections. Our results did not show any significant difference at days 14 and 21 (data not shown). In contrast, significant differences were observed when synovial lymphocytes were quantified at day 7 after intra-articular BSA injections (Fig. 4). As shown in Fig. 4, the intra-articular administration of BSA on pre-immunized animals exerted a significant decrease of synovial CD8 + T cells when compared to basal values (*p* = 0.025). In contrast, the percentage of CD4 + T cells as well as the CD4/CD8 ratio was significantly increased (*p* = 0.025 and *p* = 0.026, respectively). It is important to note that, in order to have a control for intra-articular injections, PBS was intra-articularly injected in pre-sensitized animals and no significant differences were observed when compared to basal values (Fig. 4). Moreover, in order to establish a proper negative control, PBS and BSA were intra-articularly injected in non-immunized

animals. No differences were observed in terms of CD4 + T cells, CD8 + T cells, CD4/CD8 ratio (Additional file 1) and biochemical parameters (Additional file 2).

Altogether, our results demonstrated that intra-articular administration of BSA on pre-immunized animals elicited a significant increase of synovial leukocytes as well as a redistribution of synovial T cell subsets towards a CD4-driven response.

Local administration of BSA on pre-sensitized animals modifies the cytokine profile of synovial fluid

Once evaluated the changes in the leukocyte counts as well as in the percentages of synovial CD4+ and CD8+ T cells, we aimed to evaluate the inflammatory environment by quantifying a wide range of cytokines. The following cytokines were quantified by Luminex technology: IFNα, IFNγ, IL-1b, IL-4, IL-6, IL-8, IL-10, IL-12p40 and TNFα.

The synovial fluids from immunized animals only showed detectable and significant differences on IL-12p40 cytokine (data not shown for the rest of cytokines). This cytokine was quantified at days 7, 14 and 21 after intra-articular BSA injections.

Our results showed significant differences on IL-12p40 at day 7 after intra-articular BSA-immunization (*p* ≤ 0.05) and non-significant differences (but a trend to increase) were found at day 14. Finally, non-significant differences were observed after 21 days (Fig. 5).

Arthroscopy as a diagnostic procedure in synovitis

Carpal joints from BSA-immunized animals were evaluated by minimally invasive procedures. Arthroscopy was performed at day 14 after intra-articular BSA or PBS injections. A total of 8 arthroscopic evaluations were performed and four out of four carpal joints where BSA was intra-articularly injected showed a slightly red to orange color (Fig. 6d). In contrast, those control carpal joints where PBS was injected, showed clear, colorless or straw colored synovia (Fig. 6c).

Apart from the macroscopic observation, aspirated synovial fluids from control and BSA were classified according to synovial nucleated cells. This classification

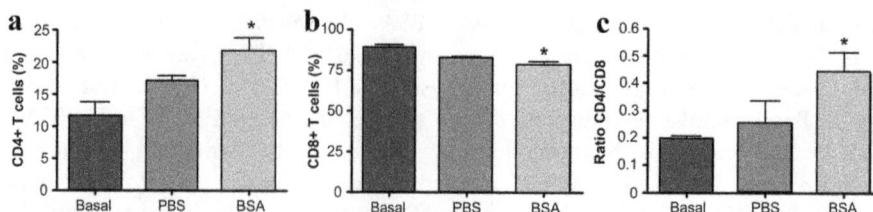

Fig. 4 Distribution of synovial lymphocyte subsets. Synovial fluid lymphocytes were collected for flow cytometric analysis just before intra-articular injection (basal) and 7 days after. The graphic shows the percentage of CD4+ T cells (**a**) CD8+ T cells (**b**) and their ratio **c**. Values show the mean ± SD (*n* = 3). *Statistically significant difference (*p* ≤ 0.05) compared to basal level

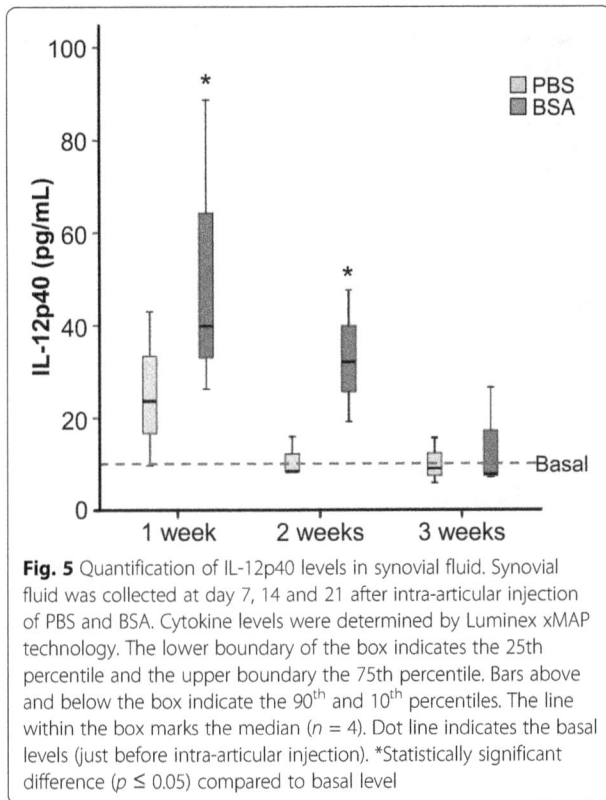

Fig. 5 Quantification of IL-12p40 levels in synovial fluid. Synovial fluid was collected at day 7, 14 and 21 after intra-articular injection of PBS and BSA. Cytokine levels were determined by Luminex xMAP technology. The lower boundary of the box indicates the 25th percentile and the upper boundary the 75th percentile. Bars above and below the box indicate the 90th and 10th percentiles. The line within the box marks the median ($n = 4$). Dot line indicates the basal levels (just before intra-articular injection). *Statistically significant difference ($p \leq 0.05$) compared to basal level

is based on a previous report from El-Gabalawy [19] where synovial fluid can be classified as Normal, if it contains fewer than 180 nucleated cells/mm^3; Non-inflammatory, when synovial fluid contains less than 2000 cells/mm^3, and Inflammatory, when synovial fluid contains 2000–50,000 cells/mm^3. Our results demonstrated that, synovial fluid from control joints can be classified as Normal or Non-inflammatory and those synovial fluids where BSA was injected could be considered as Inflammatory (Fig. 6e).

Monitoring of synovitis by pressure platform gait analysis

The kinematic gait parameters were evaluated by a pressure platform. The pre-sensitized animals were biomechanically evaluated at day 7 after intra-articular injections of BSA or PBS. The parameters evaluated were impulse (Kg x sec) and the vertical maximum force (Kg). In terms of animal management, our experience demonstrated that kinematic parameters could be easily quantified with the porcine model (Fig. 7a). Our results showed that, the impulses in the forelimbs with BSA showed an enormous inter-individual variability (Fig. 1c) and no significant difference was observed in terms of vertical maximum force (Fig. 7b). Finally, it is important to note that because of ethics and animal welfare, this kinematic analysis had to be performed under analgesia.

Discussion

Synovitis is an inflammation of the joint lining. This inflammation is painful and usually linked to osteoarthritis, rheumatoid arthritis or infections [3, 4, 6]. To alleviate pain and discomfort, the synovitis can be successfully treated with anti-inflammatory medications such as non-steroidal anti-inflammatory drugs [9] or biological therapies [10, 11, 14, 20]. At the present, new therapies are currently being investigated to improve their clinical efficacy and to reduce the adverse effects commonly associated to non-steroidal anti-inflammatory drugs.

Clinically relevant animal models are essential to evaluate therapeutic strategies to target inflammation and to predict outcome of clinical trials. The anatomical similarities between pigs and humans, particularly for surgical procedures, makes this animal model a valuable tool to evaluate the safety, feasibility and dosage pattern of new therapies for synovitis. Based on that, the main objective of our work has been focused in the development of an experimentally-induced synovitis model to be used for the evaluation and follow up of synovitis from different perspectives. It is important to note that, the synovitis in the animal is triggered by a T cell-mediated response induced by BSA, which is somehow comparable to the T cell-mediated response in the synovial tissue of clinically active rheumatoid arthritis patients [21].

It is interesting to note that immunologically induced synovitis models have been previously described in pigs. In this sense, Möller et al. succeeded in inducing a reliable and reproducible synovitis using turkey egg albumin (more appropriate than chicken egg albumin) [18]. This animal model was proposed to be useful to investigate the potential applicability of laser treatment in arthroscopic synovectomy. In contrast to our BSA-induced synovitis model, in the turkey egg albumin model from Möller et al. the synovitis examination was performed in terms of macroscopic observations (joint profile, synovial fluid and membrane) as well as in terms of histologic findings (synovial membrane, stratum synoviale and fibrosum). Our antigen-induced synovitis model provides the methodologies and procedures for monitoring the inflammation in terms of immune biomarkers. Moreover, similarly to the model from Möller et al. this animal model allowed us the evaluation of synovitis by arthroscopic inspection.

First of all, the BSA pre-sensitization in the porcine model was optimized and adapted taking as a reference previous reports with rabbits and dogs [22–24]. Similarly to antigen-induced synovitis model developed in other animals, our results demonstrated that BSA emulsified with complete Freund's adjuvant was strongly efficient to promote a rapid and maintained antigen-specific humoral response. Moreover, based on the kinetic of the

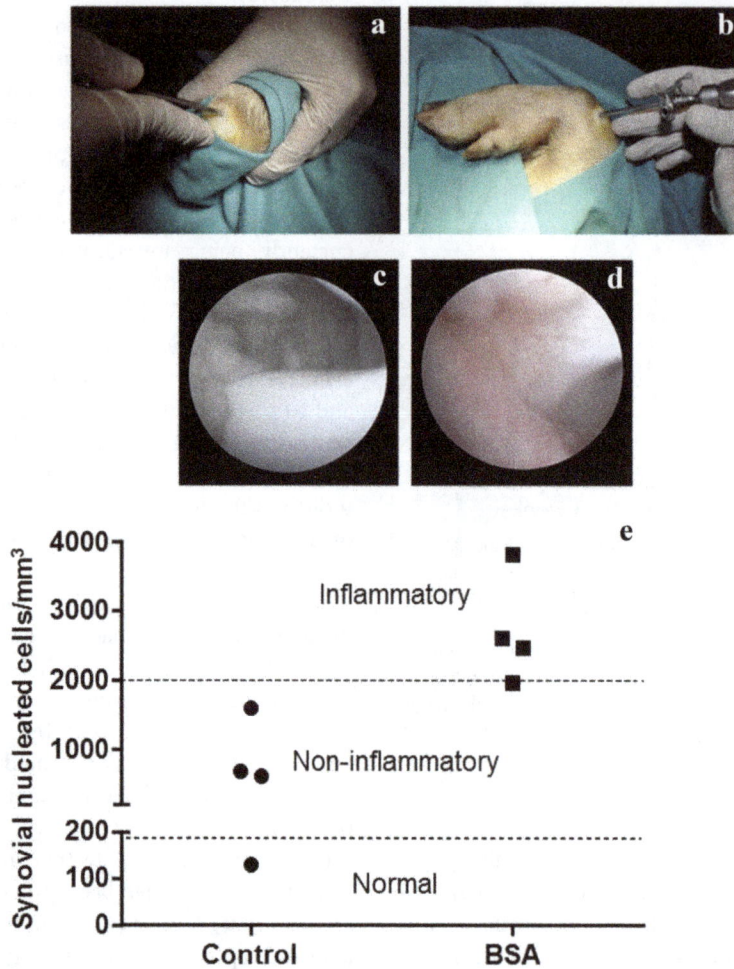

Fig. 6 Surgical approach and arthroscopic analysis. Two weeks after intra-articular injection of PBS or BSA, an arthroscopic evaluation was performed. Figure shows the access to the articular cavity **a**, the arthroscopic procedure **b** representative image of arthroscopy in the control joint **c** and representative image of arthroscopy in the BSA-injected joint **d**. Synovial fluid classification according to nucleated cells/mm^3 **e**. Synovial fluid is classified as "normal" if it contains less than 180 nucleated cells/mm^3 or "non-inflammatory" when synovial fluid contains less than 2000 cells/mm^3. On the contrary, when synovial fluid contains 2000–50,000 cells/mm^3 it is classified as "inflammatory" [19]

humoral response against BSA, and taking into account that the anti-BSA titers did not significantly increased after second and third immunizations, it would be interesting to evaluate in future experiments a different pre-sensitization protocol based on a single BSA-immunization. Apart from humoral response against BSA, and in contrast to other studies using antigen-induced synovitis models, here we focused our interest on the cellular response. In this sense, we analyzed the CD4+ and CD8+ T cell subsets on the peripheral blood from BSA-immunized animals. Our results demonstrated that BSA-immunization induced slight changes (non-statistically significant) on T cell subsets. However, the absence of significant changes would be the consequence of analgesic and anti-inflammatory treatment with buprenorphine (required by ethical guidelines) during immunization.

Once demonstrated that the immunization protocol triggered a humoral response against BSA, we aimed to induce an inflammatory response in synovial tissue. Our results demonstrated that, intra-articular administration of BSA significantly induced changes on synovial leukocyte counts. Moreover, the flow cytometry analysis showed significant changes in the distribution of synovial CD4+ and CD8+ T cells. Based on that, and taking into account that the presence of large numbers of activated CD4+ T cells in synovial tissue is important in the pathogenesis of chronic synovitis [25], here we suggest that synovial T cell distribution could be suitable biomarker in the evolution of synovitis.

Additionally, although the functional phenotype of synovial CD4+ T cells could not be evaluated (because of the limited availability of synovial lymphocytes), the significant increase of synovial CD4+ T cells may reflect

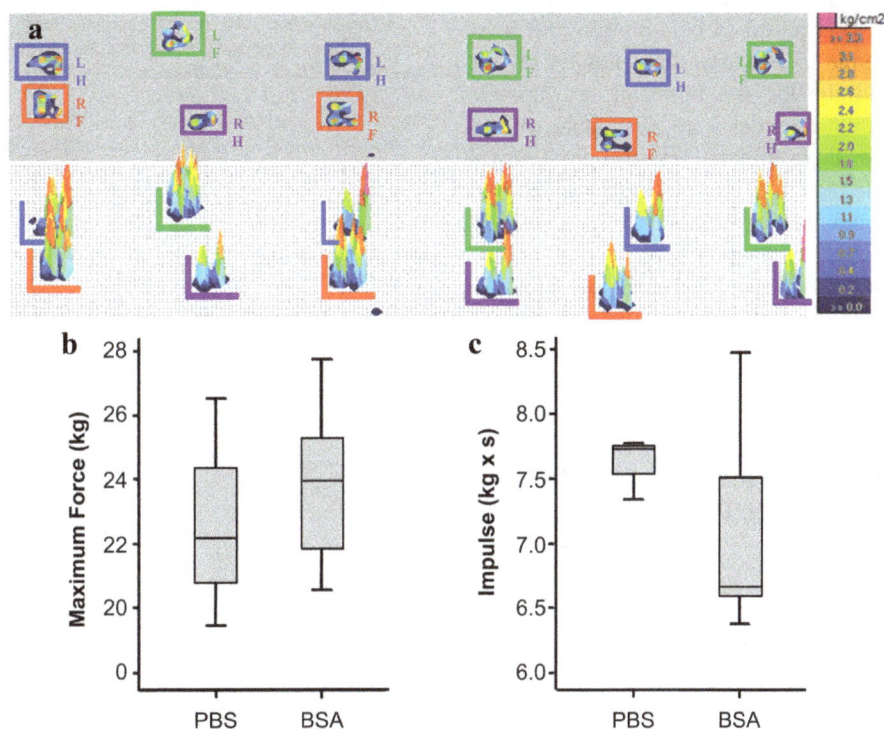

Fig. 7 Pressure platform gait analysis. Seven days after intra-articular injection of PBS or BSA, a pressure platform gait analysis was performed to evaluate plantar pressure distributions. **a** Above, a representative image of the gait analysis (*LF: left forelimb; LH: left hind limb; RF: right forelimb; RH: right hind limb*) is represented. Below, the pressure of each limb is shown. The legend on the right shows the equivalence between numeric and colorimetric values. Maximum forces **b** and impulses **c** in control and BSA-injected limbs (*n* = 4). The lower boundary of the box indicates the 25th percentile and the upper boundary the 75th percentile. Bars above and below the box indicate the 90th and 10th percentiles. The line within the box marks the median. No significant differences were found between PBS and BSA injected joints

an increase of 'type 1' polarity (TH1) with CD4+ CD45RO+ phenotype and IFNγ expression. This assumption is based on previous reports which demonstrated that synovial CD4+ T cells from rheumatoid arthritis patients were predominantly of 'type 1' polarity [26–28].

Additionally, in order to identify soluble factors to be used as synovitis biomarker in this animal model, we aimed to characterize a large panel of cytokines in the synovial fluids from immunized animals. It is important to note that, from an immunological and mechanistic point of view, it was important to define if local inflammatory response is dominated by a Th1 or Th2 response [29]. Based on that premise, the following panel of cytokines was quantified: IFNα, IFNγ, IL-1b, IL-4, IL-6, IL-8, IL-10, IL-12p40 and TNFα. Our results showed that, probably because of the detection limit of commercially available swine immune reagents, only IL-12p40 could be efficiently quantified in the synovial fluids. The IL-12p40 is a subunit of IL12p70 [30] which is mainly produced by monocytes, macrophages and dendritic cells [31]. The presence of this cytokine initiates the differentiation of Naïve CD4+ T cells towards a Th1 response [32], so according to the observed increase of IL-12p40, here we hypothesize that this

antigen-induced synovitis model is dominated by a local Th1 response.

It is important to discuss the importance of synovial biomarkers in the evaluation of the disease course and monitoring of treatments. In this sense, several inflammatory cytokines have been defined as biomarkers in patients with rheumatoid arthritis and osteoarthritis [33]. Other authors have also identified the Cartilage Oligometric Matric Proteinin in synovial fluid as a biomarker to predict the development of osteoarthritis [34]. The levels of C-terminal telopeptides of type II collagen and hyaluronan have also been defined as potential biomarkers of synovitis [35, 36]. Here we hypothesize that IL-12p40 could be considered as immunological biomarker in the evaluation of synovitis in this animal model. Supporting this statement, similar changes have been observed in the synovial tissue of rheumatoid arthritis patients where increased IL-12p40 levels have been detected [37].

Apart from the identification of immunological biomarkers in the evaluation of disease progression, this paper aimed to have a multi-criteria assessment in the evaluation of synovitis. Arthroscopic evaluations and pressure platform gait analyses were performed to have additional elements in the monitoring of synovitis. Firstly, arthroscopy was found to be a simple and feasible surgical technique to evaluate the synovitis in this animal model. Additionally, the kinematic parameters quantified in the animal model were a valuable tool to evaluate the functional parameters (impulse and vertical forces). This porcine model, in contrast to the sheep that become nervous and more difficult to handle [38], demonstrated several advantages in terms of animal handling being particularly suitable for gait analysis. Unfortunately, our results did not reveal any significant difference in terms of impulse or vertical forces when forelimbs were compared in the animal model. In this case, the absence of differences would not necessarily imply that the kinetic was unaffected, so we should clarify that ethical consideration and animal welfare guidelines forced us to perform the pressure gait analysis in animals under analgesia.

Conclusions

Taking into consideration that the establishment of an animal model is an absolute prerequisite in preclinical research, this paper describes the development and characterization of a clinically relevant porcine model of synovitis. This antigen-induced inflammation model triggered a cell-mediated response allowing us the identification of immunological parameters to be used as biomarkers in the monitoring of synovitis and newly developed therapies. Moreover, here we demonstrated that, our antigen-induced model of synovitis can also be evaluated by standard arthroscopic instruments and kinetic studies.

Additional files

Additional file 1: Distribution of synovial lymphocyte subsets in control samples. Synovial fluid lymphocytes were collected from non pre-immunized animals. Flow cytometric analysis was performed on synovial fluids at day 7 after PBS (0.5 ml) or BSA injections (0.5 ml of BSA at 20 mg/ml). The graphic shows the percentage of CD4+ T cells (A), CD8+ T cells (B) and their ratio (C). Values show the mean ± SD (n = 3). (JPEG 154 kb)

Additional file 2: Biochemical analysis of synovial fluid in non-pre-immunized animals (n = 3). (DOCX 14 kb)

Abbreviations

BSA: Bovine Serum Albumin; FCA: Freund Complete Adjuvant; MSCs: Mesenchymal Stem Cells; PBLs: Peripheral Blood Lymphocytes; PBS: Phosphate Buffer Saline; SF: Synovial Fluid; SFLs: Synovial Fluid Lymphocytes; Th1: T helper 1

Acknowledgements

Technical and human support provided by Facility of Bioscience Applied Techniques of SAIUEx (financed by UEX, Junta de Extremadura, MICINN, FEDER and FSE). In vivo experiments were performed by the ICTS "Nanbiosis", more specifically by the Unit 14 (Cell Therapy), Unit 22 (Animal housing), Unit 21 (Experimental Operating Rooms) and Unit 24 (Medical Imaging) at CCMIJU. In vitro experiments were performed by the ICTS "Nanbiosis", more specifically by the Unit 14 at CCMIJU.

Funding

This work was supported in part by one grant from Junta de Extremadura (Ayuda a grupos catalogados de la Junta de Extremadura, GR15175) and two grants from Junta de Extremadura to JGC (TA13042 and IB13123 co-financed by FEDER/FSE). Project "Large Animal Biopole (LAB-POLE)" financed by FEDER (Programa Operativo Fondos Tecnológicos). The funders had no role in study designs, data collection and analysis, decision to publish or preparation of the manuscript.

Authors' contribution

FJV and FMSM equally contributed and should be regarded as co-first authors. FJV, FMSM and JGC conceived and designed the experiments. FJV, RBD, FMSM, RT, VA, MTMB, AC and JGC performed the experiments and analyzed the data. FJV, RB, RT, JGC and FMSM wrote the manuscript. All authors read and approved the final manuscript.

Competing interests

The authors declare that they have no competing interests.

Consent to publication

Not applicable.

Author details

[1]Stem Cell Therapy Unit, Minimally Invasive Surgery Centre, 10071, Caceres, Spain. [2]Immunology Unit, Department of Physiology, University of Extremadura, 10071, Caceres, Spain. [3]Anaesthetic Unit, inimally Invasive Surgery Centre, 10071, Caceres, Spain. [4]Interactive 3D Unit, Minimally Invasive Surgery Centre, 10071, Caceres, Spain. [5]CIBER de Enfermedades Cardiovasculares, Caceres, Spain.

References

1. Ene R, Sinescu RD, Ene P, Cirstoiu MM, Cirstoiu FC. Synovial inflammation in patients with different stages of knee osteoarthritis. Romanian J Morphol Embryol. 2015;56:169–73.
2. Eynard AR, Valentich MA, Rovasio RA. Histología y embriología del ser humano: bases celulares y moleculares. 4ª ed. Buenos Aires: Médica Panamericana; 2008.
3. Terao C, Hashimoto M, Yamamoto K, Murakami K, Ohmura K, Nakashima R, et al. Three groups in the 28 joints for rheumatoid arthritis synovitis–analysis using more than 17,000 assessments in the KURAMA database. PLoS One. 2013;8:e59341.
4. El-Gabalawy H. The challenge of early synovitis: multiple pathways to a common clinical syndrome. Arthritis Res. 1999;1:31–6.
5. Scanzello CR, Goldring SR. The role of synovitis in osteoarthritis pathogenesis. Bone. 2012;51:249–57.
6. Kastrissianakis K, Beattie TF. Transient synovitis of the hip: more evidence for a viral aetiology. Eur J Emerg Med. 2010;17:270–3.
7. Firestein GS, Zvaifler NJ. How important are T cells in chronic rheumatoid synovitis? Arthritis Rheum. 1990;33:768–73.
8. Tamer TM. Hyaluronan and synovial joint: function, distribution and healing. Interdiscip Toxicol. 2013;6:111–25.
9. Nouri A, Walmsley D, Pruszczynski B, Synder M. Transient synovitis of the hip: a comprehensive review. J Pediatr Orthop B. 2014;23:32–6.
10. Lippross S, Moeller B, Haas H, Tohidnezhad M, Steubesand N, Wruck CJ, et al. Intraarticular injection of platelet-rich plasma reduces inflammation in a pig model of rheumatoid arthritis of the knee joint. Arthritis Rheum. 2011;63:3344–53.
11. Baltzer AWA, Moser C, Jansen SA, Krauspe R. Autologous conditioned serum (Orthokine) is an effective treatment for knee osteoarthritis. Osteoarthr Cartil. 2009;17:152–60.
12. Casado JG, Gomez-Mauricio G, Alvarez V, Mijares J, Tarazona R, Bernad A, et al. Comparative phenotypic and molecular characterization of porcine

mesenchymal stem cells from different sources for translational studies in a large animal model. Vet Immunol Immunopathol. 2012;147:104–12.

13. Blazquez R, Sanchez-Margallo FM, de la Rosa O, Dalemans W, Alvarez V, Tarazona R, et al. Immunomodulatory potential of human adipose Mesenchymal stem cells derived Exosomes on in vitro stimulated T cells. Front Immunol. 2014;5:556.

14. Tanaka Y. Human mesenchymal stem cells as a tool for joint repair in rheumatoid arthritis. Clin Exp Rheumatol. 2015;33:S58–62.

15. Hassan EA, Lambrechts NE, Moore GE, Weng H-Y, Heng HG, Breur GJ. Development of a model to induce transient synovitis and lameness in the hip joint of dogs. Am J Vet Res. 2015;76:869–76.

16. Brahn E, Trentham DE. Experimental synovitis induced by collagen-specific T cell lines. Cell Immunol. 1989;118:491–503.

17. Largo R, Roman-Blas JA, Moreno-Rubio J, Sánchez-Pernaute O, Martínez-Calatrava MJ, Castañeda S, et al. Chondroitin sulfate improves synovitis in rabbits with chronic antigen-induced arthritis. Osteoarthr Cartil. 2010;18(Suppl 1):S17–23.

18. Möller KO, Wethling H, Abel HH, Lind BM, Karcher K, Schramm U, et al. Studies on an immunologically induced synovitis model in pigs and sheep. Clin Orthop. 1999:228–36.

19. El-Gabalawy HS. Chapter 53: synovial fluid analyses, synovial biopsy, and synovial pathology. In: Kelleys Textbollk Rheumatol. 9th ed. Philadelphia: Elsevier Inc; 2013. p. 753–69.

20. Williams LB, Koenig JB, Black B, Gibson TWG, Sharif S, Koch TG. Equine allogeneic umbilical cord blood derived mesenchymal stromal cells reduce synovial fluid nucleated cell count and induce mild self-limiting inflammation when evaluated in an LPS induced synovitis model. Equine Vet J. 2015;48:619–25.

21. Arend WP, Firestein GS. Pre-rheumatoid arthritis: predisposition and transition to clinical synovitis. Nat Rev Rheumatol. 2012;8:573–86.

22. Goldlust MB, Rich LC, Brown WR. Immune synovitis in rabbits. Effects of differing schedules for intra-articular challenge with antigen. Am J Pathol. 1978;91:329–44.

23. Ohashi F, Shimada T, Sakurai M, Ishihara S, Kuwamura M, Yamate J, et al. The production of arthritis in beagles by an immunological reaction to bovine serum albumin. Exp Anim. 1996;45:299–307.

24. Sharma ML, Bani S, Singh GB. Anti-arthritic activity of boswellic acids in bovine serum albumin (BSA)-induced arthritis. Int J Immunopharmacol. 1989;11:647–52.

25. Striebich CC, Falta MT, Wang Y, Bill J, Kotzin BL. Selective accumulation of related CD4+ T cell clones in the synovial fluid of patients with rheumatoid arthritis. J Immunol. 1998;161:4428–36.

26. McInnes IB, Leung BP, Liew FY. Cell-cell interactions in synovitis. Interactions between T lymphocytes and synovial cells. Arthritis Res. 2000;2:374–8.

27. Chan H-C, Ke L-Y, Liu C-C, Chang L-L, Tsai W-C, Liu H-W, et al. Increased expression of suppressor of cytokine signaling 1 mRNA in patients with rheumatoid arthritis. Kaohsiung J Med Sci. 2010;26:290–8.

28. van Roon JAG, Glaudemans CAFM, Bijlsma JWJ, Lafeber FPJG. Differentiation of naive CD4+ T cells towards T helper 2 cells is not impaired in rheumatoid arthritis patients. Arthritis Res Ther. 2003;5:R269–76.

29. Muraille E, Leo O, Moser M. TH1/TH2 paradigm extended: macrophage polarization as an unappreciated pathogen-driven escape mechanism? Front Immunol. 2014;5:603.

30. Croxford AL, Kulig P, Becher B. IL-12-and IL-23 in health and disease. Cytokine Growth Factor Rev. 2014;25:415–21.

31. Gee K, Guzzo C, Che Mat NF, Ma W, Kumar A. The IL-12 family of cytokines in infection, inflammation and autoimmune disorders. Inflamm Allergy Drug Targets. 2009;8:40–52.

32. Brombacher F, Kastelein RA, Alber G. Novel IL-12 family members shed light on the orchestration of Th1 responses. Trends Immunol. 2003;24:207–12.

33. Rosengren S, Firestein GS, Boyle DL. Measurement of inflammatory biomarkers in synovial tissue extracts by enzyme-linked immunosorbent assay. Clin Diagn Lab Immunol. 2003;10:1002–10.

34. Kühne SA, Neidhart M, Everson MP, Häntzschel H, Fine PR, Gay S, et al. Persistent high serum levels of cartilage oligomeric matrix protein in a subgroup of patients with traumatic knee injury. Rheumatol Int. 1998;18:21–5.

35. Rousseau J-C, Delmas PD. Biological markers in osteoarthritis. Nat Clin Pract Rheumatol. 2007;3:346–56.

36. Vilím V, Vytásek R, Olejárová M, Machácek S, Gatterová J, Procházka B, et al. Serum cartilage oligomeric matrix protein reflects the presence of clinically diagnosed synovitis in patients with knee osteoarthritis. Osteoarthr Cartil. 2001;9:612–8.

37. Möttönen M, Isomäki P, Luukkainen R, Lassila O. Regulation of CD154-induced interleukin-12 production in synovial fluid macrophages. Arthritis Res. 2002;4:R9.

38. Kim J, Breur GJ. Temporospatial and kinetic characteristics of sheep walking on a pressure sensing walkway. Can J Vet Res. 2008;72:50–5.

11

Identification and characterization of two CD4 alleles in Microminipigs

Tatsuya Matsubara[1,2], Naohito Nishii[1,2*], Satoshi Takashima[2], Masaki Takasu[1,2], Noriaki Imaeda[2], Kayo Aiki-Oshimo[2], Kazuaki Yamazoe[1,2], Michinori Kakisaka[3], Shin-nosuke Takeshima[3], Yoko Aida[3], Yoshie Kametani[4], Jerzy K. Kulski[4,5], Asako Ando[4] and Hitoshi Kitagawa[1,2]

Abstract

Background: We previously identified two phenotypes of CD4+ cells with and without reactions to anti-pig CD4 monoclonal antibodies by flow cytometry in a herd of Microminipigs. In this study, we analyzed the coding sequences of CD4 and certified the expression of CD4 molecules in order to identify the genetic sequence variants responsible for the positive and negative PBMCs reactivity to anti-pig CD4 monoclonal antibodies.

Results: We identified two CD4 alleles, *CD4.A* and *CD4.B*, corresponding to antibody positive and negative, respectively, by nucleotide sequencing of PCR products using CD4 specific primer pairs. In comparison with the swine CD4 amino-acid sequence [GenBank: NP_001001908], CD4.A had seven amino-acid substitutions and CD4.B had 15 amino-acid substitutions. The amino-acid sequences within domain 1 of CD4.B were identical to the swine CD4.2 [GenBank: CAA46584] sequence that had been reported previously to be a modified CD4 molecule that had lost reactivity with an anti-pig CD4 antibody in NIH miniature pigs. Homozygous and heterozygous *CD4.A* and *CD4.B* alleles in the Microminipigs herd were characterised by using the RFLP technique with the restriction endonuclease, *Bse*RI. The anti-pig CD4 antibody recognized pig PBMCs with *CD4.AA* and *CD4.AB*, but did not recognized those with *CD4.BB*. We transfected HeLa cells with the FLAG-tagged CD4.A or CD4.B vectors, and certified that transfected HeLa cells expressed FLAG in both vectors. The failure of cells to react with anti-CD4 antibodies in CD4.B pigs was associated to ten amino-acid substitutions in domain 1 and/or one amino-acid substitution in joining region 3 of CD4.B. We also found exon 8 was defective in some *CD4.A* and *CD4.B* resulting in the loss of the transmembrane domain, which implies that these CD4 proteins are secreted from helper T cells into the circulation.

Conclusions: We identified that amino-acids substitutions of domain 1 in CD4.B gave rise to the failure of some CD4 expressing cells to react with particular anti-pig CD4 monoclonal antibodies. In addition, we developed a PCR-RFLP method that enabled us to simply identify the CD4 sequence variant and the positive and negative PBMCs reactivity to our anti-pig CD4 monoclonal antibodies without the need to use flow cytometric analysis.

Keywords: CD4 polymorphism, PCR-RFLP, Amino-acid substitution, Microminipigs

Background

The CD4 molecule is a cell-surface glycoprotein receptor expressed by helper T cells, monocytes, macrophages, and dendritic cells; and its structure consists of four immunoglobulin-like domains (D 1 to D 4) as part of the extracellular domain, a transmembrane domain, and a cytoplasmic tail [1, 2]. The extracellular domain binds to the monomorphic region of MHC class II to increase the affinity of the T cell receptor to the antigen peptide-MHC class II complex [3, 4]. The cytoplasmic portion of CD4+ recruits tyrosine kinase, Lck, and the kinase enhances signal transduction in T cell activation [5, 6].

Microminipigs are extra-small and novel miniature pigs developed for biomedical research in Japan [7]. Recently, swine leukocyte antigen (SLA) haplotypes were assigned in a herd of Microminipigs in order to further investigate their immunological characteristics [8] during

* Correspondence: nishii@gifu-u.ac.jp
[1]United Graduate School of Veterinary Sciences, Gifu University, Gifu 501-1193, Japan
[2]Department of Veterinary Medicine, Faculty of Applied Biological Sciences, Gifu University, 1-1 Yanagido, Gifu 501-1193, Japan

disease and infections. In the process of analyzing helper T cell function, we found that some pigs had CD4+ cells that could not be detected by flow cytometry while using three anti-pig CD4 monoclonal antibodies of the clones 74-12-4, MIL17, and PT90A [9]. The pedigree analysis indicated that the CD4-undetectable trait might be recessive, suggesting gene variation [9]. Failure of CD4 cells to react with an anti-pig CD4 antibody was reported previously in the NIH miniature swine [10] and the presence of partial nucleotide sequences and 10 amino-acid substitutions in exon 3 and 4 of two kinds of CD4 alleles (CD4.1, CD4.2) in these miniature swine might be the cause of helper T cells not reacting with the anti-pig CD4 antibody [11]. On the other hand, because Microminipigs have no consanguinity with NIH miniature swine, the cause for the failure of CD4 cells to react with the anti-pig CD4 antibody in Microminipigs might be different from NIH miniature swine. Hence, we need to clarify the variations in the CD4 nucleotide and amino acid sequences for the positive and negative antibody phenotypes in Microminipigs.

In this study, in order to clarify the reasons for the failure of the anti-pig CD4 antibodies to react with and detect peripheral CD4+ cells and to assess whether sequence variations within the CD4 molecules of Microminipigs might cause immunological alterations, we 1) sequenced and analyzed the coding sequence (CDS) of CD4 using genomic DNA and reverse transcribed (RT)-PCR products of CD4 mRNA in Microminipigs,, 2) developed a simple PCR-RFLP method to identify the CD4 sequence variant and the positive and negative PBMCs reactivity to anti-pig CD4 monoclonal antibodies, and 3) examined the expression of the CD4 alleles transfected into HeLa cells.

Methods
Microminipigs
Microminipigs were raised in a conventional environment at Fuji Micra Inc. (Fujinomiya, Japan) or Gifu University. This study was carried out along the Gifu University Laboratory Animal Guidelines.

Flow cytometric analysis
Flow cytometry was performed as previously [9]. Briefly, peripheral blood mononuclear cells (PBMCs) of 231 Microminipigs were isolated using Lymphoprep (Axis Shield, Oslo, Norway), stained with a FITC-conjugated anti-pig CD4a antibody (clone 74-12-4, BD Biosciences, San Jose, CA), and analyzed using FACSCalibur (BD Biosciences) to classify the pigs with and without CD4 affinity for the 74-12-4 antibody. The data was analyzed with FlowJo version 7.6.5 software (FlowJo, Ashland, OR). The antibody reactivity with the CD4 protein was measured as the MFI (median of fluorescence intensity) of CD4+ cells in PBMCs.

Direct sequencing of CD4 coding region
Genomic DNA was extracted from peripheral blood, pieces of tail or ear tissues of 11 Microminipigs (reactive CD4: six pigs, non-reactive CD4: five pigs) using a Wizard Genomic DNA Purification Kit (Promega Corporation, Madison, WI). CD4 gene-specific primer pairs for amplification and sequencing of the coding region (exons 2 to 10) were designed as shown in Table 1 based on a swine reference sequence [Genbank: NC_010447]. The PCR cycling parameters included an initial denaturation step of 4 min at 94 °C, 35 cycles consisting of 30 s at 94 °C, 30 s at 60 °C, 30 s at 72 °C, and a final extension step of 7 min at 72 °C. Sequencing was performed with ABI PRISM 3100 (Life Technologies, Carlsbad, CA) using Big Dye Terminator ver. 3.1 (Life Technologies). The nucleotide and deduced amino-acid sequence results were aligned using GENETYX version 10 (GENETYX, Tokyo, Japan) with three swine CD4 sequences: [GenBank: NM_001001908, GenBank: X65629 (CD4.1), GenBank: X65630 (CD4.2)].

Table 1 CD4 exonic primer sets for DNA sequencing

Amplification exon	Forward primer sequence	Reverse primer sequence	Length of PCR product size (bp)
2	5'-GTACCTGTGGGTGTCAGTTTAGAG-3'	5'-CTTACCCAGCACCAGATATTTTTC-3'	383
3	5'-CTCAGACTCAAACTGGGATGATTG-3'	5'-GATCCCAGAGTTTACTAGGAGCTG-3'	366
4	5'-AATGAGCAACTCAGATCAGAAGAGT-3'	5'-CTTATCCATCTCTGGACGGTTG-3'	363
5	5'-CTTCTCCTTGGGGATAGTGCAT-3'	5'-ACACTACAGCCACGAGCAGAG-3'	358
6	5'-GCCTAGAGCTAGATGGGAATTTAAG-3'	5'-GATTCCAGCCTCAGTTCAAACC-3'	617
7	5'-CTTTAGAGCAGACAAGTGCTAGGAA-3'	5'-ACCATACCCATAACCCACTGACTC-3'	373
8	5'-AGCATAAGGATCAGACCCAAGTGT-3'	5'-TAACTCTGTGGCTTCTTGTCTCTC-3'	400
9	5'-GTTAATTCTGGGACAGATGGCTTC-3'	5'-CTCTCTTCACCCCTCCTCTTTG-3'	238
10-1	5'-CCATCTCTGTGCAGGAAAAGTC-3'	5'-AGCTGAGCTGCTTGGGTGATA-3'	698
10-2	5'-ACTGACGGAGCCACAGACTC-3'	5'-GGCTATCAACTTTCGCAGGA-3'	668

CD4 genotyping by PCR-restriction fragment length polymorphism (PCR-RFLP) method

The PCR-RFLP technique in association with the restriction enzyme *Bse*RI was used to identify and differentiate between the two CD4 alleles. PCR amplification was performed on genomic DNA to amplify CD4 exon 3, and the PCR products were digested with an enzyme, *Bse*RI (New England Biolabs Inc., Ipswich, MA). The allele-specific bands were analyzed by 2 % agarose gel electrophoresis.

We determined the hereditary pattern of CD4 alleles of sibs from heterozygous parents by using the PCR-RFLP method to genotype 64 piglets, 35 males and 29 females, born from 17 matings. In addition, CD4 genotypes and phenotypes were assigned in 143 Microminipigs by the PCR-RFLP methods and flow cytometry as described above. The percentage and MFI of CD4+ cells in PBMCs were also compared between the two CD4 genotypes.

Detection of CD4 mRNA by analyzing RT-PCR products

Peripheral blood samples of Microminipigs were collected into Paxgene Blood RNA tubes (PreAnalytiX, Hombrechtikon, Switzerland). Total RNA was extracted using a PAXgene Blood RNA Kit (PreAnalytiX). Complementary DNA (cDNA) was synthesized from oligo dT primers using total RNA and the reverse transcriptase kit, ReverTra Ace (TOYOBO, Osaka, Japan).

To characterise the expressed CD4 mRNA, RT-PCR amplification was performed between exon 1 and 4 or exon 1 and 5 by using two specific primer pairs (Table 2) that were designed from the nucleotide sequence information of two CD4 alleles, *CD4.A* and *CD4.B*, obtained from Microminipigs and the swine CD4 reference sequence [GenBank: NM_001001908]. RT-PCR was performed using the same conditions as those used for sequencing amplification. The RT-PCR products were digested with *Bse*RI, and electrophoresed in 2 % agarose gel.

Transfection of two kinds of CD4 alleles into HeLa cells

We chose HeLa cells for the analysis of CD4 expression analysis in Microminipigs because the same cells have been used for the analysis in human [12, 13]. To verify the differences in the antibody reactivity of CD4 alleles, HeLa cells were transfected with the FLAG-tagged CD4 vectors (CD4-FLAG) constructed by adding FLAG to C-

terminus of the two different CD4 alleles. PBMCs were isolated from two pigs genotyped to two types of CD4 homozygotes using the Lymphoprep kit (Axis Shield) and their total RNAs were extracted with ISOGEN (NIPPON GENE, Tokyo, Japan). cDNA was synthesized by SuperScript III First-Strand Synthesis System (Life Technologies) using a sequence specific reverse primer (5′-TCAGGTGAGGGAATAGTTCTTCTGTTGCCG-3′). RT-PCR was performed with PrimeSTAR Max DNA Polymerase (TaKaRa Bio Inc., Otsu, Japan) and a CD4 specific primer pair containing *Xho*I and *Not*I recognition sequences and FLAG sequences (Forward: 5′-TATCTCGAGATGGACCCAGGAACCTCTCT-3′; Reverse: 5′- TATGCGGCCGCTCACTTGTCATCGTCCTTGTAATCGGTGAGGGAATAGTTCTTCTTCTGTTGC-3′). The RT-PCR products of CD4-FLAG were cloned into the mammalian expression vector pCAGGS [14], and the integrity of the constructed vectors were confirmed by DNA sequencing using the following five primers; Forward 1: 5′-GCAGGGACTTCCTTTGTCCCAAAT-3′; Forward 2: 5′- TATCTCGAGATGGACCCAGGAACCTCTCT-3′; Forward 3: 5′-AGTCACCCTACAGTGCAATGGAAAG-3′; Reverse 1: 5′- TATGCGGCCGCTCACTTGTCATCGTCCTTGTAATCGGTGAGGGAATAGTTCTTCTTCTGTTGC-3′; Reverse 2: 5′-TGTCCTTCCGAGTGAGAGACACAA-3′. The constructed plasmids were transfected into HeLa cells using Lipofectamine 2000 (Life Technologies) according to the manufacturer's instructions. After culturing for 20 h, the transfected HeLa cells were stained with a rabbit anti-FLAG polyclonal antibody (Sigma-Aldrich, St. Louis, MO) followed by the Alexa Fluor 488 goat anti-rabbit IgG antibody (Life Technologies). The PE-conjugated mouse anti-pig CD4a monoclonal antibody (clone 74-12-4, SouthernBiotech, Birmingham, UK) was used for the CD4 molecule detection. The cells were also stained with Hoechst 33342 (ImmunoChemistry Technologies, Bloomington, IN). Fluorescence imaging was conducted using scanning laser confocal microscope FV1000-D IX81 (Olympus, Tokyo, Japan).

Statistical analysis

In the hereditary analysis, the observed and theoretical values were assessed by the chi-squared test using Excel 2007 (Microsoft, Seattle, WA) with an add-in software Statcel 3 (OMS, Tokorozawa, Japan). Theoretical values were determined on the basis of the Punnett square. A difference of $P < 0.05$ was considered as significant.

Results

PCR amplification of CD4 gene sequences between exons 2 and 10 was performed on 11 Microminipigs, six pigs that were CD4 antibody reactive and five pigs that were CD4 antibody unreactive. DNA sequencing and analysis of the 11 PCR products identified three

Table 2 Primers for RT-PCR to detect the expression of CD4 mRNA

Name	Forward primer sequence	Reverse primer sequence	Length of PCR products (bp)
Primer 1	5′-GTAAGAGAAGCAGAGGGGAAGAG-3′	5′-GATTCTTGATGATCAGGGGAAAG-3′	400
Primer 2	5′-GTAAGAGAAGCAGAGGGGAAGAG-3′	5′-CATTCTTGCTTTTATTCCCTGGAC-3′	595

homozygous and three heterozygous allelic sequences from the six CD4 antibody reactive samples, and five homozygous allelic sequences from the five CD4 antibody unreactive samples. We aligned the eight homozygous allelic sequences against the swine CD4 reference sequence [GenBank: NM_001001908] and identified two distinct allelic nucleotide sequences between exons 2 and 10 of the CD4 genes that we classified as alleles CD4.A and CD4.B (Additional file 1). In comparison with the [GenBank: NM_001001908] sequence, the CD4.A [DDBJ: LC064059] and CD4.B [DDBJ: LC064060] alleles had 15 and 22 nucleotide substitutions between exon 2 and 10 regions, respectively (Table 3). Nucleotide sequences identical to CD4.A have not been found in GenBank, and so far appear to be unique to the Microminipigs. In contrast, the nucleotide sequences of CD4.B were identical to that of the partial CD4.2 sequence that reported only exons 3 and 4 in the CD4-undetectable NIH miniature swine [GenBank: X65630] [11].

In comparing the derived CD4 protein sequences with the swine CD4 amino-acid reference sequence [GenBank: NP_001001908], the CD4.A and CD4.B protein sequences had seven and 15 amino-acid substitutions, respectively, in the regions of exons 2 to 10 (Fig. 1, Table 4). In CD4.A, there was one amino-acid substitution in three of the four extracellular domains as well as in the joining regions 1 and 4, and two amino-acid substitutions in the transmembrane domain. In CD4.B, there were ten amino-acid substitutions in domain 1, one in domain 3, one each in joining regions 3 and 4, and two in the transmembrane domain, some of which may change the polarity or charge of the amino-acid side chains. There was no amino-acid substitution in the cytoplasmic region of either CD4.A or CD4.B.

Three CD4 genotypes in Microminipig herd were assigned as CD4.AA, AB, and BB by the PCR-RFLP method using BseRI (Fig. 2). The restriction enzyme patterns of CD4.AA, AB and BB showed a single band (366 bp), three bands (366, 260, and 106 bp), and two bands (260 and 106 bp), respectively. The matings of 17 pairs of heterozygous parents revealed that the inheritance pattern of CD4 genotypes was autosomal (Table 5). As shown with the flow cytometry results in Table 6, PBMCs with CD4.AA and AB reacted with the antibody clone 74-12-4. In contrast,

PBMCs with CD4.BB were unreactive with the antibody. The MFI of CD4.AB was approximately half the intensity of CD4.AA, even though the percentage of CD4+ cells in PBMCs were not different between the two CD4 alleles (Fig. 3).

CD4 gene expression was analyzed by RFLP using the RT-PCR sequence products that were amplified between exons 1 and 4 (Fig. 4a) or between exons 1 and 5 (Fig. 4b). RFLP distinguished the genotypes CD4.AA, CD4.BB and CD4.AB in both cases. In Fig. 4a, the RT-PCR products were detected as a single 400 bp-band by electrophoresis. After BseRI digestion, the single band remained in CD4AA, whereas two digested bands of 303 bp and 97 bp were obtained in CD4.BB. Combinatorial band patterns of CD4.AA and CD4.BB were observed in CD4.A/B. In Fig. 4b, the undigested RT-PCR products were detected as a single 595 bp band. After the BseRI digestion, the single 595 bp band remained in CD4.AA, whereas two digested bands of 300 bp and 295 bp were obtained in CD4.BB, and the combinatorial band patterns of CD4.AA and CD4BB were observed in CD4.A/B. Consequently, these results suggested that PBMCs with heterozygous CD4 genotype coexpressed CD4.A and CD4.B alleles at the mRNA level.

In validating the expression vector sequences, the insertion sequences of CD4.A-FLAG and CD4.B-FLAG were found to be identical to the genomic exon sequences described above (Additional file 1) except for the added FLAG sequence. Moreover, we also found a spliced form that lacked the CD4 exon 8 in both of the two CD4 alleles. These spliced forms with the exon 8 deficiency gave rise to a stop codon at the N-terminus of transmembrane domain as a result of a frameshift from the beginning of the exon 8 region, whereas amino-acid sequences of the external domains in the spliced forms were identical to those of the CD4.A and CD4.B derived from the nucleotide sequencing using genomic DNA (Fig. 5). Therefore, we used the constructs with complete sequences of CD4-FLAG for expression in HeLa cells. These alternative spliced forms were submitted to DDBJ (http://www.ddbj.nig.ac.jp) as CD4.A exon 8 deficiency [DDBJ: LC064061] and CD4.B exon 8 deficiency [DDBJ: LC064062].

Figure 6 shows the transient expression of CD4-FLAG without the exon 8 deficiency in HeLa cells. The CD4.A and FLAG proteins in CD4.A-FLAG were detected with the anti-pig CD4 antibody and anti-FLAG antibody. In contrast, the CD4.B in CD4.B-FLAG was unreactive with the anti-pig CD4 antibody even though FLAG was detected with the anti-FLAG antibody. These results show that we expressed the CD4.B protein in HeLa cells, but that we could not detect it with the anti-CD4 antibody.

Table 3 The number of nucleotide substitutions in CD4.A and CD4.B CDS compared to [GenBank: NM_00100908]

Allele	Exon	2	3	4	5	6	7	8	9	10
	The number of nucleotide substitutions									
CD4.A		0	1	1	2	3	3	5	1	0
CD4.B		0	12	1	1	3	0	5	1	0

```
                                            Exon 2 ↓ Exon 3                                      CDR1
                                                              ................. Domain 1    <--- ----- --->
                                     _____ Leader Sequence _____
NP_001001908        1   MDPGTSLRHLFLVLQLAMLPAASGTQEKYLVLGKAGDLAELPCHSSQKKNLPFNWKNSNQ   60
CD4.A               1   ..........................................................S...   60
CD4.B               1   ..........................................................S...D.  60
CAA46583(CD4.1)     1   -------------------------------..........................S...D.  27
CAA46584(CD4.2)     1   -------------------------------..........................S...D.  27

                             CDR2        ↓ Exon 4                                        CDR3
                        ......... <--- ---->                                         <--- --- ---
NP_001001908       61   TKILGGHGSFWHTASVTELTSRLDSKKNMWDHGSFPLIIKNLEVTDSGIYICEVEDKRIE   120
CD4.A              61   ............................................................   120
CD4.B              61   (I)..(R)S.(R)NL..(K).....S...................................   120
CAA46583(CD4.1)    28   (I)..(R)S.(R)NL..(K).....S...................................    87
CAA46584(CD4.2)    28   (I)..(R)S.(R)NL..(K).....S...................................    87

                        __ __ >|Exon 5
                        _ JR 1  ↓                                            Domain 2 ...............
NP_001001908      121   VQLLVFRLTASVTRVLLGQSLTLTLEGPSGSHPTVQWKGPGNKSKNDVKSLLLPQVGLED   180
CD4.A             121   .............A..............................................   180
CD4.B             121   ............................................................   180
CAA46583(CD4.1)    88   ...........------------------------------------------------- --    99
CAA46584(CD4.2)    88   ...........------------------------------------------------- --    99

                        ..............._____ JR 2   ↓ Exon 6          Domain 3 ...................
NP_001001908      181   SGLWTCTVSQDQKTLVFRSNIFVLAFQKVPSTVYVKEGDQVALSFPLTFEAESLSGELMW   240
CD4.A             181   .........................................V..................   240
CD4.B             181   .........................................V..................   240
CAA46583(CD4.1)    99   ------------------------------------------------------------    99
CAA46584(CD4.2)    99   ------------------------------------------------------------    99

                        ......................
NP_001001908      241   RQTKGASSPQSWITFSLKDRKVTVQKSLQNLKLRMAEKLPLQITLLQALPQYAGSGNLTL   300
CD4.A             241   ............................................................   300
CD4.B             241   ............................................................   300
CAA46583(CD4.1)    99   ------------------------------------------------------------    99
CAA46584(CD4.2)    99   ------------------------------------------------------------    99

                        .........._____ JR 3   ↓ Exon 7 ...........         Domain 4 ...........
NP_001001908      301   VLPEGRLHREVNLVVMRATQSKNEVTCEVLGPTPPKVVLSLKLGNQSMKVSDQQKLVTVL   360
CD4.A             301   .......................................................(R).....   360
CD4.B             301   ..................I.........................................   360
CAA46583(CD4.1)    99   ------------------------------------------------------------    99
CAA46584(CD4.2)    99   ------------------------------------------------------------    99

                        ..................._____ JR 4   ↓ Exon 8 ...........  TM Domain ...............
NP_001001908      361   DPEAGMWRCLLRDKDKVLLESQVEVLPTAFTRAWPELLASVIGGIIGLLFLAGFCIACVK   420
CD4.A             361   ..............................................(K)...(E)..................V...   420
CD4.B             361   ..............................................(K)...(E)..................V...   420
CAA46583(CD4.1)    99   ------------------------------------------------------------    99
CAA46584(CD4.2)    99   ------------------------------------------------------------    99

                        ↓ Exon 9             ↓ Exon 10
                        _____ Cytoplasmic Domain
NP_001001908      421   CWHRRRRAERMSQIKRLLSEKKTCQCAHRQQKNYSLT                          457
CD4.A             421   ....................................                          457
CD4.B             421   ....................................                          457
CAA46583(CD4.1)    99   ------------------------------------                           99
CAA46584(CD4.2)    99   ------------------------------------                           99
```

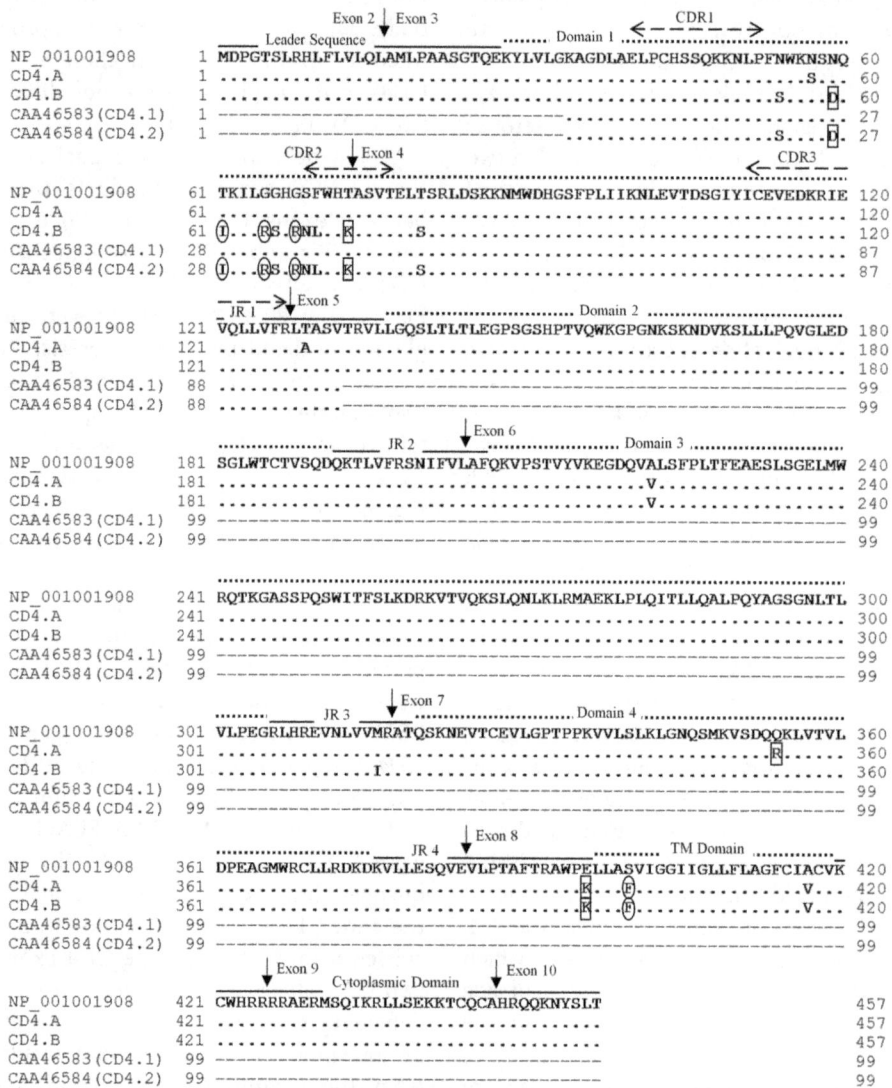

Fig. 1 Comparison of amino-acid sequences of porcine CD4 alleles. Deduced amino-acid sequences of CD4.A and CD4.B were compared with those of the swine CD4 reference sequence [GenBank: NP_001001908]. Amino-acid sequences of two CD4 alleles reported in NIH miniature swine [GenBank: CAA46583 (CD4.1), CAA46584 (CD4.2)] also were compared with CD4.A and CD4.B. (-) indicates gaps or absence of sequence corresponding to [GenBank: NP_001001908]. (.) indicates having identical sequence with that of [GenBank: NP_001001908]. Arrow indicates the putative boundary of each exon. Regions of leader sequence, four extracellular Ig-like domains (Domain 1-4), joining region (JR 1-4), transmembrane (TM) domain, and cytoplasmic domain are also shown. <——> indicates CDR1-3 like region in domain 1. An outlined circle indicates that the amino-acid side chain has changed the polarity in association with amino-acid substitution. An outlined square indicates that the amino-acid side chain has changed the charge in association with amino-acid substitution

Table 4 The number of amino-acid substitutions in CD4.A and CD4.B compared to [GenBank: NP_001001908]

CD4 type	Regions of CD4 molecule									
	D 1	JR 1	D 2	JR 2	D 3	JR 3	D 4	JR 4	TM	CP
	The number of amino-acid substitutions									
CD4.A	1	1	0	0	1	0	1	1	2	0
CD4.B	10	0	0	0	1	1	0	1	2	0

D 1-4: domain 1-4; JR 1-4: joining region 1-4; *TM* transmembrane domain; *CP* cytoplasmic domain

Discussion

The CD4 exonic sequences of the Microminipig CD4 gene were analyzed using the DNA isolated from CD4+ cells that were CD4-reactive and non-reactive to the 74-12-4 antibody, and two corresponding alleles, *CD4.A* and *CD4.B*, respectively, were identified. Although the CD4 gene is thought to be highly conserved, CD4 polymorphisms were reported previously in human, bovine, and ovine [15–17]. Also, two CD4 partial allelic sequences were reported in NIH miniature swine (*CD4.1*: X65629;

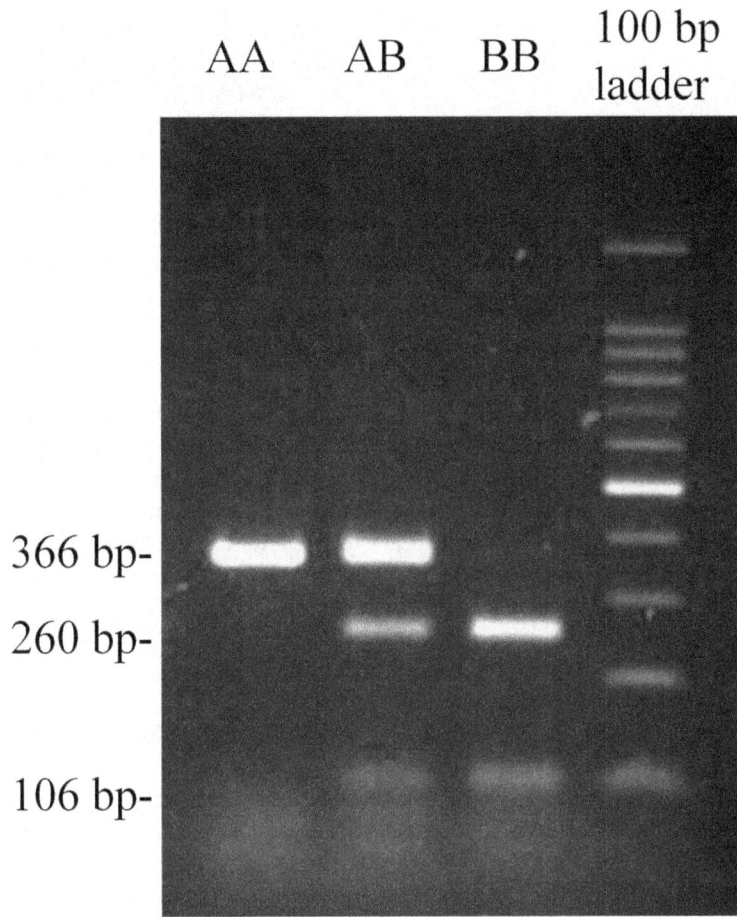

Fig. 2 Electrophoretic pattern of PCR-RFLP of genomic DNA. The lanes are AA: *CD4.AA*; AB: *CD4.AB*; BB: *CD4.BB*; and the 100 bp ladder. The 366 bp-fragment was amplified from genomic DNA using primer pair for exon 3 (See Table 1). The PCR product was digested with *Bse*RI. PCR fragments with genotype of *CD4.AA*, *CD4.AB*, and *CD4.BB* showed single fragment (366 bp), three fragments (366, 260, and 106 bp), and two fragments (260 and 106 bp), respectively

CD4.2: X65630) [11]. The nucleotide sequences of exons 3 and 4 of *CD4.B* in Microminipigs were identical to those of *CD4.2* in NIH miniature swine. We could not conclude that *CD4.B* is identical to the complete CD4 gene sequence of NIH miniature swine because only the nucleotides of exons 3 and 4 were sequenced for *CD4.2*.

Table 5 CD4 genotypes of piglets delivered from the matings of CD4 heterozygous pigs

CD4 genotype	The number of piglets		Theoretical value	
	Male	Female	Male	Female
AA	10	9	8	8
AB	16	13	16	16
BB	9	7	8	8
Total	35	29	32	32

The hereditary pattern corresponds to the theoretical value on the basis of autosomal heredity in heterozygous by analysis of chi-squared test ($P > 0.05$). Hence, the hereditary pattern of CD4 genotypes is autosomal in mode

However, the Microminipig breed is the result of crosses with western breeds, but it has no consanguinity with the NIH miniature swine [7]. Although the *CD4.B* of Microminipigs and *CD4.2* of NIH miniature swine might have a co-ancestor, the origins of *CD4.B* and *CD4.2* remain uncertain.

In comparing the amino-acid sequence alignments of CD4.A and CD4.B with the swine CD4 amino-acid reference sequence [GenBank: NP_001001908], we identified one amino-acid substitution in domain 4 of the extracellular region of CD4.A that involve alterations in the charge of the amino-acid side chain, and consequently a structural change in this domain of CD4. Domains 3 and 4 of CD4 play an important role in interacting with the T cell receptor-CD3 complex to influence signal transduction in T cell activation and function [18]. Therefore, the amino-acid substitution on domain 4 of CD4.A might affect signal transduction and T cell function during the interaction of CD4 with the T cell receptor-CD3

Table 6 The relationship between CD4 genotype and affinity to anti-pig CD4 antibody

CD4 genotype	Number	CD4 reactivity	Number
AA	24	Reactive	95
AB	71		
BB	48	Non-reactive	48

CD4 genotype was assigned by PCR-RFLP method using *Bse*RI. CD4 reactivity was veriified by flow cytometry. CD4+ cells in PBMCs could not be detected with the antibody when they carried the *CD4.BB* genotype

complex. The five amino-acid substitutions observed in domain 1 of CD4.B also alter the polarity or charge of amino-acid side chains and might elicit a structural alteration in this domain of the CD4. The domain 1 of the CD4 combines with the monomorphic region of the MHC molecule in the presentation of antigenic determinants to activate selected lymphocytes [3, 4]. Moreover, the amino-acid substitutions in the region of domain 1 in CD4.B correspond to the CDR2-like region of CD4.2 in NIH miniature swine and the CDR2-like region of CD4 in humans that bind to MHC class II molecules and the HIV envelope glycoprotein gp120 [11]. No clinical abnormalities have been observed as yet with the *CD4.B* genotype in Microminipigs, although the affinity of CD4.B to MHC class II might be different from that of CD4.A [9]. In this regard, the PCR-RFLP technique using *Bse*RI has allowed us to identify the three CD4 genotypes *CD4.AA*, *AB* and *BB* that correlated with CD4 reactivity to anti-pig CD4 antibodies. This simple CD4 genotyping method might be useful for selectively breeding *CD4.A* or *CD4.B* homozygous pigs and for developing association studies of immunity to infections and immunologically-related diseases.

Our PCR-RFLP study has demonstrated that both *CD4.A* and *CD4.B* are co-expressed in PBMC of heterozygous pigs. Moreover, the study on the expression of CD4-FLAG in HeLa cells confirmed that the amino-acid substitutions in CD4.B were associated with the loss of affinity to anti-CD4 antibody. On the other hand, the seven amino-acid substitutions observed within CD4.A reacted with the anti-CD4 antibody and one or other of them are likely to be linear or sequential epitopes recognized by the anti-CD4 antibody. Therefore, one or more of the ten amino-acid substitutions in domain 1 and/or the one amino-acid substitution in joining region 3 of CD4.B, which are not found in CD4.A, may have replaced the antigenic determinant and caused the lose of affinity for the anti-pig CD4 antibodies.

The detection of reduced levels of MFI in CD4 cells with *CD4.AB* in the Microminipigs appears to be due to the anti-CD4 antibody reacting with CD4.A, but not with the CD4.B molecules, if both types of CD4 proteins are coexpressed on the surface of helper T cells. Moreover, in CD4-FLAG insertion sequencing, the *CD4.A* and *CD4.B* alleles also had exon 8 deficiency forms that lacked the subsequent of transmembrane domain in the deduced amino-acid sequences. Thus, if the CD4 transcripts are without a transmembrane domain then the translated proteins might be secreted into the serum rather than be bound within the cellular membrane. The alternative spliced forms of CD4 CDS in swine have not been reported previously even though there are such variants registered in GenBank [GenBank: XM_005652591, GenBank: XM_005652592, GenBank: KC333254, GenBank: AY515293]. However, the lack of CD4 transmembrane region was reported for a mutant mouse model that secreted soluble CD4 without expression

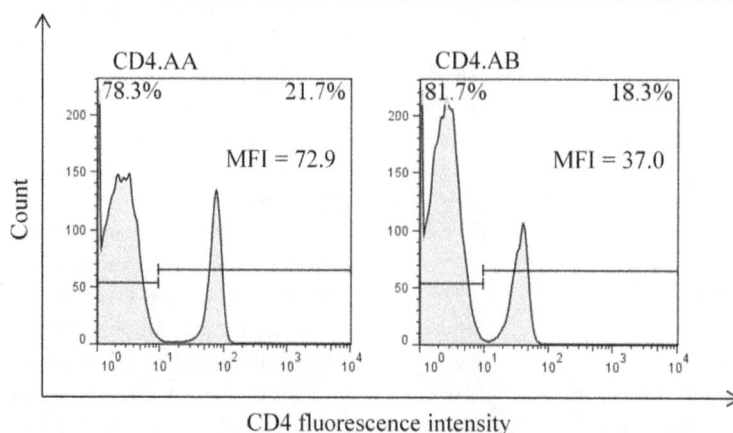

Fig. 3 The percentage and MFI of CD4+ cells in PBMCs with *CD4.AA* and *CD4.AB*. CD4 genotypes in 2-month old Microminipigs assigned by PCR-RFLP. PBMCs were stained with FITC-conjugated anti-pig CD4 antibody and assessed by flow cytometry as described in Materials and Methods. The MFI of CD4+ cells with *CD4.AB* was almost half of those with *CD4.AA*, even though there was no significant difference in the percentage of CD4+ cells between *CD4.AA* and *CD4.AB*

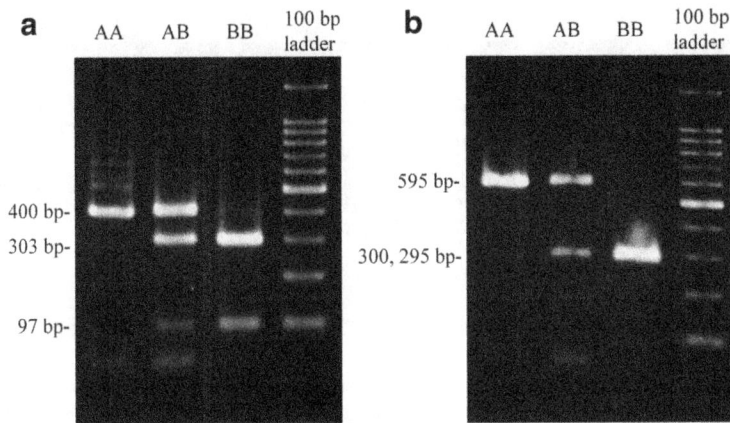

Fig. 4 Electrophoretic pattern of RT-PCR products after enzyme digestion with *Bse*RI. The lanes are AA: *CD4.AA*; AB: *CD4.AB*; BB: *CD4.BB*; and the 100 bp ladder. The 400 bp (**a**) and 595 bp (**b**) of the CD4 sequence were amplified from cDNA using primer sets shown in Table 2 and the amplified products were digested with *Bse*RI. **a** After digestion with *Bse*RI, *CD4.AA*, *CD4.AB*, and *CD4.BB* showed a 400 bp-fragment (400 bp), three fragments of 400, 303 and 97 bp, and two fragments of 303 and 97 bp, respectively. **b** After digestion with *Bse*RI, *CD4.AA*, *CD4.AB*, and *CD4.BB* showed a 595 bp-fragment, three fragments of 595, 300 and 295 bp, and two fragments of 300 and 295 bp, respectively

of membrane-bound CD4 [19]. This mouse model was used to show that soluble CD4 impaired a delayed-type hypersensitivity response by inhibiting IFN-γ production, and prohibited over-activation of CD4+ T cells by competitive inhibition of the binding of CD4 on the T-cell surface to MHC class II [20]. So, if the exon 8 deficiency forms are translated to the protein, the secreted CD4 might be also associated with prohibiting over-activation of CD4+ T cells in swine. Thus, further studies are needed to elucidate the significance of the expression of CD4 exon 8 deletions.

In NIH miniature swine, the functional differences of CD4 between CD4.1 and CD4.2 were investigated, but no differences were detected in antibody production against staphylococcal nuclease immunization and in

the allogeneic mixed lymphocyte reaction [21]. In this regard, additional studies will be needed in Microminipigs to elucidate the functional significance or immunological importance of polymorphisms of the CD4 gene including the possible alternative spliced forms of the expressed gene. Because the CD4 molecule interacts with the MHC class II complex in antigen recognition [3, 4] the polymorphisms of both CD4 and MHC class II will need to be considered in future studies. The Microminipigs with defined SLA haplotypes [8] could be a useful animal model for further research on the interaction between CD4 allomorphs and MHC molecules in disease, infection and transplantation studies.

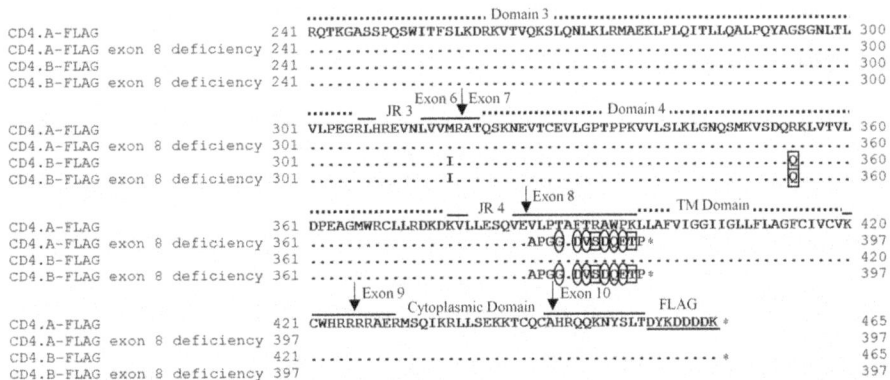

Fig. 5 Alignment of amino-acid sequences of CD4.A-FLAG and CD4.B-FLAG and their exon 8 deficiency forms. (.) indicates having identical sequence to CD4.A-FLAG. Arrow indicates the putative boundary of each exon. (*) indicates the stop codon. The regions of two extracellular Ig-like domains (Domain 3, 4), joining region (JR 3, 4), transmembrane (TM) domain, cytoplasmic domain and FLAG are also shown. Exon 8 deficiency forms gave rise to a stop codon at the N-terminus of TM domain as a result of a frameshift from the beginning of the exon 8 region, even though amino-acid sequences of their external CD4 domains in the spliced forms were identical to those of CD4.A-FLAG and CD4.B-FLAG. Thus, we used the constructs with complete sequences of CD4.A-FLAG and CD4.B-FLAG for the expression study in HeLa cells

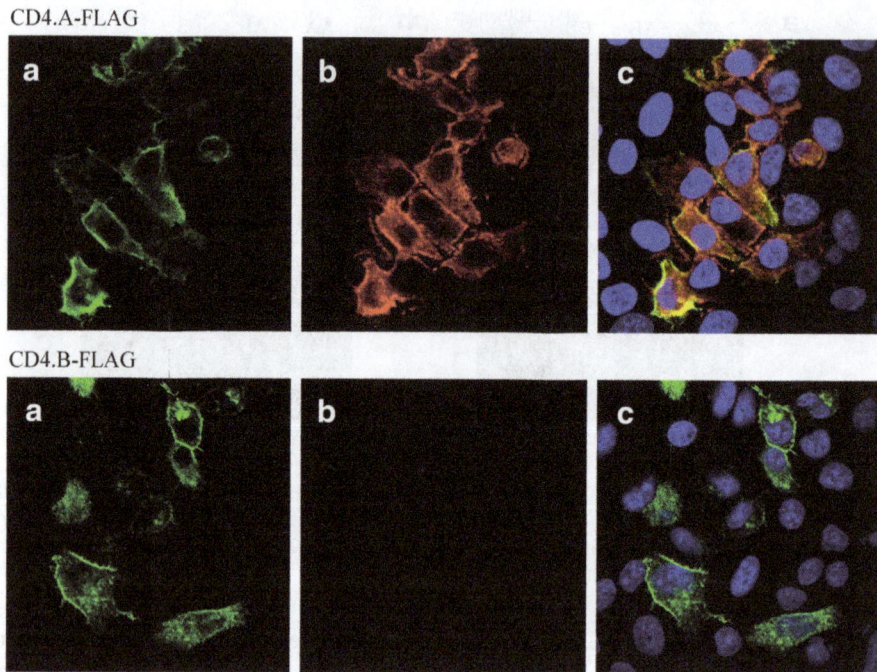

Fig. 6 Expression of the CD4-FLAG vectors in HeLa cells. We expressed only the constructs CD4-FLAG with complete sequences in HeLa cells as described in Fig. 5. **a** Cells stained with rabbit anti-FLAG antibody followed by Alexa Fluor 488 goat anti-rabbit IgG antibody. **b** Cells stained with PE conjugated mouse anti-pig CD4 antibody. **c** Cells stained with the overlay of three fluorophore signals; anti-FLAG antibody, anti-pig CD4 antibody, and Hoechst 33342

Conclusions

Two CD4 alleles, named as *CD4.A* and *CD4.B*, were identified in Microminipigs, and these two alleles were found to express an exon 8 deficiency, indicating the potential for alternative spliced forms. The loss of reactivity of antigenic epitopes to an anti-CD4 antibody probably resulted because of amino-acid substitutions in CD4.B. These CD4 polymorphisms could be genotyped and identified simply by the PCR-RFLP technique using *Bse*RI in Microminipigs.

Additional file

Additional file 1: Alignment of CD4 CDS based on swine CD4 reference sequence [GenBank: NM_00100908]. Nucleotide sequences of *CD4.A* and *CD4.B* were aligned based on swine CD4 reference sequence [GenBank: NM_00100908], and two CD4 alleles reported in NIH miniature swine were also aligned [GenBank: X65629 (*CD4.1*), GenBank: X65630 (*CD4.2*)]. (−) indicates having no sequence corresponding to [GenBank: NM_00100908]. (.) indicates having identical sequence with that of [GenBank: NM_00100908]. An arrow indicates an exon boundary. (TIF 1208 kb)

Acknowledgement

We wish to express our appreciation to assistance of Fuji Micra Inc. for sample collection.

Funding

The authors received no financial support for this study.

Authors' contributions

TM participated in performing sequencing of CD4 and flow cytometry, and certifying the expression of CD4 mRNA and molecule, collected samples, analyzed data, and drafted the manuscript. NN, ST, and KOA participated in experimental design, performed sequencing of CD4 and certifying the expression mRNA, and drafted the manuscript. MT participated in sample collection and performed flow cytometry. NI contributed collecting samples and extracting DNA. KY drafted the manuscript. MK, ST, and YA conceived the expression study of CD4 molecule, participated in experimental design, coordinated experiments. YK contributed flow cytometric analysis and drafted the manuscript. JK drafted the manuscript. AA contributed sequencing analysis and drafted the manuscript. HK participated in experimental design, coordinated experiments, and drafted the manuscript. All authors read and approved the final manuscript.

Competing interests

The authors declare that they have no competing interests.

Consent for publication

Not applicable.

Author details

[1]United Graduate School of Veterinary Sciences, Gifu University, Gifu 501-1193, Japan. [2]Department of Veterinary Medicine, Faculty of Applied Biological Sciences, Gifu University, 1-1 Yanagido, Gifu 501-1193, Japan. [3]Viral Infectious Diseases Unit, RIKEN, Wako 351-0198, Japan. [4]Department of Molecular Life Science, Division of Basic Medical Science and Molecular

Medicine, Tokai University School of Medicine, Isehara 259-1193, Japan.
[5]School of Psychiatry and Clinical Neurosciences, The University of Western Australia, Crawley, WA 6009, Australia.

References

1. Kwong PD, Ryu SE, Hendrickson WA, Axel R, Sweet RM, Folena-Wasserman G, et al. Molecular characteristics of recombinant human CD4 as deduced from polymorphic crystals. Proc Natl Acad Sci U S A. 1990;87:6423–7.

2. Maddon PJ, Molineaux SM, Maddon DE, Zimmerman KA, Godfrey M, Alt FW, et al. Structure and expression of the human and mouse T4 genes. Proc Natl Acad Sci U S A. 1987;84:9155–9.

3. König R, Huang LY, Germain RN. MHC class II interaction with CD4 mediated by a region analogous to the MHC class I binding site for CD8. Nature. 1992;356:796–8.

4. Miceli MC, Parnes JR. Role of CD4 and CD8 in T cell activation and differentiation. Adv Immunol. 1993;53:59–122.

5. Veillette A, Bookman MA, Horak EM, Samelson LE, Bolen JB. Signal transduction through the CD4 receptor involves the activation of the internal membrane tyrosine-protein kinase p56lck. Nature. 1989;338:257–9.

6. Holdorf AD, Lee KH, Burack WR, Allen PM, Shaw AS. Regulation of Lck activity by CD4 and CD28 in the immunological synapse. Nat Immunol. 2002;3:259–64.

7. Kaneko N, Itoh K, Sugiyama A, Izumi Y. Microminipig, a non-rodent experimental animal optimized for life science research: preface. J Pharmacol Sci. 2011;115:112–4.

8. Ando A, Imaeda N, Ohshima S, Miyamoto A, Kaneko N, Takasu M, et al. Characterization of swine leukocyte antigen alleles and haplotypes on a novel miniature pig line, Microminipig. Anim Genet. 2014;45:791–8.

9. Matsubara T, Nishii N, Takashima S, Takasu M, Imaeda N, Aiki-Oshimo K, et al. Identification of a CD4 variant in Microminipigs not detectable with available anti-CD4 monoclonal antibodies. Vet Immunol Immunopathol. 2015;168:176–83.

10. Sundt 3rd TM, LeGuern C, Smith CV, Sachs DH. Identification of a CD4 polymorphism in swine. Transplant Proc. 1991;23:419–20.

11. Gustafsson K, Germana S, Sundt 3rd TM, Sachs DH, LeGuern C. Extensive allelic polymorphism in the CDR2-like region of the miniature swine CD4 molecule. J Immunol. 1993;151:1365–70.

12. Pelchen-Matthews A, Armes JE, Marsh M. Internalization and recycling of CD4 transfected into HeLa and NIH3T3 cells. EMBO J. 1989;8:3641–9.

13. Maddon PJ, Dalgleish AG, McDougal JS, Clapham PR, Weiss RA, Axel R. Human immunodeficiency virus infection and syncytium formation in HeLa cells expressing glycophospholipid-anchored CD4. J Virol. 1991;65:3276–83.

14. Niwa H, Yamamura K, Miyazaki J. Efficient selection for high-expression transfectants with a novel eukaryotic vector. Gene. 1991;108:193–9.

15. Tokito S, Kishi S, Yamamoto R, Takenaka T, Nakauchi H. Single amino acid substitution in the V3 domain of CD4 is responsible for OKT4 epitope deficiency. Immunogenetics. 1991;34:208–10.

16. Morrison WI, Howard CJ, Hinson CJ, MacHugh ND, Sopp P. Identification of three distinct allelic forms of bovine CD4. Immunology. 1994;83:589–94.

17. Boscariol R, Pleasance J, Piedrafita DM, Raadsma HW, Spithill TW. Identification of two allelic forms of ovine CD4 exhibiting a Ser183/Pro183 polymorphism in the coding sequence of domain 3. Vet Immunol Immunopathol. 2006;113:305–12.

18. Vignali DA, Carson RT, Chang B, Mittler RS, Strominger JL. The two membrane proximal domains of CD4 interact with the T cell receptor. J Exp Med. 1996;183:2097–107.

19. Nagase H, Wang CR, Yoshimoto T, Sugishita C, Shiroishi T, Matsuzawa A, et al. Novel mutant mice secreting soluble CD4 without expression of membrane-bound CD4. Eur J Immunol. 1998;28:403–12.

20. Wang CR, Hino A, Yoshimoto T, Nagase H, Kato T, Hirokawa K, et al. Impaired delayed-type hypersensitivity response in mutant mice secreting soluble CD4 without expression of membrane-bound CD4. Immunology. 2000;100:309–16.

21. Sundt 3rd TM, LeGuern C, Germana S, Smith CV, Nakajima K, Lunney JK, et al. Characterization of a polymorphism of CD4 in miniature swine. J Immunol. 1992;148:3195–201.

12

A first immunohistochemistry study of transketolase and transketolase-like 1 expression in canine hyperplastic and neoplastic mammary lesions

Giovanni Pietro Burrai[1], Alessandro Tanca[2], Tiziana Cubeddu[1], Marcello Abbondio[2], Marta Polinas[1], Maria Filippa Addis[2] and Elisabetta Antuofermo[1*]

Abstract

Background: Canine mammary tumors represent the most common neoplasm in female dogs, and the discovery of cancer biomarkers and their translation to clinical relevant assays is a key requirement in the war on cancer. Since the description of the 'Warburg effect', the reprogramming of metabolic pathways is considered a hallmark of pathological changes in cancer cells. In this study, we investigate the expression of two cancer-related metabolic enzymes, transketolase (TKT) and transketolase-like 1 (TKTL1), involved in the pentose phosphate pathway (PPP), an alternative metabolic pathway for glucose breakdown that could promote cancer by providing the precursors and energy required for rapidly growing cells.

Results: TKT and TKTL1 protein expression was investigated by immunohistochemistry in canine normal ($N = 6$) and hyperplastic glands ($N = 3$), as well as in benign ($N = 11$) and malignant mammary tumors ($N = 17$). TKT expression was higher in hyperplastic lesions and in both benign and malignant tumors compared to the normal mammary gland, while TKTL1 levels were remarkably higher in hyperplastic lesions, simple adenomas and simple carcinomas than in the normal mammary glands ($P < 0.05$).

Conclusions: This study reveals that the expression of a key PPP enzyme varies along the evolution of canine mammary neoplastic lesions, and supports a role of metabolic changes in the development of canine mammary tumors.

Keywords: Canine mammary tumors, Immunohistochemistry, Transketolase, Transketolase-like 1

Background

Cancer is the leading cause of death in companion animals, and mammary tumor, the most common neoplasm in female dog, represents a serious issue in worldwide veterinary practice [1, 2]. The etiopathogenesis of canine mammary tumors (CMT) is still unclear. Despite several authors reported genetic alterations of oncogenes and tumor suppressor genes, biological and morphological heterogeneity of CMTs has challenged veterinary pathologists since the early days of diagnostic pathology [3, 4].

As in humans, the identification of prognostic markers represents a major area of investigation in canine mammary cancer and an increasing number of potential prognostic factors, both clinicopathological and molecular, have been investigated [2, 4, 5]. However, classical clinicopathological features are not always sufficient to predict the biological behavior of CMTs. A few studies employed proteomic approaches to identify proteins related to the development and the aggressiveness of canine mammary tumors [6–9].

In a previous study performed by our group, several proteins showing an increased abundance in both tumor and non-tumor bearing canine mammary glands have been identified. We focused our attention on the enzyme transketolase (TKT) [9]. TKT, a dimeric protein

* Correspondence: eantuofermo@uniss.it
[1]Department of Veterinary Medicine, University of Sassari, Via Vienna 2, 07100 Sassari, Italy
Full list of author information is available at the end of the article

composed of two monomers of about 68 kDa belonging to the family of transferases, is a thiamin diphosphate-dependent enzyme that catalyzes a reversible reaction by the transfer of two carbon atoms from an aldose to a ketose in the non-oxidative branch of the pentose phosphate/hexose monophosphate shunt pathway (PPP) [10–12]. The PPP pathway has been shown to generate *de novo* ribose-5-phosphate (R5P) and NADPH, and therefore is thought to play a major role in the proliferation of cancer cells [12, 13]. Constraining TKT activity, and consequently the PPP, using glycolytic pathway inhibitors such as oxythiamine or oxybenfothiamin, was shown to induce cell apoptosis and to inhibit cell proliferation by the reduction of the major RNA backbone, R5P, and the main antioxidant NADPH [14–17].

The human genome, in addition to TKT, encodes for two further TKT-related proteins, termed transketolase-like 1 (TKTL1) and transketolase-like 2 (TKTL2), which share 61 and 66% amino acid sequence homology with TKT, respectively [11]. A marked difference between TKT and TKTL1 is a deletion of 38 amino acids of the N-terminal catalytic domain in the latter, suggesting that TKTL1 is incapable of binding to the thiamine pyrophosphate and carrying out the TKT reaction [10, 17].

Furthermore, TKTL1 has been extensively investigated in cancers, and it has been supposed to be a catalytically active mutant form of human TKT, through formation of heterodimers with other TKT isoforms and/or by activation of other thiamine derivatives [13, 15].

TKTL1 is overexpressed in a range of human malignancies including breast, colon, ovary, lung, nasopharynx, gastric, renal, cervical, lung and liver cancers, and increased TKTL1 levels were shown to be associated with reduced survival for patients with cancers of the colon, oropharynx, bladder and with oral squamous cell carcinomas [18–24].

To date, no studies have characterized the protein expression of TKT and TKTL1 and their potential role in the onset of canine mammary tumors. Here, we investigate the expression of TKT and TKTL1 in canine mammary tissues by immunohistochemistry, exploring hyperplastic lesions as well as benign and malignant tumors, including simple and complex types.

Methods

Tissue collection

Thirty-seven fresh mammary samples were obtained from 35 female dogs that underwent surgery for mammary neoplasia at the Sassari Veterinary Hospital. Dogs belonged to the following breeds: Mixed breed (20), Yorkshire Terrier (7), German Shepherd (3) Dachshund (2), Pinscher (1) Labrador Retriever (1), Poodle (1). The dog ages ranged from 5 to 15 years (median 11.5 years).

Experiment permission was not required from the University's Animal Care Ethics Committee because all the samples were retrieved from the archive of the pathology laboratory and were used for diagnostic purposes. Immediately after the surgical resection, the specimens were divided into two aliquots and stored in appropriate conditions based on the downstream analyses to be performed.

For histological examination, 10% formalin fixed samples were dehydrated in graded alcohol, embedded in paraffin wax, 3 µm-sectioned and stained with haematoxylin and eosin (H&E). Mammary samples were classified according to the World Health Organization criteria for canine mammary neoplasms [25]. In addition, canine mammary hyperplastic lesions were further evaluated as previously described by Antuofermo et al. and Mouser et al. [26, 27]. Lesions were imaged using Nikon Eclipse 80i and digital computer images were recorded with a Nikon Ds-fi1 camera.

Western immunoblotting analysis, carried out in order to validate antibody specificity, employed complementary tissues from 3 normal mammary glands and 3 simple tubulopapillary carcinomas that had been snap frozen upon collection and archived at −80 °C. After thawing, tissues were included in the Optimal Cutting Temperature medium (Tissue-Tek, Sakura Finetek, Torrance, CA, USA) and cut into 10 serial cryosections (Leica CM 1950, Heidelberg, Germany). Cryostat sections were histologically evaluated in order to confirm the presence of neoplastic lesions. Furthermore, HeLa cells (human fibroblasts derived from uterine cervix carcinoma) and ovine milk were retrieved to be used as positive and negative controls, respectively.

Western immunoblotting

Proteins were extracted by incubating tissue and cell line samples in SDS-buffer as illustrated elsewhere [28]. Then, about 3 micrograms of each protein extract were separated by electrophoresis in a polyacrylamide gel (AnyKD, Bio-Rad, Hercules, CA, USA), blotted onto nitrocellulose membranes and blocked overnight with 3% bovine serum albumin (BSA) in phosphate-buffered saline (PBS) plus 0.05% Tween 20. TKT was detected upon sequential incubation with a mouse monoclonal anti-TKT primary antibody (1:10000 dilution in PBS plus 3% BSA and 0.05% Tween 20; clone ab112997, Abcam, Cambridge, UK) and a secondary antibody directed against mouse immunoglobulin (1:250000 dilution in PBS plus 1% BSA and 0.05% Tween 20; A9044, HRP, Sigma-Aldrich, Saint Louis, MO, USA). TKTL1 protein was detected upon sequential incubation with a rabbit polyclonal anti-TKTL1 primary antibody (1:2000 dilution in PBS plus 3% BSA and 0.05% Tween 20; clone LS-4019, LSBio, Seattle, WA, USA) and a secondary antibody directed against rabbit immunoglobulin (1:250000 dilution in PBS plus 1% BSA and 0.05% Tween 20; A9169, HRP, Sigma-Aldrich). The immunoreactivity was detected using a chemiluminescent peroxidase substrate (Sigma-Aldrich) and displayed with the VersaDoc Imaging System (Bio-Rad).

Immunohistochemistry

To analyze the expression of TKT and TKTL1, histological sections (3 μm thick) from formalin-fixed, paraffin-embedded canine mammary tissue were mounted on positively charged Superfrost slides (Fisher Scientific). Slides were immersed for 20 min in a 98 °C preheated solution (WCAP, citrate pH 6, BiOptica, Milan, Italy) that simultaneously allows dewaxing, rehydration and antigen unmasking. Briefly, slides were mounted in a sequenza chamber (Shandon, Runcorn, UK) and tissues were then blocked for endogenous peroxidase with a 15 min incubation in Dako REAL Peroxidase-Blocking Solution (S2023, Dako, Glostrup, DK), and for nonspecific binding with 2.5% normal horse serum (ImmPRESS reagent kit, Vector Labs, Burlingame, CA, USA) for 30 min at room temperature.

Then, sections were incubated overnight at 4 °C with a mouse monoclonal anti-TKT antibody (clone ab112997, Abcam) and rabbit polyclonal anti-TKTL1 (clone LS-B4019, LSBio) at 1:150 and 1:100 dilution, respectively.

Then, sections were incubated for 20 min at room temperature with an anti-mouse/rabbit secondary antibody (MP-7500, ImmPRESS reagent kit, Vector Laboratories, Burlingame, CA, USA). 3,3′-Diaminobenzidine (DAB) (ImmPACT DAB, Vector Laboratories, Burlingame, CA, USA) was used as chromogen. All washing steps were performed three times with Tris-buffered saline (TBS) with 0.1% Tween 20 (BiOptica, Milano, Italy). Tissues were counterstained with haematoxylin, dehydrated and mounted with Eukitt Mounting Medium (BiOptica, Milan, Italy). A canine testis served as positive control, while negative controls were carried out by replacing the primary antibody with normal mouse or rabbit serum (ThermoFisher Scientific, Monza, Italy).

Evaluation of immunohistochemical data

The extent of TKT immunopositivity was evaluated considering the nuclear signal, while the TKTL1 was quantified by estimating the cytoplasmic immunostaining. Immunoreactivity was semi-quantitatively scored considering the number of positive cells in 10 HPF (grade 0: no positive cells, 1: <10%; 2: 11–30%; 3: 31–60%; 4:> 60%) and the intensity of staining graded as weak (1), moderate (2), and strong (3). Then, a combined immunoreactivity score (IRS), ranging from 1 to 12, was calculated for each specimen by multiplying the values of these two categories.

The slides were reviewed independently by two authors (GPB, EA) and a consensus score was obtained for each case on a multiheaded microscope.

Statistical Analysis

Statistical analysis of immunohistochemical expression data was carried out using nonparametric Kruskal-Wallis ANOVA followed by Dunn's post hoc test. Spearman correlation analysis was performed to evaluate associations of TKT and TKTL1 protein levels. Data were analyzed with Stata version 11.2 (StataCorp, 2009), and results were considered significant when $P \leq 0.05$.

Results

Histological classification of lesions

Histologically, the lesions represent a morphologically heterogeneous group of samples and were classified as follows: normal mammary glands ($n = 6$), ductal hyperplasias ($n = 3$), benign tumors ($n = 11$; 6 simple adenomas and 5 complex adenomas), and carcinomas ($n = 17$; 11 simple tubulo-papillary carcinomas and 6 complex carcinomas). In addition, the 11 simple carcinomas were further characterized as well differentiated (2), moderately differentiated (5) and solid or undifferentiated type according to Pena and colleagues [29].

Expression of TKT in canine mammary tissues

Antibody reactivity was assessed on three normal mammary glands and three simple tubulo-papillary carcinomas (one well-differentiated and two moderately differentiated) by Western immunoblotting. Reactive bands were observed at the expected molecular weight range (around 65 kDa), with different signal intensities, in normal and in mammary tumor tissues, as well as in the positive control; no signal was detected in the negative control (Fig. 1). A band of lower molecular weight (approx. 50 kDa) was also present in mammary tumor samples, with different signal intensities, and was absent from both the positive and the negative control.

Upon immunohistochemical analysis, TKT expression was found in all tissue types, normal mammary glands ($n = 4/6$, 66%; IRS = 0, range 0–4), hyperplastic lesions ($n = 3/3$, 100%; IRS = 6, range 1–9), complex adenomas ($n = 5/5$, 100%; IRS = 4, range 1–9), simple adenomas (n 6/6, 100%; IRS = 5, range 1–9) complex carcinomas ($n = 6/6$, 100%; IRS = 6, range 1–12) and simple carcinomas ($n = 11/11$, 100%; IRS = 1, range 1–9) (Fig. 2) (Additional file 1). Furthermore, statistical significant differences were noticed within the different histological lesions (Additional file 2). In comparison with normal mammary tissue, a significantly increased expression was observed in hyperplastic as well as neoplastic lesions, suggesting a pivotal role of TKT during the evolution of mammary carcinogenesis process ($P < 0.001$).

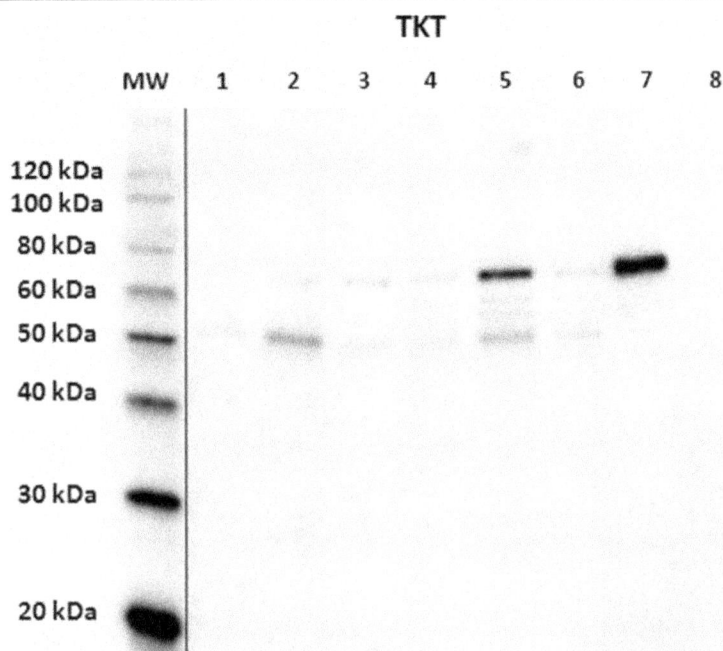

Fig. 1 Western immunoblotting verification of anti-transketolase antibody reactivity in canine mammary tissues. *Lanes 1–3*: normal mammary glands; *lanes 4–6*: simple tubulo-papillary carcinomas. *Lane 7*: reactive control; *lane 8*: negative control; MW: molecular weight (MW) marker (MagicMark™ XP Western Protein Standard, Invitrogen). Standard MWs are displayed on the left side

In addition, a statistically significant difference between normal mammary gland and simple carcinomas (IRS =1) ($P < 0.01$) was observed, corroborating the data obtained by mass spectrometry in our previous work, where TKT was found as differently expressed between tumor and normal gland both in formalin fixed and fresh frozen mammary tissues [9].

Moreover, simple carcinomas (IRS = 1) showed IRS values lower than hyperplastic lesions (IRS = 6) or benign and malignant tumors, both of simple and complex type, suggesting a possible existence of an additional pathway responsible for the onset of more aggressive mammary neoplasms ($P < 0.05$). As a partial confirmation of this hypothesis, moderately differentiated carcinomas (grade II) showed lower IRS values compared to poorly differentiated simple carcinomas (grade III) ($P < 0.05$).

Expression of TKTL1 in canine mammary tissues

Antibody reactivity against TKTL1 was assessed as above, on the same 3 normal mammary glands and 3 simple tubulo-papillary carcinomas (1 well-differentiated and 2 moderately differentiated) by Western immunoblotting. Reactive bands were observed for TKTL1 at a slightly lower molecular weight (approx. 58 kDa) than TKT, with different signal intensities in normal and in mammary tumor tissues, as well as in the positive control; again, no signal was detected in the negative control. A further reactive band of lower molecular weight (approx. 53 kDa) was visible in canine mammary tissue samples, with different signal intensities, and was absent from the positive and the negative control (Fig. 3).

Immunohistochemically, TKTL1 expression was found in all tissue types, normal mammary glands (n = 5/6, 83%; IRS = 1, range 0–12), hyperplastic lesions (n = 3/3, 100%; IRS = 12, range 9–12), complex adenomas (n = 5/5, 100%; IRS = 1, range 0–6), simple adenomas (n = 6/6, 100%; IRS = 8, range 1–12), complex carcinomas (n = 5/6, 83%; IRS = 1, range 0–12) and simple carcinomas (n = 11/11, 100%; IRS = 3, range 1–12) (Fig. 4) (Additional file 1).

In particular, hyperplastic lesions (IRS = 12), as well simple adenomas (IRS = 8) and simple carcinomas (IRS = 3), showed higher values than the normal mammary glands ($P < 0.001$).

Of interest, hyperplastic lesions showed the highest values of TKTL1 expression when compared to all the other lesions, suggesting a possible role of the PPP in the early stage of neoplastic transformation ($P = 0.001$).

Comparing the expression of TKTL1 among the various tumors, it is also worthy of note that the simple type adenomas and carcinomas tend to show a higher expression compared to the complex forms, whether they are benign (IRS = 1) and malignant (IRS = 1), indicating therefore a predominant role of TKTL1 in the epithelial cells compared to the myoepithelial component ($P < 0.001$). This hypothesis is further supported by the higher TKTL1 expression in simple adenomas than in complex carcinomas ($P < 0.001$) (Additional file 3).

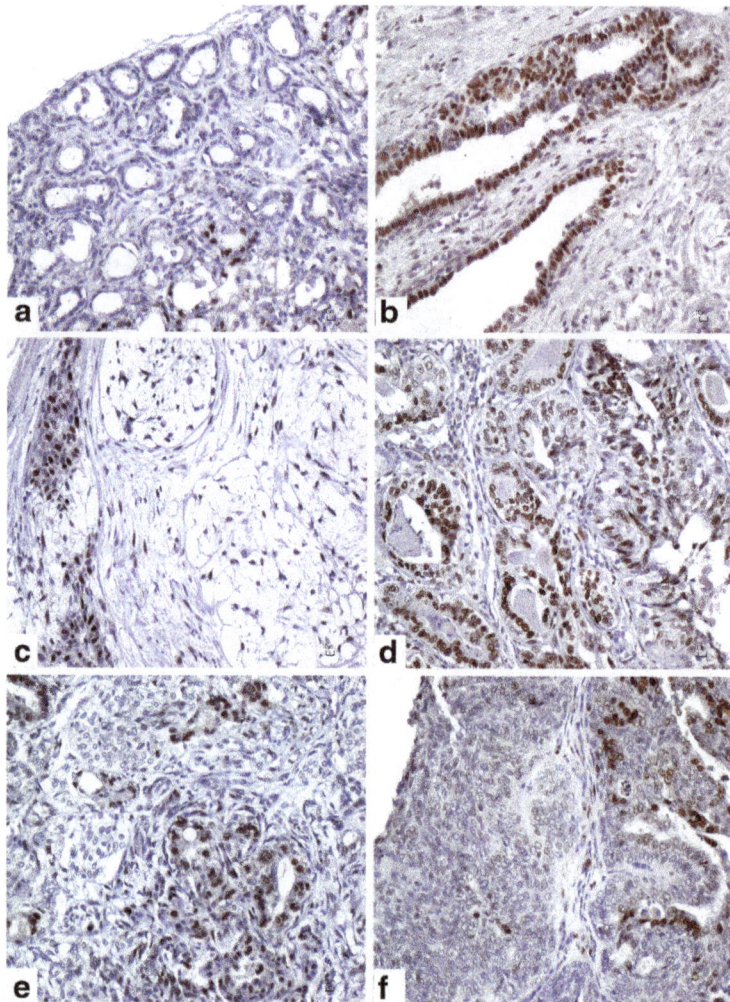

Fig. 2 Transketolase immunohistochemical expression in canine mammary glands. Nuclear expression of TKT in epithelial cells of normal mammary gland (IRS = 1) (**a**), hyperplastic mammary gland (IRS = 9) (**b**), complex adenoma (IRS = 4) (**c**), simple adenoma (IRS = 6) (**d**), complex carcinoma (IRS = 4) (**e**) and simple carcinoma (IRS = 2) (**f**)

Significant positive correlations were observed between TKT and TKTL1 expression in normal mammary gland ($\rho = 0.59$, $P < 0.05$), while a negative correlation was observed for complex adenomas ($\rho = -0.39$, $P = 0.003$).

Discussion

Reprogramming of metabolic pathways is considered a hallmark of pathological changes in cancer cells [30]. Since the description of the so-called 'Warburg effect', it has been known that neoplastic cells use the anaerobic degradation of glucose even in the presence of oxygen [31, 32].

This observation kept scientific focus on glycolysis and highlighted other aspects of glucose metabolism that could promote cancer by providing the precursors and energy required for a rapidly growing cell, such as adenosine 5′-triphosphate (ATP) and carbon intermediates [33].

Noteworthily, an alternative metabolic pathway for glucose breakdown is the pentose phosphate/hexose monophosphate shunt pathway [34].

The main purpose of the PPP is to generate R5P, which is used in the nucleotides synthesis, and NADPH, that neutralizes reactive oxygen species (ROS) enabling cancer cells to survive oxidative stress [35]. This can benefit cancer cells by facilitating cell proliferation, tumor invasion and resistance to apoptosis, which in turn promotes tumor invasion [36].

Thus, in this study, we sought to analyze by immunohistochemistry the expression of TKT, a key enzyme in the non-oxidative part of the PPP, and TKTL1, a TKT isoform frequently reported in human tumor related pathways, in a retrospective patient cohort with invasive canine mammary tumor as well as in normal and hyperplastic mammary glands. As a result, the expression of TKT was observed in all examined mammary tissues.

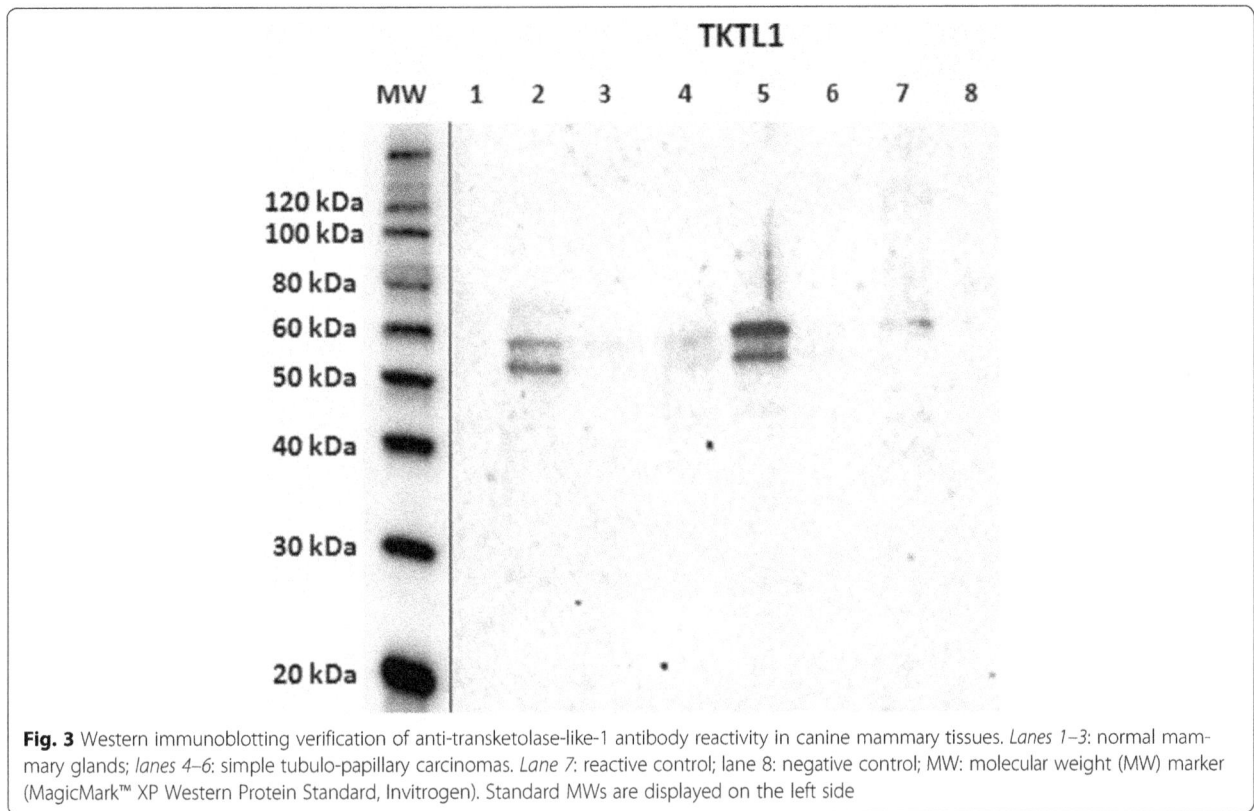

Fig. 3 Western immunoblotting verification of anti-transketolase-like-1 antibody reactivity in canine mammary tissues. *Lanes 1–3*: normal mammary glands; *lanes 4–6*: simple tubulo-papillary carcinomas. *Lane 7*: reactive control; lane 8: negative control; MW: molecular weight (MW) marker (MagicMark™ XP Western Protein Standard, Invitrogen). Standard MWs are displayed on the left side

Furthermore, the increased protein expression in hyperplastic lesions and in both benign and malignant tumors compared to normal mammary gland suggests a significant involvement of the PPP and, consequently a role of TKT during the canine mammary carcinogenesis process. The increased expression of TKT found in mammary tumors and in hyperplastic lesions of the dog appears to be substantially in agreement with those reported in recent studies carried out in human and veterinary medicine, in which there was an increased expression of TKT in cancer tissues and in progestin-induced canine mammary hyperplasia compared to non-tumor tissues, respectively [12, 36, 37].

In addition, our results lead to hypothesize that a pathway that synthesizes antioxidants, the PPP, is necessary to tumor development, particularly in hyperplastic lesions where TKT is an up regulated gene and reaches the highest protein expression values, thus confirming what has been described in the mouse mammary tumor model by Lu and colleagues [36, 38]. In fact, as elegantly proposed by Gatenby and Gilles in 2004, hyperplastic lesions are exposed to a hypoxic environment and acquire the glycolytic phenotype with the production of hydrogen ions (H+); this leads to the consequent acidification of the extracellular space, resulting in cellular toxicity due the increase of ROS [39]. Thus, an increase of PPP down-streaming molecules, such as NADHP, is necessary to counteract and mitigate oxidative stress, especially in hyperplastic lesions.

In this study, simple carcinomas showed a lower expression of TKT when compared to the others lesions, with a significant reduction of the enzyme in the most undifferentiated forms (i.e. simple carcinoma grade III). The underexpression trend of TKT in the more aggressive neoplasm suggests that probably a further molecular pathway exists that limits or inhibits the protein expression in the most aggressive and life-threatening mammary neoplastic histotype. For example, it was revealed that the tumor suppressor p53, often expressed in canine carcinomas, can inhibit the PPP by binding to glucose-6-phosphate dehydrogenase (G6PD), the rate-limiting enzyme in the oxidative branch of the PPP, which ultimately results in decreased transketolase expression [40, 41]. Moreover, additional and more focused studies are needed in order to confirm this hypothesis.

As a partial confirmation of the validity of our results and of the important role played by the TKT in the carcinogenic process, several studies report that the use of transketolase competitive inhibitors, such as oxythiamine, in experimental models significantly reduces the tumor cell proliferation rate [14, 16, 42].

Compelling evidence has proved that TKTL1 is a cancer related molecule and that it plays a key role in the onset of different neoplastic disease. Its overexpression

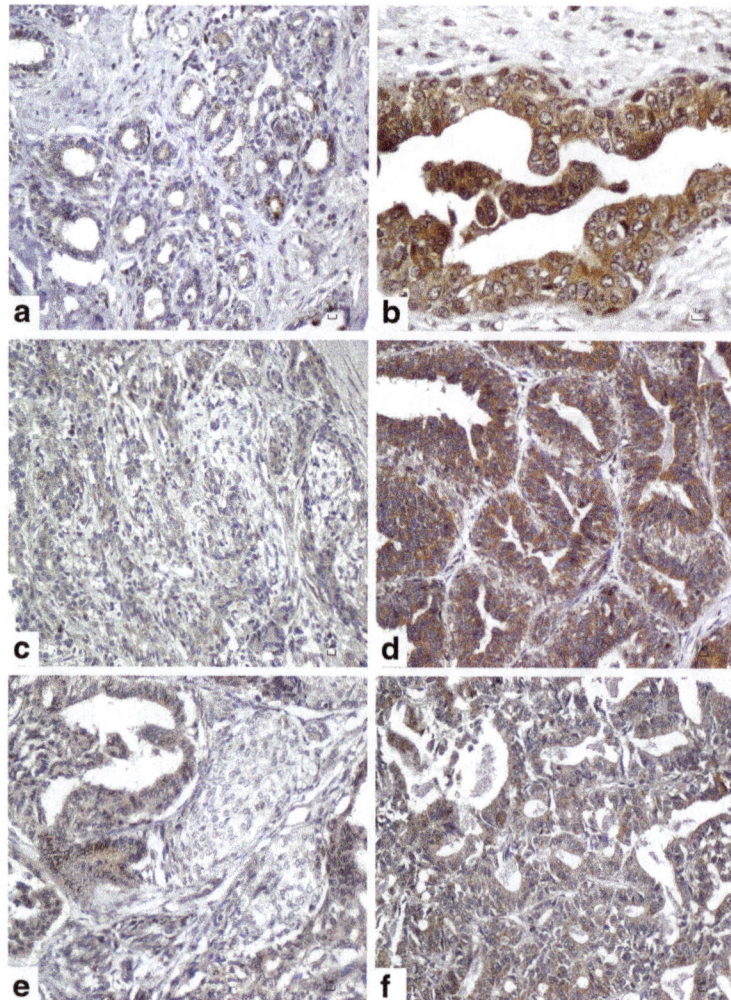

Fig. 4 Transketolase like-1 immunohistochemical expression in canine mammary glands. Cytoplasmic expression in epithelial cells of normal mammary gland (IRS = 1) (**a**), hyperplastic mammary gland (IRS = 12) (**b**), complex adenoma (IRS = 1) (**c**), simple adenoma (IRS = 8) (**d**), complex carcinoma (IRS = 4) (**e**) and simple carcinoma (IRS = 6) (**f**)

predicts poor patient survival, tumor recurrence and resistance to chemo and radiation therapy in many cancers [18–24].

In our work, TKTL1 was expressed in most of the hyperplastic and neoplastic lesions and in 83% of non-neoplastic mammary tissue. Furthermore, the statistical analysis of different histological types showed an increased TKTL1 expression in hyperplastic lesions and in both benign and malignant simple tumors, in agreement with other reports in women breast cancer [18, 43]. However, in contrast to what described by these authors, TKTL1 expression in mammary tissues of the dog showed higher values in hyperplastic lesions and a reduction of the immunoreactivity as the degree of malignancy increased. This indicates that the protein could play a crucial role in the stepwise progression

from early hyperplastic lesions to fully malignant CMT. In fact, hyperplastic lesions have been considered as risk factors for subsequent development of invasive mammary cancer both in human and in canine species [26, 44, 45]. In this perspective, we might speculate that the selective block of TKTL1 through the targeting of PPP metabolic pathway could limit neoplastic development in its early stages represented by hyperplastic and benign tumors, arresting tumor progression in its *"primum movens"*.

In addition, TKTL1 was more expressed in simple canine neoplasms, both benign and malignant, when compared to complex types, suggesting a predominant role of TKTL1 in epithelial cells *vs* the myoepithelial component. Moreover, to our knowledge, no studies have investigated the role of TKT or TKTL1 in myoepithelial cells, both in human and canine tumors, and consequently, definitive and conclusive hypothesis cannot be drawn.

Conclusions

In conclusion, this is the first study investigating the expression of TKT and TKT-like enzymes in canine mammary tumors and hyperplastic lesions. We observed increased expression of TKT and TKTL1 in the proposed multistep carcinogenesis of CMT, thus indicating that PPP is a cancer metabolism-related pathway also in canine mammary tumors. TKTL1 has recently been used as a biomarker in a blood test based on the epitope detection in monocytes (EDIM) technology, allowing for the non-invasive detection of neoplasia and tumor recurrence, and thereby it has been proposed as a therapeutic target [42]. Similar efforts to identify important metabolic changes during canine mammary cancer progression hold the potential for providing putative diagnostic and prognostic biomarkers, as well as new therapeutic targets, also in canine species.

Additional files

> **Additional file 1:** Immunohistochemical evaluation of TKT and TKTL1. Immunoreactivity scores (IRS) of normal mammary glands ($n = 6$), ductal hyperplasias ($n = 3$), benign tumors ($n = 11$), and carcinomas ($n = 17$), considering the number and the stain intensity of positive cells per high power field (HPF). (XLSX 18 kb)
>
> **Additional file 2:** Graphical representation (box-plot) of TKT immunohistochemical evaluation. Immunoreactivity scores (IRS) of normal mammary glands ($n = 6$), ductal hyperplasias ($n = 3$), benign tumors ($n = 11$) and carcinomas ($n = 17$), with statistical differences between lesions. Different letters (a, b, c, d) indicate significant differences ($P < 0.05$), red line (median values), Kruskal-Wallis ANOVA followed by Dunn's post hoc test. (TIF 1566 kb)
>
> **Additional file 3:** Graphical representation (box-plot) of TKTL1 immunohistochemical evaluation. Immunoreactivity scores (IRS) of normal mammary glands ($n = 6$), ductal hyperplasias ($n = 3$), benign tumors ($n = 11$) and carcinomas ($n = 17$), with statistical differences between lesions. Different letters (a, b, c, d) indicate significant differences ($P < 0.05$), red line (median values), Kruskal-Wallis ANOVA followed by Dunn's post hoc test. (TIF 970 kb)

Abbreviations

ATP: Adenosine 5'-triphosphate; BSA: Bovine serum albumin; CMT: Canine mammary tumors; EDIM: Epitope detection in monocytes; G6PD: Glucose-6-phosphate dehydrogenase; H&E: Haematoxylin and eosin; IRS: Immunoreactivity score; PBS: Phosphate-buffered saline; PPP: Pentose phosphate pathway; R5P: Ribose-5-phosphate; ROS: Reactive oxygen species; TKT: Transketolase; TKTL1: Transketolase-like 1; TKTL2: Transketolase-like 2

Acknowledgements

The authors would like to thank Dr. Veronica Vitiello and Dr. Marina Antonella Sanna for their histological support and assistance.

Funding

This work was financially supported by Fondazione Banco di Sardegna Grant Number: RF 851/2010.0153.

Authors' contributions

GPB. designed the study, performed the immunohistochemistry experiment, analyzed the data and drafted the manuscript; AT, TC, MA, MFA carried out immunoblotting and critical revised the manuscript for important intellectual content; MP carried out immunohistochemistry experiment and critical revised the manuscript; EA designed and supervised the study, analyzed the data and drafted the manuscript. All authors read and approved the final manuscript.

Competing interests

The authors declare that they have no competing interests.

Consent for publication

Not applicable

Author details

[1]Department of Veterinary Medicine, University of Sassari, Via Vienna 2, 07100 Sassari, Italy. [2]Porto Conte Ricerche, S.P. 55 Porto Conte/Capo Caccia Km 8.400, Loc, 07041 Tramariglio, Alghero, Italy.

References

1. Lana SE, Rutteman GR, Withrow SJ. Tumors of the mammary gland. In: Withrow SJ, MacEwen EG, editors. Small animal clinical oncology. Philadelphia: Elsevier Saunders; 2007. p. 619–36.
2. Sleeckx N, de Rooster H, Kroeze EJBV, Van Ginneken C, Van Brantegem L. Canine mammary tumours, an overview. Reprod Domest Anim. 2011;46: 1112–31.
3. Klopfleisch R, von Euler H, Sarli G, Pinho SS, Gartner F, Gruber AD. Molecular carcinogenesis of canine mammary tumors: news from an old disease. Vet Pathol. 2011;48:98–116.
4. Visan S, Balacescu O, Berindan-Neagoe I, Catoi C. In vitro comparative models for canine and human breast cancers. Clujul Med. 2016;89:38–49.
5. Matos AJF, Baptista CS, Gartner MF, Rutteman GR. Prognostic studies of canine and feline mammary tumours: the need for standardized procedures. Vet J. 2012;193:24–31.
6. Klopfleisch R, Klose P, Weise C, Bondzio A, Multhaup G, Einspanier R, et al. Proteome of metastatic canine mammary carcinomas similarities to and differences from human breast cancer. J Proteome Res. 2010;9:6380–91.
7. Klose P, Weise C, Bondzio A, Multhaup G, Einspanier R, Gruber AD, et al. Is there a malignant progression associated with a linear change in protein expression levels from normal canine mammary gland to metastatic mammary tumors? J Proteome Res. 2011;10:4405–15.
8. Kycko A, Reichert M. Proteomics in the search for biomarkers of animal cancer. Curr Protein Pept Sci. 2014;15:36–44.
9. Tanca A, Pagnozzi D, Burrai GP, Polinas M, Uzzau S, Antuofermo E, et al. Comparability of differential proteomics data generated from paired archival fresh-frozen and formalin-fixed samples by GeLC-MS/MS and spectral counting. J Proteomics. 2012;77:561–76.
10. Meshalkina LE, Drutsa VL, Koroleva ON, Solovjeva ON, Kochetov GA. Is transketolase-like protein, TKTL1, transketolase? BBA-Mol Basis Dis. 1832; 2013:387–90.
11. Mitschke L, Parthier C, Schroder-Tittmann K, Coy J, Ludtke S, Tittmann K. The crystal structure of human transketolase and new insights into its mode of action. J Biol Chem. 2010;285:31559–70.
12. Xu IM, Lai RK, Lin SH, Tse AP, Chiu DK, Koh HY, et al. Transketolase counteracts oxidative stress to drive cancer development. Proc Natl Acad Sci U S A. 2016;113:E725–34.
13. Zastre JA, Sweet RL, Hanberry BS, Ye S. Linking vitamin B1 with cancer cell metabolism. Cancer Metab. 2013;1:16.
14. Boros LG, Puigjaner J, Cascante M, Lee WNP, Brandes JL, Bassilian S, et al. Oxythiamine and dehydroepiandrosterone inhibit the nonoxidative synthesis of ribose and tumor cell proliferation. Cancer Res. 1997;57:4242–8.

15. Jayachandran A, Lo PH, Chueh AC, Prithviraj P, Molania R, Davalos-Salas M, et al. Transketolase-like 1 ectopic expression is associated with DNA hypomethylation and induces the Warburg effect in melanoma cells. BMC Cancer. 2016;16:134.

16. Wang J, Zhang X, Ma D, Lee WN, Xiao J, Zhao Y, et al. Inhibition of transketolase by oxythiamine altered dynamics of protein signals in pancreatic cancer cells. Exp Hematol Oncol. 2013;2:18.

17. Coy JF, Dubel S, Kioschis P, Thomas K, Micklem G, Delius H, et al. Molecular cloning of tissue-specific transcripts of a transketolase-related gene: Implications for the evolution of new vertebrate genes. Genomics. 1996;32:309–16.

18. Foldi M, Stickeler E, Bau L, Kretz O, Watermann D, Gitsch G, et al. Transketolase protein TKTL1 overexpression: a potential biomarker and therapeutic target in breast cancer. Oncol Rep. 2007;17:841–5.

19. Fritz P, Coy JF, Murdter TE, Ott G, Alscher MD, Friedel G. TKTL-1 expression in lung cancer. Pathol Res Pract. 2012;208:203–9.

20. Krockenberger M, Honig A, Rieger L, Coy JF, Sutterlin M, Kapp M, et al. Transketolase-like 1 expression correlates with subtypes of ovarian cancer and the presence of distant metastases. Int J Gynecol Cancer. 2007;17:101–6.

21. Langbein S, Zerilli M, zur Hausen A, Staiger W, Rensch-Boschert K, Lukan N, et al. Expression of transketolase TKTL1 predicts colon and urothelial cancer patient survival: Warburg effect reinterpreted. Brit J Cancer. 2006;94:578–85.

22. Schultz H, Kahler D, Branscheid D, Vollmer E, Zabel P, Goldmann T. TKTL1 is overexpressed in a large portion of non-small cell lung cancer specimens. Diagn Pathol. 2008;3:35.

23. Staiger WI, Coy JF, Grobholz R, Hofheinz RD, Lukan N, Post S, et al. Expression of the mutated transketolase TKTL1, a molecular marker in gastric cancer. Oncol Rep. 2006;16:657–61.

24. Wu HT, Allie N, Myer L, Govender D. Anaplastic nephroblastomas express transketolase-like enzyme 1. J Clin Pathol. 2009;62:460–3.

25. Misdorp W. Histological classification of mammary tumors of the Dog and the Cat. Washington: Armed Forces Institute of Pathology in cooperation with the American Registry of Pathology and the World Health Organization Collaborating Center for Worldwide Reference on Comparative Oncology; 1999.

26. Antuofermo E, Miller MA, Pirino S, Xie J, Badve S, Mohammed SI. Spontaneous mammary intraepithelial lesions in dogs - a model of breast cancer. Cancer Epidemiol Biomark. 2007;16:2247–56.

27. Mouser P, Miller MA, Antuofermo E, Badve SS, Mohammed SI. Prevalence and classification of spontaneous mammary intraepithelial lesions in dogs without clinical mammary disease. Vet Pathol. 2010;47:275–84.

28. Burrai GP, Tanca A, De Miglio MR, Abbondio M, Pisanu S, Polinas M, et al. Investigation of HER2 expression in canine mammary tumors by antibody-based, transcriptomic and mass spectrometry analysis: is the dog a suitable animal model for human breast cancer? Tumor Biol. 2015;36:9083–91.

29. Pena L, De Andres PJ, Clemente M, Cuesta P, Perez-Alenza MD. Prognostic value of histological grading in noninflammatory canine mammary carcinomas in a prospective study with two-year follow-up: relationship with clinical and histological characteristics. Vet Pathol. 2013;50:94–105.

30. Hanahan D, Weinberg RA. Hallmarks of cancer: the next generation. Cell. 2011;144:646–74.

31. Warburg O. On respiratory impairment in cancer cells. Science. 1956;124: 269–70.

32. Warburg O. On the origin of cancer cells. Science. 1956;123:309–14.

33. Heiden MGV, Cantley LC, Thompson CB. Understanding the Warburg effect: the metabolic requirements of cell proliferation. Science. 2009;324:1029–33.

34. Payen VL, Porporato PE, Baselet B, Sonveaux P. Metabolic changes associated with tumor metastasis, part 1: tumor pH, glycolysis and the pentose phosphate pathway. Cell Mol Life Sci. 2016;73:1333–48.

35. Phan LM, Yeung SC, Lee MH. Cancer metabolic reprogramming: importance, main features, and potentials for precise targeted anti-cancer therapies. Cancer Biol Med. 2014;11:1–19.

36. Rao NA, van Wolferen ME, Gracanin A, Bhatti SF, Krol M, Holstege FC, Mol JA. Gene expression profiles of progestin-induced canine mammary hyperplasia and spontaneous mammary tumors. J Physiol Pharmacol. 2009; 60 Suppl 1:73–84.

37. Lin CC, Chen LC, Tseng VS, Yan JJ, Lai WW, Su WP, et al. Malignant pleural effusion cells show aberrant glucose metabolism gene expression. Eur Respir J. 2011;37:1453–65.

38. Lu X, Bennet B, Mu E, Rabinowitz J, Kang YB. Metabolomic changes accompanying transformation and acquisition of metastatic potential in a syngeneic mouse mammary tumor model. J Biol Chem. 2010;285:9317–21.

39. Gatenby RA, Gillies RJ. Why do cancers have high aerobic glycolysis? Nat Rev Cancer. 2004;4:891–9.

40. Riganti C, Gazzano E, Polimeni M, Aldieri E, Ghigo D. The pentose phosphate pathway: an antioxidant defense and a crossroad in tumor cell fate. Free Radic Biol Med. 2012;53(3):421–36.

41. Dolka I, Krol M, Sapierzynski R. Evaluation of apoptosis-associated protein (Bcl-2, Bax, cleaved caspase-3 and p53) expression in canine mammary tumors: an immunohistochemical and prognostic study. Res Vet Sci. 2016; 105:124–33.

42. Grimm M, Teriete P, Schmitt S, Biegner T, Stenzl A, Hennenlotter J, et al. A biomarker based detection and characterization of carcinomas exploiting two fundamental biophysical mechanisms in mammalian cells. Oncol Res Treat. 2014;37:3–4.

43. Schmidt M, Voelker HU, Kapp M, Krockenberger M, Dietl J, Kammerer U. Glycolytic phenotype in breast cancer: activation of Akt, up-regulation of GLUT1, TKTL1 and down-regulation of M2PK. J Cancer Res Clin Oncol. 2010; 136:219–25.

44. Ellis IO. Intraductal proliferative lesions of the breast: morphology, associated risk and molecular biology. Modern Pathol. 2010;23:S1–7.

45. Pare R, Yang T, Shin JS, Tan PH, Lee CS. Breast cancer precursors: diagnostic issues and current understanding on their pathogenesis. Pathology. 2013;45:209–13.

13

Lymphocytic, cytokine and transcriptomic profiles in peripheral blood of dogs with atopic dermatitis

Alicja Majewska[1]*(iD), Małgorzata Gajewska[1], Kourou Dembele[2], Henryk Maciejewski[3], Adam Prostek[1] and Michał Jank[4]

Abstract

Background: Canine atopic dermatitis (cAD) is a common chronic and pruritic skin disease in dogs. The development of cAD involves complex interactions between environmental antigens, genetic predisposition and a number of disparate cell types. The aim of the present study was to perform comprehensive analyses of peripheral blood of AD dogs in relation to healthy subjects in order to determine the changes which would be characteristic for cAD.

Results: The number of cells in specific subpopulations of lymphocytes was analyzed by flow cytometry, concentration of chosen pro- and anti-inflammatory cytokines (IL-4, IL-10, IL-13, TNF-α, TGF-β1) was determined by ELISA; and microarray analysis was performed on RNA samples isolated from peripheral blood nuclear cells of AD and healthy dogs. The number of Th cells ($CD3^+CD4^+$) in AD and healthy dogs was similar, whereas the percentage of Tc ($CD3^+CD8^+$) and Treg ($CD4^+CD25^+$ $Foxp3^+$) cells increased significantly in AD dogs. Increased concentrations of IL-13 and TNF-α, and decreased levels of IL-10 and TGF-β1 was observed in AD dogs. The level of IL-4 was similar in both groups of animals. Results of the microarray experiment revealed differentially expressed genes involved in transcriptional regulation (e.g., transcription factors: *SMAD2, RORA*) or signal transduction pathways (e.g., *VEGF, SHB21, PROC*) taking part in T lymphocytes lineages differentiation and cytokines synthesis.

Conclusions: Results obtained indicate that $CD8^+$ T cells, beside $CD4^+$ T lymphocytes, contribute to the development of the allergic response. Increased IL-13 concentration in AD dogs suggests that this cytokine may play more important role than IL-4 in mediating changes induced by allergic inflammation. Furthermore, observed increase in Treg cells in parallel with high concentrations of TNF-α and low levels of IL-10 and TGF-β1 in the peripheral blood of AD dogs point at the functional insufficiency of Treg cells in patients with AD.

Keywords: Canine atopic dermatitis, Peripheral blood, Lymphocytes, Cytokines, Microarray

Background

Canine atopic dermatitis (cAD) is a chronic and recurrent inflammatory and pruritic skin disease which affects 10 % of canine population. This disease is one of the most prevalent skin diseases in dogs, with characteristic clinical features most commonly associated with IgE-mediated hypersensitivity to environmental allergens. Its pathogenesis is associated with a complex of interactions between environmental factors, genetic predisposition, defective skin barrier and immunological hyperreactivity [1, 2]. AD develops as a result of defective innate and adaptive immune responses. The inflammatory reaction is caused by biphasic T cell polarization. The initial acute T-helper 2 (Th2) response is characterized by predominant secretion of interleukins: IL-4, IL-5 and IL-13 resulting in recruitment of eosinophils into inflammatory site, and activation of B lymphocytes, which are stimulated to produce IgE. The allergen-specific IgE binding to mast cells causes degranulation of these cells. The secreted inflammatory mediators lead to inflammation. In human AD (hAD) acute phase leads to Th1-driven chronic phase. The activation of Th1 cells causes IFN-γ and IL-2, IL-12 secretion [3]. In dogs only the initial Th2 type response is typically found, and it is difficult to recognize the typical Th1 type response, but rather a mixed Th1-Th2 response is observed [4, 5]. Until recently studies have been focused

* Correspondence: alicja_majewska@sggw.pl
[1]Department of Physiological Sciences, Faculty of Veterinary Medicine, Warsaw University of Life Sciences-SGGW, Warsaw, Poland
Full list of author information is available at the end of the article

on the imbalance of Th1 and Th2 cells, but now in human, as well as veterinary medicine multiple lymphocyte phenotypes are considered to play a role in the immune response during AD. Th9 and Th17 cells control local tissue inflammation secreting proinflammatory cytokines and chemokines [6, 7]. In scientific literature information about the role of $CD8^+$ T cytotoxic (Tc) cells is scarce. Some studies indicate that $CD8^+$ T cells may contribute to development of human AD skin lesion, because they infiltrate to the skin very early, prior other leukocyte subsets [8]. However, Olivry et al. [9] and Sinke et al. [10] reported infiltration of $CD4^+$ and $CD8^+$ T cells in both lesional and non-lesional cAD skin, but $CD4^+$ T cells was predominant in lesional skin. Regulatory T cells (Tregs) are a heterogenic subpopulation of lymphocytes. In humans two main Treg cells subsets are distinguished: naturally occurring thymic selected Tregs characterized by the expression of $CD4^+CD25^+$ $Foxp3^+$ and type -1 IL-10 secreting Tregs (Trl1) induced in the periphery under tolerogenic conditions. Tregs are characterized by the ability to secrete anti-inflammatory cytokines, such as IL-10 and TGF-β, resulting in suppression of allergen induced specific T cells activation, and also suppression of effector cells of allergic inflammation, such as must cells, basophils, and eosinophils, as well as IgE production [7, 11–13]. Although many studies have been exploiting the functions of the subpopulations of Treg cells and their activity, the knowledge is still insufficient and requires further investigation. While a broad array of molecules have been implicated in Treg cell mediated suppression in vitro these pathways remain mostly unexplored in vivo. In the case of human Treg cells it has been shown that they are highly heterogenous and difficult to identify [14]. Moreover, rigorous analyses of the functional properties of these cells have been hindered by the lack of reliable surface markers. Natural Treg cells are arguably the best characterized Treg type in humans. In the case of cAD we know even less.

Cytokines play the major role in development, differentiation and function of cells (lymphocytes, mast cells, dendritic cells, and eosinophils), which take part in the immune response. During allergic inflammation, already secreted and newly synthesized cytokines are released contributing to the pathology observed in allergic diseases. They exert their effects by binding to specific cell surface receptors and inducing the expression of relevant target genes.

Until now research on cAD has been focused on lymphocytes and other leukocytes subsets, as well as cytokines and inflammatory mediators in regard to their contribution to the developing immune response in patients. Some studies aimed to reveal the molecular mechanism of cAD on transcriptomic level [15–17], and the majority of these studies were carried out on the

lesional and non-lesional skin samples, allowing to analyze site directly affected by inflammation. On the other hand use of blood samples as the investigated material gives an overview of organism's reaction on allergen. Furthermore, collection of blood samples is easier and less painful for a dog. Thus, in the present study we aimed to determine a comprehensive picture of the state of organism affected by cAD in order to investigate complex interactions between multiple genes and environmental factors inducing this disease. For this purpose we analyzed the profile of peripheral blood lymphocytes, plasma levels of cytokines and the transcription profile of peripheral blood nuclear cells in AD and clinically healthy dogs.

Methods
Animals
This study complies with national and institutional guidelines on the use of animals in clinical research according to the Polish legal act from January 21st, 2005 (Ustawa o doświadczeniach na zwierzętach z dnia 21 stycznia 2005 r. (Dz. U. z 2005 r. Nr 33, poz. 289 z późn.zm.)), concerning experiments performed on client owned animals. All dogs were patients of Small Animal Clinic at Warsaw University of Life Sciences. Before enrolling a dog into the study an informed consent from its owner was obtained and a high standard of care was adhered to throughout each examination. In the case of AD dogs research was carried out as part of routine veterinary diagnostic procedure. Dogs included in control group were blood donors from *"Milusia"* Veterinary Blood Bank who were submitted to the Small Animal Clinic for routine checkup.

Twenty privately owned dogs of various breeds, with cAD (13 females and seven males) were included in this study. The breeds were: Labrador retriever (3), Golden retriever (2), American Staffordshire terrier (2), Boxer (2), West Highland white terrier, American Bulldog, French Bulldog, Bull Terrier, Small Munsterlander, Dachshund, German shepherd, crossbreeds (3). Their age ranged between 1 and 8 years (mean age: 3.8 years). Eight healthy dogs served as a control group (3 females and 5 males), their age ranging between 3 and 8 years (mean age: 4.6 years). The following breeds were included in control group: American Staffordshire terrier (2), Labrador retriever (2), Bulldog, Great Dane, Staffordshire Bull Terrier, Weimaraner.

cAD diagnosis and sample collection
Diagnosis of cAD was based on compatible history and clinical signs determined using Willemse and Prélaud diagnostic criteria, completed by Favrot criteria as follows: pruritus sine material, indoor lifestyle and the exclusion of other causes of pruritus ongoing for at least one year.

In all dogs with chronic pruritus other causative factors were excluded, i.e.,: skin parasites (Sarcoptic mange, Demodectic mange, flea allergic dermatitis). Bacterial pyoderma and *Malassezia dermatitis* were excluded on the basis of negative results of in vitro culture assays. The role of food antigens as a cause of the skin condition was assessed using elimination diets for 6–8 weeks. Clinical diagnosis of atopic dermatitis was confirmed by serological allergy testing (IDEXX allergic panel test) and intradermal skin testing (Artuvetrin test set, Netherlands). No anti-inflammatory drugs were given for at least 3 weeks prior serological test and intradermal test.

All dogs, which were classified to the investigated group had positive reactions in serological allergy testing and intradermal skin testing. Peripheral blood samples were collected just before the dogs were subjected to intradermal skin test, thus at the stage when clinical signs of AD were visible. Hematological, morphological and biochemical blood tests were conducted on samples of qualified patients. Each dog with AD, as well as the animals included in control group showed morphological parameters of blood within the reference value range.

The blood which was designated to the cytometric or transcriptomic analyses and ELISA tests was collected once, and separated into portions which were then used in particular analyses. The blood samples were collected from client-owned dogs during routine veterinary examinations.

Blood sampling and separation of peripheral blood mononuclear cells (PBMC)

Peripheral blood was collected into EDTA anticoagulant tubes. PBMC were isolated from whole blood by density gradient centrifugation in histopaque-1077 using a protocol provided with ACCUSPIN System-HISTOPAQUE-1077 (Sigma-Aldrich, St. Louis, MO, USA).

Analysis of lymphocyte subpopulations by flow cytometry

The lymphocyte subpopulations were analyzed by flow cytometry (FACS Aria II, BD Bioscience, San Jose, CA, USA). Two commercially available sets of antibodies (Dog T Lymphocyte cocktail and Dog Activated T Lymphocyte Cocktail, BD Pharmingen™, USA) were used to determine the number of T, Th, Tc, activated T cells and B lymphocytes. Dog T Lymphocyte cocktail comprised: APC-conjugated anti-CD3; PE-conjugated anti-CD4 and FITC-conjugated anti-CD8 antibodies. Dog Activated T Lymphocyte cocktail included 3 antibodies, namely: APC-conjugated anti-CD3; FITC-conjugated clone CTL 2.58 generated by using whole cell immunizations of IL-2 dependent feline T cell lines stimulated with PHA and Con A and reacting with dog T cell activation marker; and PE-conjugated LSM 11.425 antibody generated against cells derived from canine peripheral lymph nodes and used as a

prognostic tool in dog B cell lymphoma studies. Freshly isolated PBMC were suspended in 100 μL of phosphate buffered saline (PBS) and 10 μL of appropriate antibodies were added. PBMC were incubated at room temperature for 30 min in dark, next the cells were washed in PBS and analyzed using BD FACSAria™ II flow cytometer (BD Biosciences, USA). Data were collected from 20,000 lymphocytes. The population of lymphocytes was first gated based on morphological characteristics: forward scatter (FSC) and side scatter (SSC) (gate P1). Cells located in gate P1 were then analyzed in regard to their positive staining with appropriate antibodies. Unstained cells were used as negative control. The results of T and B cells were expressed as the percentage of cells within the gating area of lymphocytes (P1) and the results of Th and Tc cells are presented as the percentage of $CD3^+$ cells. The $CD4^+/CD8^+$ ratio was calculated based on the number of lymphocytes expressing $CD3^+CD4^+$ markers vs. the number of cells expressing $CD3^+CD8^+$ markers.

Treg cells analysis by flow cytometry

In order to determine the number of Treg lymphocytes freshly isolated PBMC were first stained for 30 min with antibodies against two surface markers: APC-conjugated anti-CD4 monoclonal antibody (mAb, clone: YKIX302.9; eBioscience, San Diego, CA) and FITC-conjugated anti-canine CD25 mAb (clone: P4A10; eBioscience, San Diego, CA). Appropriate isotypic controls (Rat IgG2a: APC, Mouse IgG1:FITC) were used as negative controls. Then, cells were permeabilized in fixation/permeabilization buffer for 18 h at 4 °C in the dark. After incubation cells were stained intracellularly for Foxp3 for 30 min using cross-reactive, directly conjugated anti-mouse/rat Foxp3 PE mAb (clone: FJK-16 s; eBioscience, San Diego, CA) or isotype control (Rat IgG2a: PE). Fixation and permabilization of cells was performed using a set of buffers (Foxp3/Transcription FactorStaining Buffer Set, eBioscience, San Diego, CA) recommended by the producer for (eBioscience) Foxp3 staining. The stained cells were analyzed using flow cytometry. The population of lymphocytes was first gated on the basis of FSC vs SSC. The percentage of $CD4^+CD25^+Foxp3^+$ (Treg) cells was quantified within the population of lymphocytes positively stained with anti-$CD4^+$ antibody.

Measurement of cytokine concentration in plasma by ELISA

The concentration of cytokines: IL-2, IL-4, IL-10, IL-13, TNF-α TGF-β 1and IFN-γ in plasma were determinated by ELISA. For all cytokines except IFN-γ dog specific tests from USCN Life Science (CLOUD-CLONE CORP., Wuhan, China) were used, and IFN-γ concentration was determined using Canine IFN-gamma Quantikine ELISA Kit (R&D System, Minnesota, USA). The detection limit was 5.6 pg/mL for IL-13, 5.6 pg/mL for IL-4, 5.8 pg/ml for IL-2, 5.9 pg/ml for IL-10, 6.2 pg/ml for TNF-α and TGF-β 1, 60 pg/ml for IFN-γ. ELISAs were performed according to the instructions of the kits producers.

Statistical analyses of the results of flow cytometric and ELISA analyses were performed using GraphPad Prism version 5.00 (GraphPad Software, Inc., USA). Statistical significance was calculated by unpaired t-test. Results with P value ≤ 0.05 were considered significant.

Microarray analysis

Blood samples were collected from AD and healthy dogs into Rneasy Protect Animal Blood Tubes (Qiagen, USA). Total RNA from peripheral blood nuclear cells was isolated using a Rneasy Protect Animal Blood Kit (Qiagen, USA). Additionally, contamination with DNA was eliminated by DNAse I digestion included as an additional step of the isolation protocol. The quantity of RNA was measured by NanoDrop (NanoDrop Technologies, USA). The analysis of final RNA quality and integrity was performed using Agilent 2100 Bioanalyzer (USA) and RNA 6000 Nano Kit (Agilent, Germany). To ensure optimal data quality, only RNA samples with RIN number ≥ 7.8 were included in the analysis.

The analysis of gene expression profile was performed using Canine (V2) Gene Expression Microarray, 4x44K (Agilent Technologies, USA) and Agilent Technologies Reagent Set according to the manufacturer's procedure. RNA Spike In Kit (Agilent Technologies, USA) was used as an internal control, the Low Input Quick Amp Labeling Kit was applied to amplify and label (Cy3 or Cy5) target RNA to generate complementary RNA (cRNA) for oligo-microarrays. Gene Expression Hybridization Kit was used to fragmentation and hybridization and Gene Expression Wash Buffer Kit was used for washing slides after hybridization. Acquisition and analysis of hybridization intensities were performed using Agilent DNA Microarray Scanner G2505C.

The experiment was performed using a common reference design, in which the common reference comprised a pool of equal amounts of RNA from 13 healthy dogs. These dogs did not take part in the experiment. The cRNA of common reference samples were Cy3-labelled and the cRNA of healthy dogs (control group of dogs taking part in experiment) and of AD dogs were labelled with Cy5. Twenty eight two-color microarrays were performed, one for each patient (20 microarrays with samples from AD dogs and eight from healthy dogs). On each microarray 825 ng of each sample of cRNA (Cy3-labelled common reference and Cy5-labelled control or patient) were hybridized.

Signal detection and statistical analysis

After microarray scanning, data were extracted and background subtracted using the standard procedures contained in the Agilent Feature Extraction (FE) Software version 10.7.3.1. FE performs Lowess normalization.

Prior the analysis of differential gene expression, nonspecific filtering was performed. Transcripts without expression were removed. In addition, transcripts whose median of signal in channel R and G (calculated in investigated and control samples) did not exceed 100 were identified and eliminated. This reduced the number of transcript down to 20,188.

The log2-ratio of the sample to common reference signal was calculated and the data were median-centered among all microarrays. The analysis of differential expression was performed using Limma's method (linear methods for microarrays) and R/Bioconductor package. A multiple testing correction was applied using Benjamini and Hochberg False Discovery Rate (FDR). Microarray data were deposited at the Gene Expression Omnibus data repository under the number GSE76119.

To identify signaling pathways and gene function the microarray data was analyzed using Pathway Studio 11 (Ariadne Genomics). This is a database consisting of millions of individually modeled relationships between proteins, genes, complexes, cells, tissues and diseases [18].

Real-time RT-PCR

To verify microarray results, the expression of three genes: *PIAS1* (protein inhibitor of activated STAT,1), *RORA* (RAR-related orphan receptor A) and *SH2B1* (SH2B adaptor protein 1) was analyzed using real-time PCR. The sequences of chosen genes were obtained from Ensembl or NCBI database. Primers were designed using Primer-Blast software (NCBI database) and verified using Oligo Calc: Oligonucleotide Properties Calculator (free software available online, provided by Northwestern University) to exclude sequences showing self-complementarity. To reduce chances of amplifying traces of genomic DNA, the primers were positioned in different exons. The secondary structures of the amplicon were examined using m-fold Web Server (free on-line access). Reference genes: *GAPDH* and *RPS19* were amplified using primer sequences previously published [5, 19, 20]. All primer sequences are listed in Table 1. Total RNA was reverse transcribed to first strand complementary DNA (cDNA) using the High Capacity cDNA Reverse Transcription (Applied Biosystems, USA). All analyses were performed on individual samples of total RNA using SYBR Select Master Mix (Applied Biosystems, USA) on Stratagene Mx3005P Quantitative PCR instrument for RT-PCR, following the manufacturer's protocol. For all genes annealing temperature was 58 °C. The relative expression of the target gene was quantified as mean of triplicate measurements for each biological sample. Results were calculated using the $2^{-\Delta\Delta CT}$ method [21].

Table 1 Primer sequences for real-time PCR verification of microarray result

Gene	Forward primer (5'–3')	Revers primer (5'–3')	NCBI accession number
PIAS1	TGGAGTTGATGGATGCTTGAG	GGACACTGGAGATGCTTGAT	transcript variant X1-X2: XM_005638536.2 5 XM_535524.5
RORA	AAGGCTGCAAGGGCTTTTTC	CTGCGTACAAGCTGTCTCTT	transcript varian X1- X3: XM_014109378.1 XM_535503.6 XM_014117330.1
SH2B1	CGTCCTCACTTTCAACTTCCA	GACACGACATAGCTGACAAGA	transcript variant X1-X8 XM_005621372.2 XM_005621371.2 XM_005621373.2 XM 005621374 XM_014114512.1 XM_014114513.1 XM_014114514.1 XM_014114515.1
GAPDH	GGAGAAAGCTGCCAAATATG	ACCAGGAAATGAGCTTGACA	NM_001003142.1
RPS19	CCTTCCTCAAAAAGTCTGGG	GTTCTCATCGTAGGGAGCAAG	XM_533657.3

Results

Lymphocyte subpopulations in peripheral blood of AD and healthy dogs

The number of cells in specific subpopulations of lymphocytes in peripheral blood of dogs with atopic dermatitis and control group (healthy dogs) was analyzed using flow cytometry, and are presented in Table 2. The mean percentage of lymphocytes was similar in both groups: 45.2 ± 3.3 (AD dogs) and 42.7 ± 6.5 (control). The percentage contribution of T cells ($CD3^+$) and B cells in lymphocytes population was significantly smaller in AD dogs than in control dogs ($P = 0.04$). The number of $CD3^+CD4^+$ cells within the population of T lymphocytes was almost the same in both investigated groups; whereas the percentage of $CD3^+CD8^+$ T cells was significantly higher in AD dogs than in control group ($P = 0.002$). The $CD4^+/CD8^+$ cells ratio was significantly lower ($P = 0.02$) in AD dogs than in control animals. The number of $CD4^+CD25^+$ $Foxp3^+$ Treg cells

Table 2 Percentage of lymphocyte subsets in peripheral blood of dogs with atopic dermatitis and healthy dogs

Lymphocytes subpopulations	% of cells in different subpopulations of white blood cells		
	AD dogs	Control dogs	P value
Lymphocytes	45.2 ± 3.3	42.7 ± 6.5	0.7147
$CD3^+$	$25.67^* \pm 3.02$	35.90 ± 2.65	0.0408
B cells	$3.81^* \pm 0.68$	6.24 ± 0.82	0.0373
$CD3^+ CD4^+$	67.40 ± 2.01	70.70 ± 1.94	0,1866
$CD3^+CD8^+$	$19.56^{**} \pm 0.87$	14.71 ± 1.11	0.0023
$CD4^+/CD8^+$	$3.86^* \pm 0.33$	5.31 ± 0.41	0.0132
$CD4^+CD25^+$ $Foxp3^+$	$1.54^{***} \pm 0.18$	0.48 ± 0.08	<0.0001

The results are expressed as mean percentage of positive cells ± SEM, ratio $CD4^+/CD8^+$ was calculated as the ratio of absolute number of cells within the T lymphocytes population, symbol *represents the level of significance: $P \leq 0.05$, **$P \leq 0.01$, ***$P \leq 0.001$

was increased in AD dogs in comparison to the healthy ones ($P < 0.0001$).

Cytokine profile in peripheral blood of AD and healthy dogs

The level of cytokines in plasma of AD and healthy dogs was determined based on ELISA tests, and the results obtained are presented in Fig. 1. In four out of seven analyzed cytokines significant differences were observed between the two groups of dogs. The level of IL-13 and TNF-α was significantly higher in AD dogs than in controls ($P = 0.02$); whereas L-10 was significantly lower in AD patients ($P = 0.03$). No differences were noted in the case of IL-4. In most patients IFN-γ was undetectable, only in two dogs from each investigated group this cytokine was detected on quite high level. Likewise, cytokine IL-2 was not detected in all patients, and the concentration of this interleukin was lower in AD than in control dogs ($P = 0.05$). It should be noted that IL-2 was detected in 9 out of 20 AD dogs, but the values detected exceeded the detection limit of used ELISA kit (5.8 pg/ml) only in 3 samples. Although no significant difference was noted in the level of TGF-β1 between both groups of animals, there was a tendency towards lower values of concentration of this cytokine in AD dogs ($P = 0.55$). Detailed information about the range of detected levels of cytokines and the number of dogs in which cytokines were detected are presented in Additional file 1: Table S1.

Microarrays analysis

In order to determine possible differences in gene expression in peripheral blood nuclear cells of AD and healthy dogs a microarray analysis was performed. The analysis revealed 139 differentially expressed transcripts between two investigated groups: AD and healthy dogs (FDR-adjuted P value =0.085). Among these 139 differentially expressed transcript only 59 genes have known

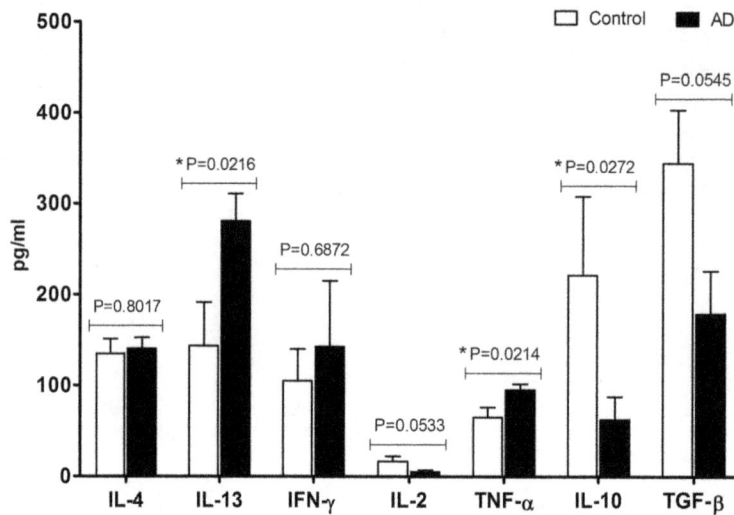

Fig. 1 Concentration of cytokines in plasma of dogs with atopic dermatitis and healthy dogs. Symbol * represents the level of significance: $P \leq 0.05$

ontology (Table 3). Even though none of the listed genes encoded proteins typically involved in the immune response, the transcripts showing differential expression between AD and healthy dogs were directly or indirectly connected with transcriptional regulation (*SMAD2*, *RORA*) or signal transduction pathways (e.g., *VEGF*, *SHB21*, *PROC*) taking part in T lymphocytes lineages differentiation and cytokines synthesis.

Validation of microarray data

To validate the microarray data we selected genes which were shown to be directly or indirectly involved in regulation of T lymphocytes differentiation, and synthesis of investigated cytokines. Thus, we chose to analyze the expression of *PIAS1*, *RORA* and *SH2B1* genes using real-time qPCR. The results obtained confirmed the decreased expression of all tested genes in AD dogs in comparison to healthy animals (Fig. 2).

Discussion

In the present study we aimed to perform comprehensive analyses of peripheral blood of AD dogs in relation to healthy subjects in order to determine the changes which would be characteristic for cAD. Therefore we analyzed the number of cells in specific subpopulations of lymphocytes, determined the concentration of chosen pro- and anti-inflammatory cytokines, and performed a microarray analysis to determine the gene expression profile of peripheral blood nuclear cells in both groups of dogs. Flow cytometric analyses revealed that the percentage contribution of CD3+ T cells and B lymphocytes in AD dogs was significantly lower than in healthy ones, the number of CD3+CD4+ T cells in both groups was similar, and the percentage of CD3+CD8+ lymphocytes

increased significantly in AD dogs. These results did not confirm previously published reports demonstrating that patients with cAD have increased number of both CD3+CD4+ and CD3+CD8+ T cells, since in our study only the subpopulation of Tc lymphocytes was increased. However, the majority of studies on dogs have focused on lymphocytes which infiltrate the atopic skin, showing the pivotal role of Th1 and Th2 cells in the development of skin inflammation. It was demonstrated that in lesional and non-lesional atopic skin the percentage of CD3+, CD4+ and CD8+ cells increased in comparison with the skin of healthy dogs, but the presence of B cells was scarce and detected only in lesional skin [9]. In canine lesional atopic skin, the predominat type of T lymphocytes was CD4+ cells; whereas, in non-lesional atopic skin an infiltration of both CD4+ and CD8+ T-cells was observed, without predominance of CD4+ T cells [9, 10]. Hennino et al. [8, 22] reported that CD8+ cells were essential for the development of AD skin inflammation in both mice and humans. In these studies AD was provoked by the epicutaneos application of house dust mites (HDM). The authors observed recruitment of CD8+ lymphocytes to the *Drematophagoides farine* exposed skin before the infiltration of other leukocytes subsets. Also in lesional skin of dogs with cutaneous adverse food reaction (CAFRs) increased number of CD3+CD4+ and CD3+CD8+ cells was observed in comparison to skin of control dogs. Furthermore, CD3+CD8+ phenotype predominated over CD3+CD4+ phenotype in these patients. The study on murine model indicated dual time-dependent role of CD8+ T cells in development of airway hyperreactivity (AHR) [23]. The authors observed that at early stage the CD8+ T cells protected the organism from systemic sensitization, but when systemic sensitization

Table 3 The list of differentially regulated genes with known ontology in AD vs healthy dogs

GeneSymbol	Description	logFC	Regulation	p-value adj.
NPTXR	neuronal pentraxin receptor	−1,09	down	0,085
CCDC54	coiled-coil domain containing 54	−1,09	down	0,085
UFL1	UFM1-specific ligase 1	−0,76	down	0,085
BBS2	Bardet-Biedl syndrome 2	−0,68	down	0,085
DCUN1D1	defective in cullin neddylation 1, domain containing 1	−0,66	down	0,085
RORA	RAR-related orphan receptor A	−0,66	down	0,085
PKIB	protein kinase (cAMP-dependent, catalytic) inhibitor beta	−0,61	down	0,085
OPN1SW	opsin 1 (cone pigments), short-wave-sensitive	−0,58	down	0,085
FAM49A	family with sequence similarity 49, member A	−0,58	down	0,085
PURA	purine-rich element binding protein A	−0,57	down	0,085
CA14	carbonic anhydrase 14-like (LOC100855809),	−0,54	down	0,085
SCN1B	sodium channel, voltage-gated, type I, beta subunit	−0,53	down	0,085
SCOC	short coiled-coil protein	−0,53	down	0,085
PIWIL4	PIWIL4 piwi-like RNA-mediated gene silencing 4	−0,53	down	0,085
WNT5B	wingless-type MMTV integration site family, member 5B	−0,53	down	0,085
FAM155B	family with sequence similarity 155, member B	−0,52	down	0,085
EPHB3	EPH receptor B3	−0,52	down	0,085
LOC100856122	olfactory receptor 4 K5-like	−0,52	down	0,085
BPIFB1	BPI fold containing family B, member 1	−0,52	down	0,085
TNKS2	tankyrase, TRF1-interacting ankyrin-related ADP-ribose polymerase 2	−0,51	down	0,085
RTN4RL1	reticulon 4 receptor-like 1	−0,51	down	0,085
TTYH2	tweety family member 2	−0,50	down	0,085
AK9	adenylate kinase 9	−0,50	down	0,085
GPR12	G protein-coupled receptor 124	−0,49	down	0,085
PCIA1	cross-immune reaction antigen	−0,49	down	0,085
VEGFA	vascular endothelial growth factor A	−0,49	down	0,085
OTOP1	otopetrin 1	−0,49	down	0,085
TTF2	transcription termination factor, RNA polymerase II	−0,49	down	0,085
FGFBP3	fibroblast growth factor binding protein 3	−0,48	down	0,085
ABHD15	abhydrolase domain containing 15	−0,48	down	0,085
PROC	protein C (inactivator of coagulation factors Va and VIIIa)	−0,47	down	0,085
EM2	transmembrane protein 25	−0,47	down	0,085
EMC1	ER membrane protein complex subunit 1	−0,47	down	0,085
TMEM52	transmembrane protein 52	−0,47	down	0,085
RHOV	ras homolog family member V	−0,47	down	0,085
TEKT1	tektin 1	−0,47	down	0,085
GDPD3	glycerophosphodiester phosphodiesterase domain containing 3	−0,47	down	0,085
ANAPC5	anaphase promoting complex subunit 5 [	−0,47	down	0,085
ABCA4	ATP-binding cassette, sub-family A (ABC1), member 4	−0,46	down	0,085
ZC3H10	zinc finger CCCH-type containing 10	−0,46	down	0,085
SMAD2	SMAD family member 2	−0,46	down	0,085
SSH3	slingshot protein phosphatase 3	−0,46	down	0,085
SH2B1	SH2B adaptor protein 1	−0,45	down	0,085
PIAS1	protein inhibitor of activated STAT, 1	−0,45	down	0,085

Table 3 The list of differentially regulated genes with known ontology in AD vs healthy dogs (Continued)

SUFU	suppressor of fused homolog (Drosophila)	−0,44	down	0,085
ALKBH4	alkB, alkylation repair homolog 4 (E. coli) A	−0,44	down	0,085
NRG2	neuregulin 2	−0,44	down	0,085
TMEM231	transmembrane protein 231	−0,44	down	0,085
OGT	OGT O-linked N-acetylglucosamine (GlcNAc) transferase	−0,44	down	0,085
RBM25	RNA binding motif protein 25	−0,43	down	0,085
SCN2B	sodium channel, voltage-gated, type II, beta subunit	−0,42	down	0,085
PTP4A2	protein tyrosine phosphatase type IVA, member 2	−0,42	down	0,085
PEX26	peroxisomal biogenesis factor 2	−0,41	down	0,085
EIF4ENIF1	eukaryotic translation initiation factor 4E nuclear import factor 1	−0,40	down	0,085
THEMIS	thymocyte selection associated	−0,39	down	0,085
ERLIN1	ER lipid raft associated 1	−0,39	down	0,085
DDX1	DEAD (Asp-Glu-Ala-Asp) box helicase 1	−0,39	down	0,085
PABPC5	poly(A) binding protein, cytoplasmic 5	−0,37	down	0,085
CDT1	chromatin licensing and DNA replication factor 1	−0,34	down	0,085

Log fold change (FC) expressed as log2
p-value adj. was adjusted by multiple testing using the Benjamini-Hochberg False discovery rate procedure (FDR) for each comparison

was established, these cells may play a bystander or proinflamatory role in the development of allergic airway disease [23]. There is only a few reports regarding the subsets of lymphocytes in peripheral blood in atopic dogs. Tarpatakiet al. [24] indicated an increase of CD4+/CD8+ ratio of T lymphocytes in AD dogs in comparison with healthy dogs. In contrast, other studies obtained results which are comparable to our data showing that the percentage of CD4+ T cells did not change in atopic dogs in relation to healthy dogs but percentage of CD8+ T cells significantly increased and as a result ratio of CD4+/CD8+ T lymphocytes in AD dogs decreased [25]. In German shepherd dogs suffering from pyoderma (GSP) the percentage of CD4+ cells decreased, CD8+ cells increased and

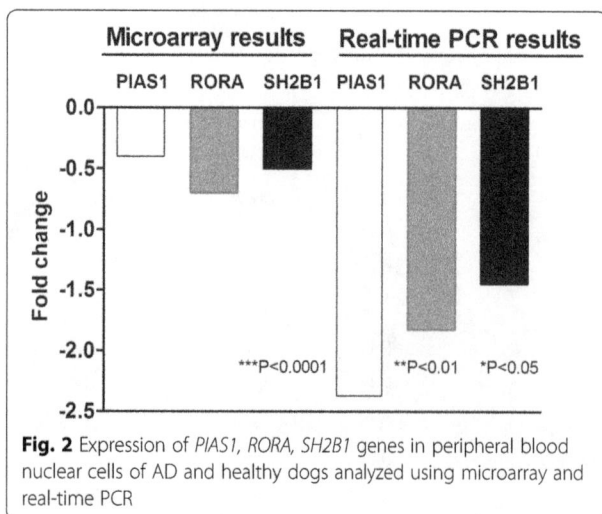

Fig. 2 Expression of PIAS1, RORA, SH2B1 genes in peripheral blood nuclear cells of AD and healthy dogs analyzed using microarray and real-time PCR

ratio CD4+/CD8+ decreased in comparison to healthy dogs [26]. Thus, the results showing a marked increase in CD8+ T cells in peripheral blood of AD dogs suggest that these lymphocytes may play an important role in skin inflammation during AD.

We also observed a significant increase in the percentage of Treg cells in dogs with AD in comparison with healthy controls. Subsets of Treg cells are responsible for healthy immune response to allergens. These cells mediate the peripheral tolerance to allergen suppressing proliferation and activity of effector cells. The population of Treg cells is heterogeneous by the expression of various surface markers and can be subdivided into several subtypes. The most known subset called naturally occurring regulatory T cells (nTreg cells) was defined based on expression of surface CD25 (IL-2Rα) and transcription factor Foxp3. It was demonstrated that in dogs CD4+CD25+ Foxp3+ cells were able to suppress the proliferation of responder CD4+ T cells in vitro [27]. Our study demonstrated that the percentage of circulating CD4+CD25+ Foxp3+ cells in atopic dogs was significantly higher compared to healthy dogs, and these results were similar to recent data of other research groups [28, 29]. On the contrary other investigations have indicated that the Treg cells are not fully efficient in atopic patients in comparison with healthy individuals. In vitro studies on T lymphocytes isolated from human grass allergic donors showed that Treg cells from these donors failed to inhibit proliferation but not cytokine production of CD4+CD25− T cells at high antigen doses, while Treg from non-atopic donors retained their regulatory properties [30]. It is possible, however, that the higher percentage of Tregs detected in AD patients in our study could be related to the chronic nature of the disease [28].

It has been shown that atopic dermatitis is affected by aberrant immune response and that imbalance in the T lymphocytes population and associated cytokine pattern play a crucial role. Cytokines are very powerful messengers, which control regulatory system in all levels: production, secretion, effect on target. During allergic inflammation, preformed and newly synthesized cytokines are released and contribute to the pathological response to allergen. These cytokines have a wide range of activities on different cell types. In our study we determined the plasma level of a few cytokines which take part in development of atopy and maintain the inflammatory state. In the initial acute phase of AD eosinophils and Th2 cells are the predominant subpopulation of immune cells, and increased production of IL-4, IL-5, IL-13 is observed. In chronic AD lesions there is a switch towards Th1 cells secreting IFN-γ and IL-12 and also IL-2. In some studies it was indicated that chronic phase is not characterized only by the presence of Th1 cells but rather by a mixed Th1 and Th2 profile [4, 5]. It results from a dynamic nature of this process.

In our study it is difficult to define the phase of immune response. The pattern of cytokines' concentration in plasma partially indicates the domination of Th-2 cells subpopulation, but the interpretation is not obvious. We noted a significantly higher level of IL-13, and slightly elevated concentration of IL-4 in AD dogs in comparison to healthy controls. Similar results were presented by Schlotter [5], who observed increased expression of IL-13 mRNA in lesional skin and non lesional skin of AD dogs, but an unchanged expression of *IL-4* gene. Increase expression of IL-13 mRNA was also noted in the skin of dogs challenged with house dust mites (HDM) allergen for 24 and 48 h, while the expression of other interleukins secreted by Th-2 cells was low and the level did not change significantly in time [31]. In addition, in humans after HDM allergen challenge secretion of IL-13 to the peripheral blood also occurred earlier and for much longer time than in the case of IL-4 [32, 33]. These results suggest that IL-13 may play more important role in atopic response than IL-4.

In the present study IFN-γ, considered as the "canonical" Th1 cytokine, was detected only in two healthy and two AD dogs. We presume that the level of IFN-γ in plasma may be a characteristic feature of each individual. In fact, among dogs exposed to immunotherapy IFN-γ was detected only in the same two dogs in which this cytokine was detected prior therapy (data not show). Similar observations were made by Hayashiya et al. [34], who detected IFN-γ mRNA expression in PBMC of nine out of ten control dogs and in two out of eight AD dogs,

and the average expression of IFN-γ mRNA was lower in AD dogs. The production of IFN-γ may be related to the stage of development of skin lesions and the type of investigated tissue. In the skin of dogs exposed to epicutaneous allergen challenge IFN-γ mRNA expression was the highest at the early time points post challenge (6 h) and after 4 days, whereas at the intermediate period the expression of this cytokine was at a low level [31]. This observation shows the dynamic nature of IFN-γ induction.

On the other hand, we noted a significantly higher concentration of TNF-α in plasma of atopic dogs then in healthy animals. This result seems to be directly connected with the state of atopic inflammation in investigated AD dogs. TNF-α is a pleiotropic cytokine, which plays a key role in bridging innate and adaptive immunity in chronic inflammatory disease [35]. Excessive secretion of this cytokine is associates with susceptibility to allergies. There are many potential sources of TNF-α: macrophages, T lymphocytes, mast cells, eosinophils and neutrophils [36]. In atopy disease TNF-α is frequently recognized as a cytokine that belongs to the Th1-type profile. TNF-α is non-specific proinflamatory mediator, inducing expression of cell adhesion molecules and eotaxins effecting recruitment of eosinophils, neutrophils, and macrophages to the sites of allergic inflammation. Furthermore, it increases the proliferation of B and T lymphocytes, and is able to induce apoptosis of keratinocytes. Additionally, TNF-α impairs the regulatory activity of natural Treg cells via the TNF-α receptor 2 (TNFR2) signaling pathway to down-modulate Foxp3 expression in allergic asthma [37]. Our results are in agreement with a previous study by Nuttall et al. [4] who observed increased expression of TNF-α mRNA in lesional skin of atopic dogs in comparison to the non-lesional and healthy control tissue.

In contrast to TNF-α concentration the level of IL-2 in plasma of AD dogs was reduced in comparison to healthy group, but the level of this cytokine was generally undetectable in majority of samples. IL-2 is secreted by Th1 cells, and it is a growth factor essential for proliferation, survival and function of both effector T cells (Teffs) and Treg cells [38–40]. Treg cells do not produce IL-2 but this interleukin is required for their activation by regulating Foxp3 expression via signaling transducer and activator of transcription 5 (STAT5) [41–44]. However, Foxp3 represses the expression of *IL-2* and activates expression of *CD25* genes (IL-2 receptor) by binding to the promoter of these genes [42–45]. Tregs also inhibit production of IL-2 in Teffs, and additionally they have a high expression of IL-2 receptors (CD25) which gives them the capacity to compete with Teffs for IL-2 [40, 44, 46, 47]. Research describing the function of IL-2 in the skin of AD dogs demonstrated that the expression of IL-2 mRNA was increased in lesional skin in comparison to non-lesional and and healthy cutaneous tissue [4]. In our study a decrease of IL-2 concentration in blood plasma of AD dogs coincided with increase number of Treg cells in these animals, suggesting the suppressive effect of Treg lymphocytes. However, AD dogs also had lower plasma levels of two anti-inflammatory cytokines: IL-10 and TGF-β1, which is contradictory to the concept of suppressive effect of the immune response. Both of these anti-inflammatory cytokines secreted by Treg cells suppress allergen-induced specific T-cell activation and allergic processes. IL-10 is synthesized by a wide range of cells besides Tregs: Th2 cells, B cells, monocytes, dendritic cells, and mast cells. It inhibits the production of proinflammatory cytokines and cytokine receptors [13, 48]. IL-10 is also a potent suppressor of allergen-specific IgE, simultaneously inducing IgG4 production by a direct influence of Tregs on B-cells. Most studies regarding cAD do not report any differences in plasma concentration of IL-10 between AD and healthy dogs [49], or in the expression of IL-10 mRNA in lesional and non-lesional skin [4], or in circulating PBMCs [34]. However, Maeda et al. [50] observed decreased *IL-10* expression in blood of cAD patients during allergen challenge, which is consistent with our results. TGF-β1 is secreted by Tregs and also similarly to IL-2 it converts naïve T cells to Treg cells by inducing the expression of Foxp3. TGF-β1 together with IL-6 contributes to the generation of Th17 cells [51]. TGF-β1 inhibits the proliferation, differentiation, and survival of both B and T lymphocytes [48]. Membrane-bound TGF-β1 shows unique and potent immunosuppressive activity towards Tregs, associated with direct contact of TGF-β1 with its receptors localized on Treg cell membrane. Upon activation of TGF-β1 receptor type II (TbRII), Treg cells become susceptible to TGF-β1 and demonstrate activation of TGF-β1 - dependent transcription factors (Smads). The Treg membrane-associated TGF-β1 might provide a sustained contact-dependent signal crucial to suppressing effector T cells and mediating cell cycle arrest, and blocking cytokine production. In addition to contact-dependent suppression of TbRII-expressing responder T cells, soluble TGF-β1 shows many direct effects on cells of the immune system, including regulation of macrophage activation, dendritic cell maturation, T-cell proliferation and cytokine generation, and B-cell antibody production [52]. Nevertheless, the role of TGF-β1 in cAD has not been fully elucidated, and the results published so far are often contradictory. Schlotter et al. [5] did not observe any difference in the expression of this cytokine in lesional and non-lesional skin of AD dogs as well as control skin samples. On the other hand Nuttall el al. [4] demonstrated lower expression of TGF-β1 in lesional and non-lesional skin in comparison to control tissue. In blood of patients undergoing allergen challenge the level of TGF-β1 mRNA decreased after four days, which is similar to our

observations [50]. Findings of the present study indicate that despite increased number of Treg cells (CD4$^+$CD25$^+$ Foxp3$^+$) detected in AD dogs the level of anti-inflammatory cytokines produced by these cells was insufficient to protect the organism against the pathological immune response.

In the last stage of our study we performed a microarray analysis in order to compare the transcriptomic profile of peripheral blood nuclear cells in AD and healthy dogs. Even though we did not detect any changes in the mRNA expression level of investigated cytokines, the genes showing differential expression between AD and healthy dogs were directly or indirectly connected with regulation of T lymphocytes lineages differentiation and synthesis, as well as secretion of the aforementioned cytokines. Pathway studio analyses enabled us to find the interactions between the differentially expressed genes and cytokines investigated in the present study (Fig. 3).

Among the differentially expressed genes which showed the highest number of interactions with other genes was *VEGFA* encoding vascular endothelial growth factor (isoform A). VEGF is known to be one of the principle mediators of angiogenesis, fibroblast stimulation and tissue remodeling in allergic conditions. It may also stimulate inflammatory cell recruitment, enhance antigen sensitization and appear crucial for adaptive Th-2 inflammation [53]. A few studies demonstrated the connection between VEGF synthesis and human AD skin lesions [54]. VEGF may play a role in the pathogenesis of AD and be involved in regulation of AD lesions development acting possibly in the persisting erythema and edema by prolonged capillary dilatation and hyperpermeability [54]. Koczy-Baron et al. [55] have shown a significant increase in VEGF plasma levels in human AD patients in comparison to controls. However, these authors did not find any correlation between the plasma levels of VEGF and the number of cells that contribute to the secretion of this growth factor (mast cells, platelets). In our study the expression of *VEGFA* was decreased in peripheral blood nuclear cells of cAD patients. It is worth noting that the difference in *VEGFA* expression was observed despite similar numbers of blood elements (platelets, white blood cells) in both investigated groups of dogs (data not shown). It is possible that the role of VEGF is predominant at the site of inflammation (skin lesions) and blood levels of this growth factor are not a suitable prognostic marker of AD. Similar conclusion was stated in the work of Koczy-Baron et al. [55]. Interestingly, *VEGF* expression is stimulated by TGF-β1-induced signaling pathway, in which Smad2 and Smad3 become activated and form heterocomplexes with Smad4, enabling their translocation to the nucleus and function as transcription

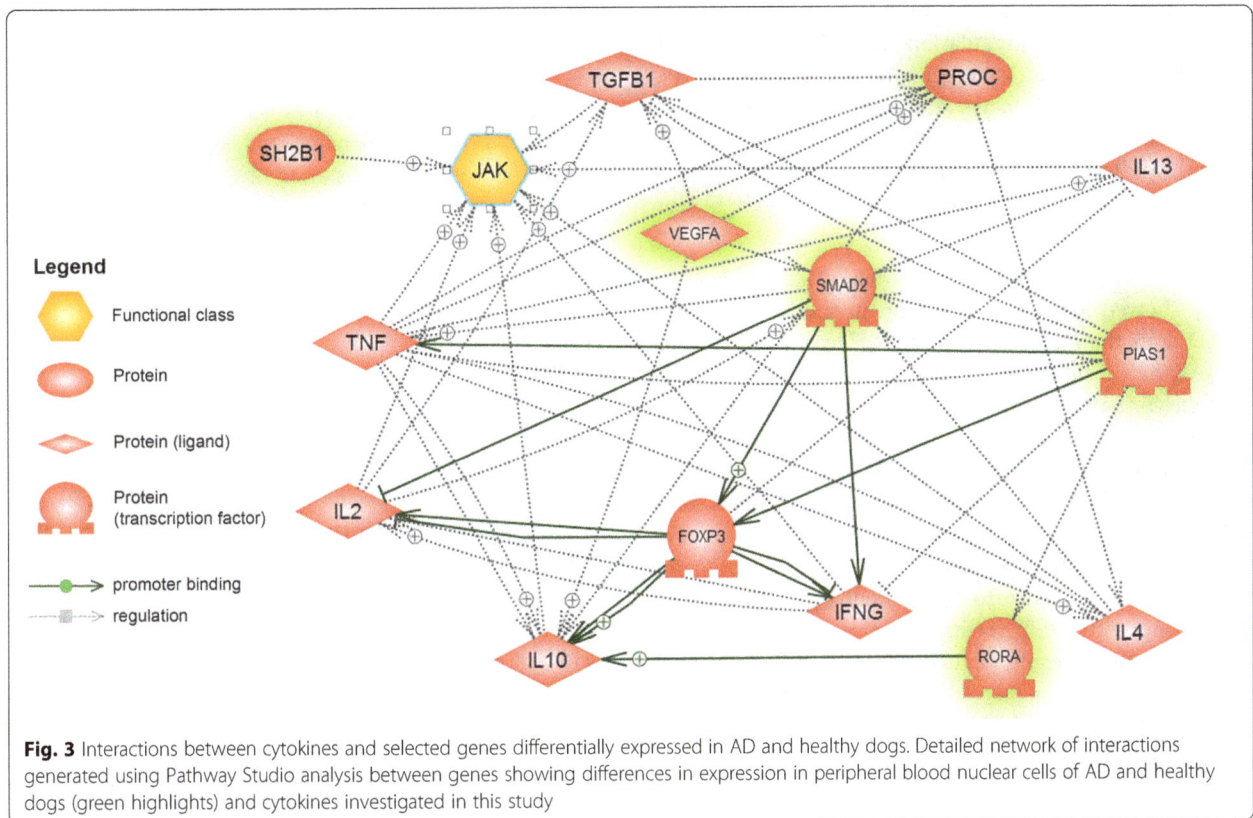

Fig. 3 Interactions between cytokines and selected genes differentially expressed in AD and healthy dogs. Detailed network of interactions generated using Pathway Studio analysis between genes showing differences in expression in peripheral blood nuclear cells of AD and healthy dogs (green highlights) and cytokines investigated in this study

activators [52, 56, 57]. In our study plasma concentration of TGF-β1 did not differ significantly between AD and healthy dogs, whereas *SMAD2* expression was downregulated in cAD patients, correlating with the decreased expression of *VEGF* detected in AD dogs. These results are in agreement with the studies showing direct relationship between the *VEGF* expression and TGF-β1-induced Smad2 signaling [58] (Fig. 3).

PIAS1 (protein inhibitor of activated STAT1) is another gene whose protein product is directly involved in regulation of transcriptional activity of Smad2 function. It has been shown that PIAS1 modulates activation of Smad2/4 complex and further promotes Smad2/4 mediated proliferation inhibition observed in some cancer cells [59]. Thus, downregulation of *SMAD2* expression observed in AD patients may be also connected with decrease levels of *PIAS1* mRNA.

RORα encoded by *RORA* gene was also among transcription factors differentially expressed in dogs with AD in comparison to controls. RORα belongs to a family of retinoid-related orphan receptors (RORs) that regulate gene transcription by binding to specific DNA response elements (ROREs) [60, 61]. RORs can function both as repressors and activators of gene transcription, interacting with corepressors, as well as coactivators of transcription. It has been demonstrated that a direct interaction of Foxp3 and RORα results in repression of RORα -mediated

transcriptional activation [62] (Fig. 3). Studies with the use of stragger (sg/sg) mice, which show a congenital deficiency of the RORα (RORα$^{sg/sg}$), demonstrated that these mice had significantly smaller spleen and the thymus, suggesting that RORα may have a role in regulation of thymopoiesis and lymphocyte development [63]. In fact, the number of mature T and B lymphocytes was significantly reduced in RORα$^{-/-}$spleen, indicating a significant role of RORα in lymphocyte development. It has been shown that Th17 differentiation is dependent on RORs, as RORs induce the expression of *IL-17* cytokine gene [64]. On the other hand, Delerive et al. [65] demonstrated that RORα1 negatively regulated the inflammatory response by interfering with NFkB signaling pathway in primary aortic smooth muscle cells. RORα1 belongs to transcription factors which induce the expression of IkB, the major inhibitory protein of NFkB activity. Since *TNF-α* expression is induced by NFkB signaling pathway, RORα1 actions contribute to attenuation of TNF-α-induced inflammatory response [65]. In our study the plasma concentration of TNF-α significantly increased, whereas *RORA* expression was downregulated in AD dogs. Furthermore, it has been recently reported that RORα is involved in transactivation of IL-10 promoter boosting the generation of protective Tr1 cells [66]. Our results relate to these recent findings, demonstrating that decreased concentration of IL-10 in dogs with AD coincided with downregulation of *RORA* expression.

Increased levels of TNF-α in AD dogs may also be connected with downregulation of *PROC* gene, which codes for protein C, a zymogen whose active form (APC – activated protein C) plays an important role in regulating anticoagulation, inflammation and cell death [67]. Several studies have demonstrated that TNF-α inhibits activation of protein C, thereby affecting the coagulation process [68–70].

Among the investigated cytokines IL-2, IL-10 and INF-γ showed lower concentration in the blood plasma of AD dogs than in healthy animals. These cytokines act via JAK/STAT signaling pathway, in which SH2B1 (SH2 domain-containing protein) protein is recognized to play a role of a potent activator of JAK2 kinase [71]. Upon ligand binding to cytokine receptors, JAKs phosphorylate themselves and their associated receptors, thereby providing multiple binding sites for signaling proteins containing SH2 or other phosphotyrosine-binding domains [72]. SH2B1 was shown to be a potent activator of JAK2 associating with JAK2 via its SH2 domain, and thereby increasing the phosphorylation of JAK2 and its downstream targets belonging to the family of STAT transcription fatcors [71, 72]. Downregulation of *SH2B1* gene expression detected in dogs with AD can be connected with the decreased levels of cytokines, which act as ligands activating the JAK/STAT signaling pathway in the immune cells of peripheral blood.

Results of the presented microarray experiment, analyzing the transcriptomic profile of peripheral blood nuclear cells in AD and healthy dogs, are not in direct correlation with the previously published studies comparing the profiles of gene expression in biopsies of lesional skin of cAD patients and normal skin samples derived from healthy dogs [15–17]. It is evident that more pronounced differences in gene expression were recognized in the cutaneous tissue, which is the direct site of inflammatory processes occurring in AD. Authors of the aforementioned studies observed increased expression of genes involved in inflammation, wound healing, immune response [15, 17], associated with alternatively activated monocyte-derived cells, IL-1 and interferon signaling pathways [16], as well as playing a role in apoptosis, barrier formation and transcriptional regulation [15]. All genes identified in our study were downregulated in AD dogs, and the protein products of differentially expressed mRNAs are involved in transcriptional regulation (transcritipon factors: Smad2, RORα) or signal transduction (VEGF, SHB21, protein C). Juxtaposing the data obtained in the present study with results published previously suggests that transcriptomic profile of peripheral blood nuclear cells does not fully reflect the inflammatory processes which are primarily induced in the cutaneous tissue. Most probably it is caused by recruitment of the activated immune cells to the site of inflammation, thus the significant changes in gene expression will be noted especially in the lesional skin. Nevertheless, obtaining biopsies from dogs with severe AD symptoms is often problematic, and blood samples are still regarded as the valuable source of information about the state of the organism. Thus, further investigation should be done to evaluate the role of detected genes in canine atopic dermatitis.

Conclusions

In the present study dogs with atopic dermatitis showed increased number of CD8+ T cells in peripheral blood, which may suggest that in addition to the commonly accepted role of the imbalance between Th1 and Th2 cells in the immune response during AD, Tc lymphocytes may also significantly contribute to the development of the immunoinflammatory response. Furthermore, observed increase in IL-13 concentration in the blood plasma of AD dogs in comparison to healthy animals, and an insignificant difference in the level of IL-4 between healthy and atopic individuals, support the hypothesis about the role of IL-13 as a more important mediator of the physiological changes induced by allergic inflammation. High concentrations of TNF-α detected in plasma of atopic dogs additionally confirmed the ongoing allergic inflammatory response in cAD patients. Although the number of detected Treg cells was higher in AD dogs than in healthy controls, the increased levels of TNF-α indicates the functional insufficiency of Treg cells in patients with AD, which may also explain the observed lower concentrations of IL-10 and TGF-β1 in the plasma of atopic dogs. Finally, microarray analysis of the difference in transcriptomic profile of peripheral blood nuclear cells of AD and healthy dogs revealed 59 genes downregulated in AD dogs. The list of differentially expressed genes did not include any cytokines taking part in allergic inflammation; however the function of identified genes was directly or indirectly connected with regulation of T lymphocytes lineages differentiation and synthesis, as well as secretion of the aforementioned cytokines.

Observed changes in the levels of chosen cytokines (especially IL-13) and the number of immune cells (e.g., CD8+ lymphocytes and Tregs) in peripheral blood of AD dogs encourage further investigations of possible correlations between cytokines profiles and particular stage of atopic dermatitis development. Such studies utilizing larger number of dogs may reveal potential blood markers helpful in AD diagnosis and determining adequate treatment of this disease.

Acknowledgements
None.

Funding
This project was funded by a grant no.: N N308 575940 from the National Science Centre, Poland. Publication of this article was funded by KNOW (Leading National Research Centre) Scientific Consortium "Healthy Animal - Safe Food", decision of Ministry of Science and Higher Education No. 05-1/KNOW2/2015.

Authors' contributions
AM: conception and design of the study, collection of research material, participation in all experiments conducted, analysis and interpretation of all data, manuscript preparation, figure preparation; MG: flow cytometric analyses and data interpretation, manuscript preparation; KD: responsible for the clinical part of the study: classification of patients; samples' collection; HM: statistical analyses of microarray data; AP: participation in ELISA analyses; MJ: participation in microarray experiment design; manuscript revision. The authors have read and approved the final version of the manuscript.

Competing interests
The authors declare that they have no competing interests.

Consent for publication
Not applicable

Author details
[1]Department of Physiological Sciences, Faculty of Veterinary Medicine, Warsaw University of Life Sciences-SGGW, Warsaw, Poland. [2]Department of Small Animal Diseases with Clinic, Faculty of Veterinary Medicine, Warsaw University of Life Sciences-SGGW, Warsaw, Poland. [3]Department of Computer Engineering, Wroclaw University of Technology, Wrocław, Poland. [4]Veterinary Institute, Faculty of Veterinary Medicine and Animal Sciences, Poznań University of Life Sciences, Poznań, Poland.

References
1. Olivry T, DeBoer DJ, Griffin CE, Halliwell RE, Hill PB, Hillier A, et al. The ACVD task force on canine atopic dermatitis: forewords and lexicon. Vet Immunol Immunopathol. 2001;81(3-4):143–6.
2. Marsélla R, Olivry T, Carlotti DN, International Task Force on Canine Atopic Dermatitis. Current evidence of skin barrier dysfunction in human and canine atopic dermatitis. Vet Dermatol. 2011;22(3):239–48.
3. Bieber T. Atopic dermatitis. N Engl J Med. 2008;358:1483–94.
4. Nuttall TJ, Knight PA, McAleese SM, Lamb JR, Hill PB. Expression of Th1, Th2 and immunosuppressive cytokine gene transcripts in canine atopic dermatitis. Clin Exp Allergy. 2002;32(5):789–95.
5. Schlotter YM, Rutten VP, Riemers FM, Knol EF, Willemse T. Lesional skin in atopic dogs shows a mixed Type-1 and Type-2 immune responsiveness. Vet Immunol Immunopathol. 2011;143(1-2):20–6. doi:10.1016/j.vetimm.2011.05.025.
6. Martinez GJ, Nurieva RI, Yang XO, Dong C. Regulation and function of proinflammatory TH17 cells. Ann N Y Acad Sci. 2008;1143:188–211.
7. Jutel M, Akdis CA. T-cell subset regulation in atopy. Curr Allergy Asthma Rep. 2011;11(2):139–45.
8. Hennino A, Jean-Decoster C, Giordano-Labadie F, Debeer S, Vanbervliet B, Rozières A, Schmitt AM, Nicolas JF. CD8+ T cells are recruited early to allergen exposure sites in atopy patch test reactions in human atopic dermatitis. J Allergy Clin Immunol. 2011;127(4):1064–7. doi:10.1016/j.jaci.2010.11.022.
9. Olivry T, Naydan DK, Moore PF. Characterization of the cutaneous inflammatory infiltrate in canine atopic dermatitis. Am J Dermatopathol. 1997;19:477–86.
10. Sinke JD, Thepen T, Bihari IC, Rutten VP, Willemse T. Immunophenotyping of skininfiltrating T-cell subsets in dogs with atopic dermatitis. Vet Immunol Immunopathol. 1997;57:13–23.
11. Akdis M, Blaser K, Akdis CA. T regulatory cells in allergy: novel concepts in the pathogenesis, prevention, and treatment of allergic diseases. J Allergy Clin Immunol. 2005;116(5):961–8.
12. Palomares O, Yaman G, Azkur AK, Akkoc T, Akdis M, Akdis CA. Role of Treg in immune regulation of allergic diseases. Eur J Immunol. 2010;40(5):1232–40.
13. Fujita H, Soyka MB, Akdis M, Akdis CA. Mechanisms of allergen-specific immunotherapy. Clin Transl Allergy. 2012;2(1):2. doi:10.1186/2045-7022-2-2.
14. Wisniewski J, Agrawal R, Woodfolk JA. Mechanisms of tolerance induction in allergic disease: integrating current and emerging concepts. Clin Exp Allergy. 2013;43(2):164–76.
15. Merryman-Simpson AE, Wood SH, Fretwell N, Jones PG, McLaren WM, McEwan NA, et al. Gene (mRNA) expression in canine atopic dermatitis: microarray analysis. Vet Dermatol. 2008;19(2):59–66.
16. Plager DA, Torres SM, Koch SN, Kita H. Gene transcription abnormalities in canine atopic dermatitis and related human eosinophilic allergic diseases. Vet Immunol Immunopathol. 2012;149(1-2):136–42.
17. Schamber P, Schwab-Richards R, Bauersachs S, Mueller RS. Gene expression in the skin of dogs sensitized to the house dust mite Dermatophagoides farinae. G3 (Bethesda). 2014;4(10):1787–95.
18. Nikitin A, Egorov S, Daraselia N, Mazo I. Pathway studio–the analysis and navigation of molecular networks. Bioinformatics. 2003;19(16):2155–7.
19. Schmitz S, Garden OA, Werling D, Allenspach K. Gene expression of selected signature cytokines of T cell subsets in duodenal tissues of dogs with and without inflammatory bowel disease. Vet Immunol Immunopathol. 2012;146(1):87–91.
20. Brinkhof B, Spee B, Rothuizen J, Penning LC. Development and evaluation of canine reference genes for accurate quantification of gene expression. Anal Biochem. 2006;356(1):36–43.
21. Livak KJ, Schmittgen TD. Analysis of relative gene expression data using real-time quantitative PCR and the 2(-Delta Delta C(T)) Method. Methods. 2001;25(4):402–8.
22. Hennino A, Vocanson M, Toussaint Y, et al. Skin-infiltrating CD8 T cells initiate atopic dermatitis lesions. J Immunol. 2007;178:5571–7.
23. Stock P, Kallinich T, Akbari O, Quarcoo D, Gerhold K, Wahn U, Umetsu DT, et al. CD8(+) T cells regulate immune responses in a murine model of allergen-induced sensitization and airway inflammation. Eur J Immunol. 2004;34(7):1817–27.
24. Tarpataki N, Terenyi M, Nagy SZ. Changes in the CD4/CD8-positive T lymphocyte ratio in the blood of atopic and non-atopic dogs. Special Issue: 7th World Congress of Veterinary Dermatology, July 24–28, 2012, Vancouver, Canada July 2012. Vet Dermatol. 2012;23 Suppl 1:58. doi:10.1111/j.1365-3164.2012.01059.x. abstract.
25. Taszkun I. Expression of CD3, CD4, CD8, CD21, and MHC II lymphocyte antigens and serum IL-10 concentration in dogs with atopic dermatitis complicated by purulent dermatitis. Bull Vet Inst Pulawy. 2013;7:365–70.
26. Chabanne L, Marchal T, Denerolle P, Magnol JP, Fournel C, Monier JC, Rigal D. Lymphocyte subset abnormalities in German shepherd dog pyoderma (GSP). Vet Immunol Immunopathol. 1995;49:189–98.
27. Pinheiro D, Singh Y, Grant CR, Appleton RC, Sacchini F, Walker KR, et al. Phenotypic and functional characterization of a CD4(+) CD25(high) FOXP3(high) regulatory T-cell population in the dog. Immunology. 2011;132(1):111–22.
28. Hauck V, Hügli P, Meli ML, Rostaher A, Fischer N, Hofmann-Lehmann R, Favrot C. Increased numbers of FoxP3-expressing CD4+ CD25+ regulatory T cells in peripheral blood from dogs with atopic dermatitis and its correlation with disease severity. Vet Dermatol. 2016;27(1):26–e9. doi:10.1111/vde.12279.
29. Beccati M, Martini V, Comazzi S, Fanton N, Cornegliani L. Lymphocyte subpopulations and Treg cells in dogs with atopic dermatitis receiving ciclosporin therapy: a prospective study. Vet Dermatol. 2016;27(1):17–e5. doi:10.1111/vde.12277.
30. Bellinghausen I, König B, Böttcher I, Knop J, Saloga J. Regulatory activity of human CD4 CD25 T cells depends on allergen concentration, type of allergen and atopy status of the donor. Immunology. 2005;116(1):103–11.
31. Marsella R, Olivry T, Maeda S. Cellular and cytokine kinetics after epicutaneous allergen challenge (atopy patch testing) with house dust mites in high-IgE beagles. Vet Dermatol. 2006;17(2):111–20.
32. Wakugawa M, Hayashi K, Nakamura K, Tamaki KJ. Evaluation of mite allergen-induced Th1 and Th2 cytokine secretion of peripheral blood mononuclear cells from atopic dermatitis patients: association between IL-13 and mite-specific IgE levels. Dermatol Sci. 2001;25(2):116–26.

33. La Grutta S, Richiusa P, Pizzolanti G, Mattina A, Pajno GB, Citarrella R, et al. CD4(+)IL-13(+) cells in peripheral blood well correlates with the severity of atopic dermatitis in children. Allergy. 2005;60(3):391–5.

34. Hayashiya S, Tani K, Morimoto M, Hayashi T, Hayasaki M, Nomura T, Une S, et al. Expression of T helper 1 and T helper 2 cytokine mRNAs in freshly isolated peripheral blood mononuclear cells from dogs with atopic dermatitis. J Vet Med A Physiol Pathol Clin Med. 2002;49(1):27–31.

35. Pasparakis M, Alexopoulou L, Episkopou V, Kollias G. Immune and inflammatory responses in TNF alpha-deficient mice: a critical requirement for TNF alpha in the formation of primary B cell follicles, follicular dendritic cell networks and germinal centers, and in the maturation of the humoral immune response. J Exp Med. 1996;184(4):1397–411.

36. Stanley AC, Lacy P. Pathways for cytokine secretion. Physiology (Bethesda). 2010;25(4):218–29.

37. Lin YL, Shieh CC, Wang JY. The functional insufficiency of human CD4 + CD25 high T-regulatory cells in allergic asthma is subjected to TNF-alpha modulation. Allergy. 2008;63(1):67–74.

38. Fontenot JD, Rasmussen JP, Williams LM, Dooley JL, Farr AG, Rudensky AY. Regulatory T cell lineage specifica-tion by the forkhead transcription factor foxp3. Immunity. 2005;22:329–41.

39. Turka LA, Walsh PT. IL-2 signaling and CD4+ CD25+ Foxp3+ regulatory T cells. Front Biosci. 2008;1(13):1440–6.

40. Nandakumar S, Miller CW, Kumaraguru U. T regulatory cells: an overview and intervention techniques to modulate allergy outcome. Clin Mol Allergy. 2009;7:5. doi:10.1186/1476-7961-7-5.

41. Zorn E, Nelson EA, Mohseni M, Porcheray F, Kim H, Litsa D, Bellucci R, Raderschall E, Canning C, Soiffer RJ, Frank DA, Ritz J. IL-2 regulates FOXP3 expression in human CD4 + CD25+ regulatory T cells through a STAT-dependent mechanism and induces the expansion of these cells in vivo. Blood. 2006;108(5):1571–9.

42. Burchill MA, Yang J, Vogtenhuber C, Blazar BR, Farrar MA. IL-2 receptor beta-dependent STAT5 activation is required for the development of Foxp3+ regulatory T cells. J Immunol. 2007;178:280.

43. Yao Z, Kanno Y, Kerenyi M, Stephens G, Durant L, Watford WT, et al. Nonredundant roles for Stat5a/b in directly regulating Foxp3. Blood. 2007;109:4368–75.

44. Sakaguchi S, Wing K, Onishi Y, Prieto-Martin P, Yamaguchi T. Regulatory T cells: how do they suppress immune responses? Int Immunol. 2009;21(10):1105–11.

45. Xie X, Stubbington MJ, Nissen JK, Andersen KG, Hebenstreit D, Teichmann SA, Betz AG. The Regulatory T Cell Lineage Factor Foxp3 Regulates Gene Expression through Several Distinct Mechanisms Mostly Independent of Direct DNA Binding. PLoS Genet. 2015;11(6):e1005251. doi:10.1371/journal.pgen.1005251. eCollection 2015.

46. Shevach EM. Mechanisms of Foxp3+ T regulatory cell-mediated suppression. Immunity. 2009;30(5):636–45.

47. Moon BI, Kim TH, Seoh JY. Functional Modulation of Regulatory T Cells by IL-2. PLoS One. 2015;10(11):e0141864. doi:10.1371/journal.pone.0141864.

48. Akdis M, Akdis CA. Mechanisms of allergen-specific immunotherapy: multiple suppressor factors at work in immune tolerance to allergens. J Allergy Clin Immunol. 2014;133(3):621–31.

49. Keppel KE, Campbell KL, Zuckermann FA, Greeley EA, Schaeffer DJ, Husmann RJ. Quantitation of canine regulatory T cell populations, serum interleukin-10 and allergen-specific IgE concentrations in healthy control dogs and canine atopic dermatitis patients receiving allergen-specific immunotherapy. Vet Immunol Immunopathol. 2008;123(3-4):337–44.

50. Maeda S, Tsuchida H, Marsella R. Allergen challenge decreases mRNA expression of regulatory cytokines in whole blood of high-IgE beagles. Vet Dermatol. 2007;18(6):422–6.

51. Zheng SG, Wang J, Horwitz DA. Cutting edge: Foxp3 + CD4 + CD25+ regulatory T cells induced by IL-2 and TGF-beta are resistant to Th17 conversion by IL-6. J Immunol. 2008;180:7112–6.

52. Wahl SM, Vázquez N, Chen W. Regulatory T cells and transcription factors: gatekeepers in allergic inflammation. Curr Opin Immunol. 2004;16(6):768–74.

53. Lee CG, Link H, Baluk P, Homer RJ, Chapoval S, Bhandari V, et al. Vascular endothelial growth factor (VEGF) induces remodeling and enhances TH2-mediated sensitization and inflammation in the lung. Nat Med. 2004;10(10):1095–103.

54. Zhang Y, Matsuo H, Morita E. Increased production of vascular endothelial growth factor in the lesions of atopic dermatitis. Arch Dermatol Res. 2006;297:425–9.

55. Koczy-Baron E, Jochem J, Kasperska-Zajac A. Increased plasma concentration of vascular endothelial growth factor in patients with atopic dermatitis and its relation to disease severity and platelet activation. Inflamm Res. 2012;61(12):1405–9.

56. Chen W, Wahl SM. TGF-beta: the missing link in CD4 + CD25+ regulatory T cell-mediated immunosuppression. Cytokine Growth Factor Rev. 2003;14(2):85–9.

57. Nakamura K, Kitani A, Fuss I, Pedersen A, Harada N, Nawata H, Strober W. TGF-beta 1 plays an important role in the mechanism of CD4 + CD25+ regulatory T cell activity in both humans and mice. J Immunol. 2004;172(2):834–42.

58. Aki S, Yoshioka K, Okamoto Y, Takuwa N, Takuwa Y. Phosphatidylinositol 3-kinase class II α-isoform PI3K-C2α is required for transforming growth factor β-induced Smad signaling in endothelial cells. J Biol Chem. 2015;290(10):6086–105.

59. Yang N, Zhao B, Rasul A, Qin H, Li J, Li X. PIAS1-modulated Smad2/4 complex activation is involved in zinc-induced cancer cell apoptosis. Cell Death Dis. 2013;4:e811. doi:10.1038/cddis.2013.33.

60. Giguere V, Tini M, Flock G, Ong E, Evans RM, Otulakowski G. Isoform-specific amino-terminal domains dictate DNA-binding properties of ROR α, a novel family of orphan hormone nuclear receptors. Genes Dev. 1994;8:538–53.

61. Jetten AM. Retinoid-related orphan receptors (RORs): critical roles in development, immunity, circadian rhythm, and cellular metabolism. Nucl Recept Signal. 2009;7:e003. doi:10.1621/nrs.07003.

62. Du J, Huang C, Zhou B, Ziegler SF. Isoform-specific inhibition of ROR alpha-mediated transcriptional activation by human FOXP3. J Immunol. 2008;180(7):4785–92.

63. Dzhagalov I, Giguère V, He YW. Lymphocyte development and function in the absence of retinoic acid-related orphan receptor alpha. J Immunol. 2004;173(5):2952–9.

64. Yang L, Anderson DE, Baecher-Allan C, Hastings WD, Bettelli E, Oukka M, et al. IL-21 and TGF-beta are required for differentiation of human T(H)17 cells. Nature. 2008;454(7202):350–2. doi:10.1038/nature07021.

65. Delerive P, Monté D, Dubois G, Trottein F, Fruchart-Najib J, Mariani J, Fruchart JC, Staels B. The orphan nuclear receptor ROR alpha is a negative regulator of the inflammatory response. EMBO Rep. 2001;2(1):42–8.

66. Farez MF, Mascanfroni ID, Méndez-Huergo SP, Yeste A, Murugaiyan G, Garo LP, et al. Melatonin Contributes to the Seasonality of Multiple Sclerosis Relapses. Cell. 2015;162(6):1338–52.

67. Mosnier LO, Zlokovic BV, Griffin JH. The cytoprotective protein C pathway. Blood. 2007;109(8):3161–72.

68. Wang L, Bastarache JA, Wickersham N, Fang X, Matthay MA, Ware LB. Novel role of the human alveolar epithelium in regulating intra-alveolar coagulation. Am J Respir Cell Mol Biol. 2007;36(4):497–503. doi:10.1165/rcmb.2005-0425OC.

69. Moxon CA, Heyderman RS, Wassmer SC. Dysregulation of coagulation in cerebral malaria. Mol Biochem Parasitol. 2009;166(2):99–108.

70. Beinsberger J, Heemskerk JW, Cosemans JM. Chronic arthritis and cardiovascular disease: altered blood parameters give rise to a prothrombotic propensity. Semin Arthritis Rheum. 2014;44(3):345–52. doi:10.1016/j.semarthrit.2014.06.006.

71. Rui L, Carter-Su C. Identification of SH2-bbeta as a potent cytoplasmic activator of the tyrosine kinase Janus kinase 2. Proc Natl Acad Sci U S A. 1999;96(13):7172–7.

72. O'Brien KB, O'Shea JJ, Carter-Su C. SH2-B family members differentially regulate JAK family tyrosine kinases. J Biol Chem. 2002;277(10):8673–81.

14

Ki-67 protein expression and tumor associated inflammatory cells (macrophages and mast cells) in canine colorectal carcinoma

M. Woldemeskel*⒤, I. Hawkins and L. Whittington

Abstract

Background: Ki67 index, tumor associated macrophages (TAMs) and mast cells (MCs) are associated with malignancies in animal and human neoplasms including colorectal carcinomas (CRC). This has not been assessed in canine CRC. Given similar genetic abnormalities between human and canine CRC, we assessed Ki-67 and mitotic indices, TAMs and MC count (MCC) in canine CRC ($n = 17$). TAMs and MCC were compared with those in adenomas ($n = 13$) and control ($n = 9$).

Results: Ki-67 index in CRC (17.13 ± 11.50) was strongly correlated ($r = 0.98$, $p < 0.05$) with mitotic index (3.52 ± 1.80). MCC was higher ($p < 0.05$) in CRC (6.30 ± 3.98) than in adenomas (0.78 ± 0.77) and control (0.35 ± 0.33). The results suggest that Ki-67 index and MCC are associated with malignancy in canine CRC. Higher average TAMs were counted in adenomas (21.30 ± 20.70) and in CRC (11.00 ± 9.82) than in the control (7.69 ± 7.26), although the differences were not significant ($p > 0.05$).

Conclusion: Ki-67 index, TAMs and MCC in canine CRC were recorded for the first time in this study. Ki-67 index and MCC are associated with malignancy in canine CRC. Quantitative assessment of MCs and Ki-67 coupled with mitotic index and other clinical parameters may help in evaluating malignancy in canine CRC. TAMs likely play a role in the development of canine colorectal tumors. Further studies to determine the clinical significance of these parameters for prognostic, chemo-preventive and chemotherapeutic purposes in canine colorectal tumors are recommended.

Keywords: Canine, Colorectal carcinoma, Ki67, Macrophage, Mast cell

Background

Colorectal cancer (CRC) is one of the most frequent and most serious malignancies in humans [1–3]. It is one of the most common malignant cancers and among the leading causes of cancer-related deaths worldwide [1, 4, 5]. Other than humans, the only domestic species that naturally develops intestinal cancer with any frequency is the dog, which shares similar environment and in some households similar diet with humans [6]. Colorectal tumors are among the most common gastrointestinal

neoplasms in the dog. Up to 60% of all canine intestinal tumors are located in the colorectum, where adenocarcinomas are relatively common [7, 8].

Ki-67 is widely applied in routine clinical work [9] and has been studied in relation to the development and progression of human CRC [2]. It was considered as an important predictive parameter in human CRC. Lumachi et al. [10] reported that there is an inverse correlation between overall survival and the percentage of Ki-67-positive tumor cells and that Ki-67 overexpression in CRC is associated with a worse outcome. However, some studies have failed to demonstrate its prognostic significance [11]. While some reported association of increased Ki-67 expression with poor prognosis [12], others [13]

* Correspondence: mwoldem@uga.edu
Department of Pathology, Tifton Veterinary Diagnostic and Investigational Laboratory, College of Veterinary Medicine, University of Georgia, 43 Brighton Rd, Tifton, GA 31793, USA

reported a good prognosis associated with Ki-67 expression. Although its prognostic value remains controversial [14], recently, Melling et al. [15] reported higher Ki-67 expression as an independent prognostic marker in human CRC.

Development of CRC has been associated with chronic inflammation of the large bowel elicited by various causes. Macrophages are among the inflammatory cells most involved in these processes [16, 17]. Pro-inflammatory cytokines released by macrophages are considered as major agents in the transition between inflammation and inflammation-related CRC [18]. Mast cells (MCs) are also among inflammatory cells involved in tumor development and progression in various human [19, 20] and animal [21–23] neoplasms. MCs can exert pro-tumor effects by influencing the microenvironment or, directly, by conditioning the fate of tumor cells including drug resistance [24]. Adenomatous polyps from which CRC develops are characterized by high mast cell count (MCC) [25] and existing polyps showed significant remission upon MC depletion in experimental mouse model [26]. It was also demonstrated that presence of MCs, particularly their ability to degranulate, is indispensable for tumor progression in a Myc- driven model of pancreatic cancer [27].

Genetic and molecular similarities as well as similar molecular and genetic pathways of cancer development and progression between human and dog CRCs have been suggested [28]. Ki-67 expression in CRC, and tumor associated macrophages and mast cells within colorectal tumors in dogs were not previously reported. We hypothesize that high Ki-67 expression and tumor associated macrophages and mast cells correlate with malignancy in canine CRC. Given genetic similarities of human and canine CRC, the objective of this study was to determine the Ki-67 index in canine CRC and assess its correlation with tumor malignancy, tumor associated macrophages (TAMs) and MCs. TAMs and MCs in canine CRC were evaluated and compared with those in colorectal adenomas and non-tumorous colorectal tissues.

Methods

Surgical biopsy specimens from colorectal tissues of 39 dogs of various breeds with carcinoma (n = 17), adenoma (n = 13) and non-neoplastic colorectal tissues from dogs with no colorectal tumors as control (n = 9) archived at the Tifton Veterinary Diagnostic and Investigational Laboratory, College of Veterinary Medicine, The University of Georgia, USA, were used in the study. The tissues were fixed in 10% buffered formalin solution, processed for routine histology, paraffin embedded, sectioned at 4–5 μm, stained with standard Hematoxylin-Eosin and Toluidine blue (Sigma, St. Louis, USA) stains and examined by light microscopy. The specimens were

evaluated by two board certified pathologists. Mitotic cells were counted in 10 high power fields (HPFs/40× objectives) and mitotic index was calculated by dividing the counts (results) by 10. Tumor malignancy was assessed based on tumor size at time of biopsy, mitotic index, necrosis and vascular invasion. MCC was made on Toluidine blue (Sigma, St. Louis, USA) stained sections. Ki-67 expression and tumor associated macrophage (TAM) count were assessed using immunohistochemistry against Ki-67 protein and macrophage marker. The average MCC and TAMs was made by counting the cells in 10 high power fields (40×).

Immunohistochemistry (IHC)

The tissue sections were subjected to IHC using antibodies against Ki-67 protein and macrophage/histiocyte marker. Immunohistochemical staining procedures for Ki-67 (Mouse-anti-KI-67, Clone 7B11; Zymed® Laboratories; Invitrogen immunodetection) and macrophage marker (Myeloid/histiocytes antigen; monoclonal-mouse, Clone MAC 387, DAKO Carpinteria, CA) were applied briefly as follows. Tissue samples were cut at 4–5 μm sections, deparaffinized by xylene-ethanol sequence, and rehydrated in graded ethanol solutions. Antigen retrieval for Ki-67 IHC was made by Heat Induced Epitope Retrieval (HIER) using a 1:10 diluted Target Retrieval Solution, pH 6 (DAKO). Heat was supplied by a Black and Decker Vegetable steamer for 25 min, followed by 10 min in the hot solution on the counter top. Endogenous peroxidase was blocked using UltraVision Hydrogen Peroxide Block for 10 min. Non-specific background staining was blocked by incubating the samples for 5 min using UltraVision Protein Block (Thermo Scientific; Lab Vision Corp, Ca, USA). Each step of incubation was followed by a thorough washing of the sections with Tris Buffered Saline (TBS) at pH 7.4. The sections were incubated for 1 h at room temperature with primary antibodies against Ki-67 and macrophage marker (Clone MAC 387) at 1:25 and 1:200 dilutions, respectively. The sections were then incubated for 10 min with a Primary Antibody Amplifier Quanto and later followed by incubation with HRP Polymer Quanto (Thermo Scientific; Lab Vision Corp, Ca, USA) for 10 min. The sections were rinsed with TBS after each step and were later incubated with DAB Quanto Chromagen and DAB Quanto Substrate mixture (DAB, Quanto) for 5 min. Finally, all sections were counterstained with Gill's Hematoxylin (Gills III- Formula, Surgipath Richmond, IL, USA). Negative control sections were made by substituting TBS for the primary antibodies.

Ki-67 expression

According to the International Ki-67 Breast Cancer Working Group [29], the Ki-67 evaluation method can be based on three patterns of Ki-67 immunostaining: homogeneous, hot spots, and a gradient of increasing staining toward the tumor edge. The most commonly used method to calculate the Ki-67 index is based on the hot spots [30]. The choice of the hot spots counting is generally based on the assumption that the areas with a high proliferation index potentially predict a more aggressive biological behavior of the neoplasm [31]. In this study, the hot-spot based counting was employed. The labeled sections were screened at 10× (lower) magnification to detect areas with distinct staining (hot-spots). In each section, the most intense three areas stained with Ki-67 were identified and at least 500 cells were counted in each area at a high power field of the microscope (40×) and also using computer assisted Image-J cell counting method. Areas with severe inflammation and necrosis were avoided. A ratio of the number of nuclei stained positively with Ki-67 antigen was determined in each area and the average of these ratios was considered as Ki-67 index as previously described [31].

Statistical analysis

The Ki-67 labelling index (%) was calculated by dividing the total Ki-67 positive cells by the total numbers of cells multiplied by 100. Mitotic index was determined by dividing the number of mitotic cells in 10 HPFs by 10. MCC and TAMs count were made in 10 high power fields (40×) of the microscope and the results were given as mean ± standard deviation (SD). Data were analyzed using analysis of variance. Correlation between the various parameters was determined using Spearman's correlation coefficient. In all cases, the results were considered statistically significant if p values were <0.05.

Results

A variety of breeds were included in the study. These included mixed breeds ($n = 6$), Labrador retriever ($n = 4$), Basset Hound ($n = 2$), Cocker Spaniel ($n = 2$), pointer ($n = 2$), unknown breed ($n = 6$) and a variety of other breeds represented only once. The average age of the dogs was 7.5 years (range was 7–12 for carcinomas, 2–11 for adenomas and 1–9 for the control). There was no statistically significant age difference between the groups.

The Ki-67 and mitotic indices (mean ± SD) in carcinomas were 17.13 ± 11.50 and 3.52 ± 1.80, respectively. A strong positive correlation ($r = 0.98$, $p < 0.05$) was recorded between the Ki-67 and mitotic indices. The Ki-67 expression was variable and in some diffuse expression (Fig. 1) was present while in other cases in which only a few Ki-67 positive cells were present, the expression was observed only in mitotic cells. Ki-67 was associated ($r = 0.71$; $P < 0.05$) with tumor malignancy based on tumor size at times of biopsy, mitotic index, necrosis and vascular invasion.

Higher average TAMs were observed in adenomas (21.30 ± 20.70) and in CRC (11.00 ± 9.82) than in non-neoplastic tissues (7.69 ± 7.26) (Fig. 2 and Table 1). The differences, however, were not statistically significant ($p > 0.05$). Although not significant ($p > 0.05$), TAMs in CRC were also, positively, but weakly correlated with mitotic ($r = 0.35$) and Ki-67 ($r = 0.25$) indices, and MCC ($r = 0.24$).

The average MCC in carcinomas, adenomas, and non-neoplastic tissues were 6.30 ± 3.98, 0.78 ± 0.77 and 0.35 ± 0.33, respectively (Fig. 3 and Table 1). The average MCC in CRC was significantly higher ($p < 0.05$) than that in adenomas and non-neoplastic tissues. No significant difference was observed between MCC in adenomas and non-neoplastic tissues ($p > 0.05$). The MCs and TAMs were accentuated on the periphery of the neoplasm in the carcinomas and were observed in the supporting stroma in the adenomas. There was a weak positive correlation ($r = 0.2$; $p > 0.05$) between Ki-67 and MCC.

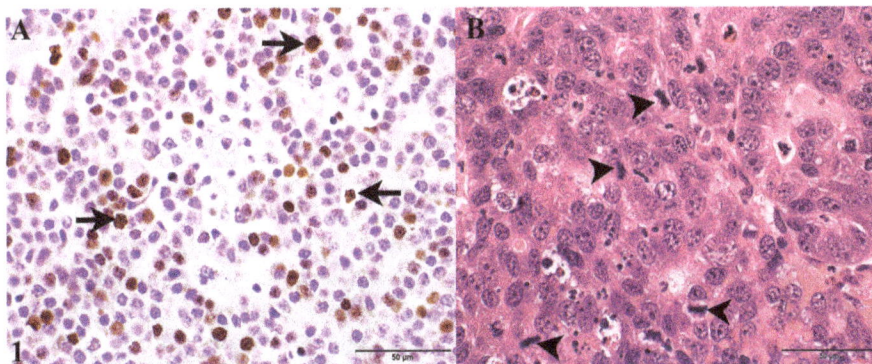

Fig. 1 Canine colorectal carcinoma. **a** Immunoreactivity of tumor cell nuclei for Ki-67 protein (arrows). Bar = 50 μm. **b** Hematoxylin-eosin stained section showing mitotic cells (arrow heads). Hematoxylin-eosin. Bar =50 μm

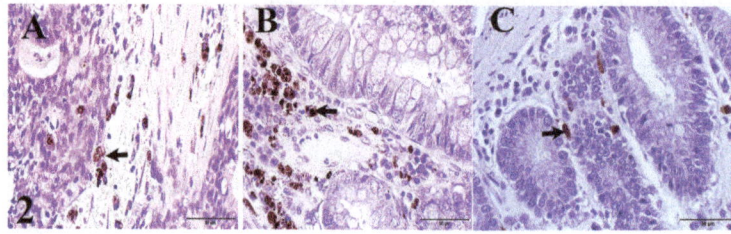

Fig. 2 Canine colorectal tissues from: **a** Carcinoma **b** Adenoma and **c** Non-neoplastic tissue (control), showing TAMs positive immunoreactivity (arrows) against macrophage marker (MAC 387). Bar = 50 μm

Discussion

Ki-67 expression has been reported in association with malignancies in various human and animal tumors. Some studies [15] reported higher Ki-67 expression as an independent prognostic marker in human CRC, while others failed to demonstrate its prognostic significance [11]. TAMs [16–18] and MCs [25] are also involved in the development and progression of human colorectal tumors.

Human and dog CRCs are suggested to share similar molecular and genetic pathways of cancer development and progression [28]. Ki-67 expression and tumor associated inflammatory cells have not previously been documented in canine CRC. Here we report Ki-67 expression, TAMs and MCC in canine CRC. Ki-67 index was strongly ($r = 0.71$; $p < 0.05$) correlated with tumor malignancy. The results suggest association of Ki-67 with malignancy in canine CRC as was previously reported for human CRC [2, 15], prostate and breast cancers [14, 32] and various animal tumors [30, 33–35]. Because, there are genetic and pathogenic similarities between canine CRC and the human disease [36], in which Ki-67 prognostic value remained controversial [1, 14], its prognostic value in canine CRC is unknown at this time. Strong correlation between Ki-67 and mitotic indexes as observed in this study was expected since both parameters indicate degree of cell proliferation. We suggest that Ki-67 should be considered for a potential use to predict prognosis coupled with other measures of malignancy and should not be used as an independent prognostic marker in canine CRC. More studies should be done to determine its value as an independent prognostic marker for canine CRC.

Table 1 Average MCC ± SD and TAMs ± SD in canine colorectal tissues

	Carcinoma ($n = 17$)	Adenoma ($n = 13$)	Control ($n = 9$)	P-value
TAMs	11.00 ± 9.82[a]	21.30 ± 20.70[a]	7.69 ± 7.26[a]	>0.05
MCC	6.30 ± 3.98[b]	0.78 ± 0.77[a]	0.35 ± 0.33[a]	<0.05

Different superscript letters in the same row indicate statistically significant differences ($p < 0.05$). *MCC* mast cell count, *TAMs* tumor associated macrophages, *SD* standard deviation

Higher TAMs were documented in the colorectal adenomas (21.30 ± 20.70) and carcinomas (11.00 ± 9.82) than non-neoplastic tissues (7.69 ± 7.26) in this study. The TAMs count, however, was not directly associated with malignancy as a higher count was documented in adenomas than in carcinomas. TAMs count in CRC was positively correlated with mitotic ($r = 0.35$) and Ki-67 ($r = 0.25$) indices although the correlations were not statistically significant ($p > 0.05$). The higher TAMs count in adenomas and carcinomas than non-tumorous tissues suggests that TAMs may play a role in initiating and maintaining canine colorectal tumors. TAMs, conditioned by the tumor microenvironment are reported to have impact on cancer development by facilitating matrix invasion, angiogenesis, and tumor cell motility [37]. Furthermore, macrophages are immunosuppressive, and prevent tumor cell attack by natural killer and T-cells during tumor progression [38]. Because canine colorectal adenomas may progress to malignancy [39], most of malignant CRC arise from benign adenomatous polyps as observed in mouse model of CRC [36] and due to higher TAMs count in adenomas, we speculate that targeting TAMs would minimize development of adenomas, which would later progress to carcinomas. Similarly, depletion of pulmonary macrophages is suggested to be a strategy for attenuating lung cancer progression in humans [40]. Detailed study with large numbers of cases should be done to determine whether an early control of TAMs would help to control the development of canine colorectal tumors.

MCC was significantly higher in CRC than adenomas and non-neoplastic tissues and was strongly correlated with Ki-67 index indicating association of MCs with malignancy as was previously reported for various human [19, 20] and animal [21–23] neoplasms. Several published studies suggest that high MCC in CRC may play a role as an unfavorable prognostic marker [41]. Increased accumulation of mast cells within tumor environments has been correlated with poor prognosis, increased metastasis and reduced survival in several types of human cancer [20, 24]. Since benign colorectal tumors are characterized by high MCC [25] and showed significant remission upon MC depletion in

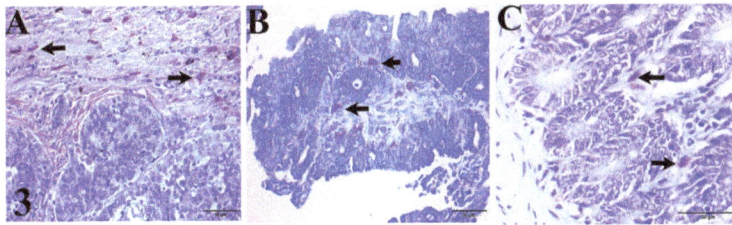

Fig. 3 Canine colorectal tissues from: **a** Carcinoma **b** Adenoma and **c** Non-neoplastic tissue (control), showing Toluidine blue stained mast cells (arrows). Toluidine blue stain. Bar = 50 μm

mice, it was suggested that MC deserve consideration as a therapeutic target in polyposis and colon cancer [26].

Conclusions

In summary, Ki-67 index, tumor associated macrophages and mast cells in canine CRC were recorded for the first time in this study. Ki-67 index, and MCC coupled with mitotic index and other clinical parameters may have a potential use in determining malignancy in canine CRC. Higher TAMs recorded in colorectal tumors than non-neoplastic tissues indicate that TAMs may play a role in the development of canine colorectal tumors. Targeting tumor associated inflammatory cells (TAMs and MCs) may be helpful in devising strategy to manage and minimize development of canine colorectal tumors. The data in this study provide a ground for further investigation of the clinical significance of the findings for chemopreventive and chemotherapeutic purposes in canine CRC.

Abbreviations
CRC: Colorectal cancer; HIER: Heat Induced Epitope Retrieval; HPF: High power field; IHC: Immunohistochemistry; MC: Mast cell; MCC: Mast cell count; SD: Standard deviation; TAM: Tumor associated macrophages

Acknowledgements
The authors would like to thank the staff of Tifton Veterinary Diagnostic and Investigational Laboratory, College of Veterinary Medicine, University of Georgia, for their technical assistance.

Funding
This work was partly funded by VMES (veterinary Medical Experiment Station) of the University of Georgia (2008).

Authors' contributions
Conceived and designed the study: WM. Histopathological and immunohistochemical analysis and sample evaluation: WM, HI, LW. Drafted the manuscript: WM. Revised the manuscript: WM and HI. The authors read and approved the manuscript.

Competing interests
The authors declare that they have no competing interests.

Consent for publication
Not applicable.

References
1. Fluge Ø, Gravdal K, Carlsen E, Vonen B, Kjellevold K, Refsum S, et al. Expression of EZH2 and Ki-67 in colorectal cancer and associations with treatment response and prognosis. Br J Cancer. 2009;101:1282–9.
2. Sousa WAT, Rodrigues LV, Silva Jr RG, Vieira FL. Immunohistochemical evaluation of p53 and Ki-67 proteins in colorectal adenomas. Arq Gastroenterol. 2012;49:35–40.
3. Mogoantă SS, Vasile I, Totolici B, Neamțu C, Streba L, Busuioc CJ, et al. Colorectal cancer - clinical and morphological aspects. Romanian J Morphol Embryol. 2014;55:103–10.
4. Birt DF, Phillips GJ. Diet, genes, and microbes: complexities of colon cancer prevention. Toxicol Pathol. 2014;42:182–8.
5. Hayashi H, Beppu T, Sakamoto Y, Miyamoto Y, Yokoyama N, Higashi T, et al. Prognostic value of Ki-67 expression in conversion therapy for colorectal liver-limited metastases. Am J Cancer Res. 2015;5:1225–33.
6. McEntee MF, Cates JM, Neilsen N. Cyclooxygenase-2 expression in spontaneous intestinal neoplasia of domestic dogs. Vet Pathol. 2002; 39:428–36.
7. Head KW, Else RW, Dubielzig RR. Tumors of the alimentary tract. In: Tumors in domestic animals, 4th Edit., Meuten DJ, eds. Iowa State Press. Ames, Iowa 2002; pp. 465-467.
8. Coleman KA, Berent AC, Weisse CW. Endoscopic mucosal resection and snare polypectomy for treatment of a colorectal polypoid adenoma in a dog. J Am Vet Med Assoc. 2014;244:1435–40.
9. Inwald EC, Klinkhammer-Schalke M, Hofstädter F, Zeman F, Koller M, Gerstenhauer M, et al. Ki-67 is a prognostic parameter in breast cancer patients: results of a large population-based cohort of a cancer registry. Breast Cancer Res Treat. 2013;139:539–52.
10. Lumachi F, Orlando R, Marino F, Chiara GB, Basso SM. Expression of p53 and Ki-67 as prognostic factors for survival of men with colorectal cancer. Anticancer Res. 2012;32:3965–7.
11. Ghiță C, Vîlcea ID, Dumitrescu M, Vîlcea AM, Mirea CS, Aşchie M, et al. The prognostic value of the immunohistochemical aspects of tumor suppressor genes p53, bcl-2, PTEN and nuclear proliferative antigen Ki-67 in resected colorectal carcinoma. Romanian J Morphol Embryol. 2012;53:549–56.
12. Chen YT, Henk MJ, Carney KJ, Wong WD, Rothenberger DA, Zheng T, et al. Prognostic significance of tumor markers in colorectal cancer patients: DNA index, S-phase fraction, p53 expression, and Ki-67 index. J Gastrointest Surg. 1997;1:266–72.
13. Allegra CJ, Paik S, Colangelo LH, Parr AL, Kirsch I, Kim G, et al. Prognostic value of thymidylate synthase, Ki-67, and p53 in patients with dukes' B and C colon cancer: a National Cancer Institute-National Surgical Adjuvant Breast and bowel project collaborative study. J Clin Oncol. 2003;21:241–50.
14. Shin IY, Sung NY, Lee YS, Kwon TS, Si Y, Lee YS, et al. The expression of multiple proteins as prognostic factors in colorectal cancer: Cathepsin D, p53, COX-2, epidermal growth factor receptor, C-erbB-2, and Ki-67. Gut Liver. 2014;8:13–23.
15. Melling N, Kowitz CM, Simon R, Bokemeyer C, Terracciano L, Sauter G, et al. High Ki67 expression is an independent good prognostic marker in colorectal cancer. J Clin Pathol. 2016;69:209–14.
16. Roncucci L, Mora E, Mariani F, Bursi S, Pezzi A, Rossi G, et al. Myeloperoxidase-positive cell infiltration in colorectal carcinogenesis as indicator of colorectal cancer risk. Cancer Epidemiol Biomark Prev. 2008;17:2291–7.
17. Mariani F, Sena P, Roncucci L. Inflammatory pathways in the early steps of colorectal cancer development. World J Gastroenterol. 2014;20:9716–31.

18. Pietrzyk L, Torres A, Maciejewsk R, Torres K. Obesity and obese-related chronic low-grade inflammation in promotion of colorectal cancer development. Asian Pac J Cancer Prev. 2015;16:4161–8.

19. Tomita M, Matsuzaki Y, Onitsuka T. Effect of mast cells on tumor angiogenesis in lung cancer. Ann Thorac Surg. 2000;69:1686–90.

20. Elpek GO, Gelen T, Aksoy NH, ErdoÄŸan A, Dertsiz L, Demircan A, et al. The prognostic relevance of angiogenesis and mast cells in squamous cell carcinoma of the oesophagus. J Clin Pathol. 2001;54:940–4.

21. Mukaratirwa S, Chikafa L, Dliwayo R, Moyo N. Mast cells and angiogenesis in canine melanomas: malignancy and clinicopathological factors. Vet Dermatol. 2006;17:141–6.

22. Sabattini S, Bettini G. An immunohistochemical analysis of canine Haemangioma and Haemangiosarcoma. J Comp Pathol. 2009;140:158–68.

23. Woldemeskel M, Sreekumari R. Mast cells in canine cutaneous hemangioma, hemangiosarcoma and mammary tumors. Vet Res Commun. 2010;43:153–60.

24. Maciel TT, Moura IC, Hermine O. The role of mast cells in cancers. F1000Prime Reports. 2015;7:09. doi:10.12703/P7-09.

25. Stockmann C, Schadendorf D, Klose R, Helfrich I. The impact of the immune system on tumor: angiogenesis and vascular remodeling. Front Oncol. 2014; 4:69. doi:10.3389/fonc.2014.00069.

26. Gounaris E, Erdman SE, Restaino C, Gurish MF, Friend DS, Gounari F, et al. Mast cells are an essential hematopoietic component for polyp development. Proc Natl Acad Sci U S A. 2007; 104: 19977-82.

27. Soucek L, Lawlor ER, Soto D, Shchors K, Swigart LB, Evan GI. Mast cells are required for angiogenesis and macroscopic expansion of Myc-induced pancreatic islet tumors. Nature Med. 2007;13:1211–8.

28. Tang J, Le S, Sun L, Yan X, Zhang M, MacLeod J, et al. Copy number abnormalities in sporadic canine colorectal cancers. Genome Res. 2010;20: 341–50.

29. Dowsett M, Nielsen TO, A'Hern R, Bartlett J, Coombes RC, Cuzick J, et al. Assessment of Ki-67 in breast cancer: recommendations from the international Ki-67 in breast cancer working group. J Natl Cancer Inst. 2011; 103:1656–64.

30. Pereira RS, Schweigert A, de Melo GD, Fernandes FV, Sueiro FAR, Machado GF. Ki-67 labeling in canine perianal glands neoplasms: a novel approach for immunohistological diagnostic and prognostic. BMC Vet Res. 2013;9:83. doi:10.1186/1746-6148-9-83.

31. Atalay T, Ak H, Celik B, Gulsen I, Seckin H, Tanik N, et al. Prognostic factors in Oligodendrogliomas: a clinical study of twenty-five consecutive patients. Asian Pac J Cancer Prev. 2015;16:5319–23.

32. Tashima R, Nishimura R, Osako T, Nishiyama Y, Okumura Y, Nakano M, et al. Evaluation of an optimal cut-off point for the Ki-67 index as a prognostic factor in primary breast cancer: a retrospective study. PLoS One. 2015;10(7):e0119565.

33. Peña LL, Nieto AI, Pérez-Alenza D, Cuesta P, Castaño M. Immunohistochemical detection of Ki-67 and PCNA in canine mammary tumors: relationship to clinical and pathologic variables. J Vet Diag Invest. 1998;10:237–46.

34. Webster JD, Yuzbasiyan-Gurkan V, Miller RA, Kaneene JB, Kiupel M. Cellular proliferation in canine cutaneous mast cell tumors: associations with c-KIT and its role in prognostication. Vet Pathol. 2007;44:298–308.

35. Bergin IL, Smedley RC, Esplin DG, Spangler WL, Kiupel M. Prognostic evaluation of Ki-67 threshold value in canine oral melanoma. Vet Pathol. 2011;48:41–53.

36. Johnson RL, Fleet JC. Animal models of colorectal cancer. Cancer Metastasis Rev. 2013;32:39. doi:10.1007/s10555-012-9404-6.

37. Coussens LM, Werb Z. Inflammation and cancer. Nature. 2002;420:860–7.

38. Noy R, Pollard JW. Tumor-associated macrophages: from mechanisms to therapy. Immunity. 2014;41:49–61.

39. Valerius KD, Powers BE, McPherron MA, Hutchison JM, Mann FA, Withrow SJ. Adenomatous polyps and carcinoma in situ of the canine colon and rectum: 34 cases (1982–1994). J Am Anim Hosp Assoc. 1997;33:156–60.

40. Fritz JM, Tennis MA, Orlicky DJ, Lin H, Ju C, Redente EF, et al. Depletion of tumor-associated macrophages slows the growth of chemically induced mouse lung adenocarcinomas. Front Immunol. 2014;5:587. doi:10.3389/fimmu.2014.00587.

41. Marech I, Ammendola M, Gadaleta C, Zizzo N, Oakley C, Gadaleta CD, et al. Possible biological and translational significance of mast cells density in colorectal cancer. World J Gastroenterol. 2014;20:8910–20.

15

Effects of vitamin E, inorganic selenium, bacterial organic selenium, and their combinations on immunity response in broiler chickens

A. M. Dalia[1,2], T. C. Loh[1], A. Q. Sazili[1], M. F. Jahromi[3] and A. A. Samsudin[1]*

Abstract

Background: Selenium (Se) and vitamin E (Vit E) can act synergistically and affect biological processes, mainly antioxidant and immunity. The use of excess dietary Vit E and Se in animals' feed could enhance immune response and induce disease resistance. Moreover, different Se sources may provide different alterations in the immune system. Accordingly, the aim of the current study was to assess the impact of dietary supplementation of Vit E, inorganic Se (sodium selenite, SS), bacterial organic Se of ADS18, and their different combinations on the plasma immunoglobulins, ceacum microbial population, and splenic cytokines gene expression in broiler chickens.

Results: Present results showed that, Se and Vit E synergistic effect was clear in plasma IgM level at day 42 and in splenic cytokines expression (TNF-a, IFN-γ, IL-2, IL-10). The combination of 0.3 mg/kg ADS18-Se with 100 mg/kg Vit E showed the highest IgM level compared to Vit E- SS complex. The combination of either SS or ADS18-Se with Vit E had no significant effect on IFN- γ and IL-10 compared to Vit E alone, while Vit E alone showed the significantly lowest TNF-a compared to the Se combinations. Supplementation of 100 mg/kg Vit E had no effect on microbial population except a slight reduction in *Salmonella* spp. The main effect of Se sources was that both sources increased the day 42 IgA and IgG level compared to NS group. ADS18-Se modulate the caecum microbial population via enhancing beneficial bacteria and suppressing the *E-coli* and *Salmonella* spp. while both Se and Vit E factors had no effect on lymphoid organ weights.

Conclusions: The inclusion of 100 mg/kg Vit E with 0.3 mg/kg ADS18-Se, effectively could support the immune system through regulation of some cytokines expression and immunoglobulin levels more than using ADS18-Se alone, while no difference was observed between using SS alone or combined with Vit E.

Keywords: Bacteria, Broiler, Selenium, Vitamin E, Immunity, Cytokines

Background

Infectious diseases are the leading causes of chick mortality. The immune system plays an important role in host defense against infectious agents. The immune system cells contain high polyunsaturated fatty acids in their cells membrane which increase their susceptibility to produce free radicals. Moreover, free radicals can be produced during the phagocytes action against the pathogens which lead to high oxidative stress [1]. It is well known that Se and Vit E can act synergistically and affect antioxidant and immunity response [2]. Vitamin E has been documented as a vital nutrient for the health, growth, and reproduction of all species of animals. This Vit is required to support the development of the nervous system and antioxidant system, as well contribute to disease resistance [3]. Selenium trace mineral plays an important role in antioxidant system through the selenoproteins, which are involved in redox regulation and antioxidant defense in all tissues and cells including the innate and adaptive immune cells [4]. The main antioxidant selenoprotein is

* Correspondence: anjas@upm.edu.my
[1]Department of Animal Science, Faculty of Agriculture, Universiti Putra Malaysia, 43400 Serdang, Selangor, Malaysia
Full list of author information is available at the end of the article

glutathione peroxidase (GSH-Px), which reduce H_2O_2 and peroxides to the water and corresponding alcohols [5]. Antioxidant enzymes prevent reactive oxygen species production, which is formed normally during the body's biological process [6]. Moreover, Se deficiency can damage the humoral immunity and cellular immunity, and deactivate B cells which results in immunoglobulin reduction [7].

The use of excess dietary Vit E and Se for enhancing the immunity and suppressing disease has been studied. Dietary Vit E and Se combination has been shown to improve the humoral immunity and provide better immunity response [8]. Vitamin E has been shown to increase antibody production by enhancing the humoral immune response or by acting as an adjuvant. Moreover, combined Vit E and Se significantly increased serum IgG and IgM levels in mice after their exposure to sodium azide which have an immune-suppressive effect [9]. In broiler chicken, higher antibody titer was observed when 0.06 mg/kg of Se was combined with 150 IU/kg Vit E in the diet, while higher cellular immunity was reported in the diet which included 300 IU/kg Vit E and 1 mg/kg Se [10]. Furthermore, the antibody titer increased when 125 mg/kg Vit E and 0.5 mg/kg Se were supplemented to the diet, and the author suggested that Se and Vit E combination improved the humoral immunity through the induction of immunoglobulins, especially IgM, which is released after the initial antigen exposure [11]. Selenium and Vit E together also may affect the proliferation of lymphoid cells and increase circulatory immunoglobulins and immune complexes, which would enhance antibody responses [8].

In the poultry industry, usually, Vit E is supplemented as α-tocopherol, which is the most abundant and bioavailable form, while dietary Se is supplemented as sodium selenite, however, recent studies demonstrated that organic Se such as seleno-aminoacids is more bioavailable than sodium selenite [12, 13]. Moreover, organic Se has the ability to accumulate Se in the animal's tissues when the received amount of Se is higher than the body requirement [14]. Organic Se can be produced biologically through microbial reduction process. *Klebsiella pneumonia* (ADS18) isolated from hot spring water and was associated with high biomass organic Se-containing protein which can be used as Se source. Although it is well recognised that Se and Vit E interaction can enhance the antioxidant system, scientific data about the effect of Vit E and organic Se combination on broiler chicken is limited, and to the best knowledge of this researcher, no study has compared the combination of Vit E with organic Se versus inorganic source and no study use the bacterial organic Se in combination with Vit E. Accordingly, the aim of the current study was to assess the impact of dietary supplementation of Vit E, inorganic Se, bacterial organic Se of ADS18, and their different combinations on the plasma immunoglobulins, ceacum microbial population, and splenic cytokines gene expression in broiler chickens.

Methods

Birds and experimental design

Two hundred and sixteen ($n = 216$) day-old female broiler chicks (Cobb, 500) were sourced from a commercial hatchery (Ayamas LI Pt. Ltd.) and housed in battery cages. Each cage was equipped with one tube feeder and one bell drinker. On arrival, the chicks were individually wing banded, weighed, and randomly divided into six dietary groups, with each group having six replicates with six chicks per replicate. The experimental design was a factorial complete randomised design of two factors; Se (2 sources) x Vit E (2 levels). The birds had access to the feed and water ad libitum. All birds were subjected to vaccination against bronchitis (IB) and Newcastle disease (ND) on day 7, and against infectious bursal disease on day 14, through the intraocular route. A basal diet was formulated based on the nutrient requirements for starter and finisher stages (Table 1). The starter and finisher diets were offered to the broiler chickens from 0 to 21 and from 22 to 42 days of age, respectively. The treatment groups included T1 = basal diet, T2 = basal diet + 100 mg/kg α-tocopherol acetate, T3 = basal diet + 0.3 mg/Kg feed sodium selenite, T4 = basal diet + 0.3 mg /kg feed ADS18 Se, T5 = basal diet + 0.3 mg/kg feed sodium selenite+ 100 mg/kg α-tocopherol acetate, T6 = 0.3 mg/kg feed ADS18 Se + 100 mg/kg α-tocopherol acetate. The organic Se of ADS18 was prepared according to the method described by Dalia et al. [15], and administered orally equivalent to the dietary 0.3 mg/kg feed, based on the feed intake of the previous day. Other groups was treated orally using distilled water. The body weight was weighed individually and daily feed intake was recorded for each replicate.

Samples and data collection

At day 21 and 42, 12 representative birds (selected randomly as 2 birds/pen) from each treatment were slaughtered for sampling in accordance with the procedures outlined in MS1500:2009 (Department of Standards Malaysia, 2009) which allows animal to be slaughtered by severing the jugular vein, without being stunned, with a razor sharp knife. In this study the slaughter was performed by a certified and highly experienced technician with a sharp knife. In this study, sustained absence of corneal reflex and rhythmic breathing were strictly monitored and checked to ensure that each individual bird was dead prior to further processing and sampling. Samples of blood, spleen, thymus, bursa of Fabricius, and ceacum digesta were collected and kept at − 80 C° for further analysis. Upon chicken slaughtering, part of spleen organ was collected in RNA-later Stabilisation

Table 1 The ingredients of the basal diet

Ingredients	Starter %	Finisher %
Corn	52.5	56.250
Palm oil (Refine)	5.00	6.00
Soybean meal (44% cp)	32.50	30.00
Fish meal (58% cp)	5.15	3.25
L-Lysine	0.25	0.25
DL-Methionine	0.25	0.25
Dicalcium phosphate 18%	1.60	1.85
Calcium carbonate	0.60	0.35
Salt (Nacl)	0.30	0.30
Mineral Premix[a]	0.15	0.15
Vitamin Premix[b]	0.10	0.10
Toxin Binder[c]	0.15	0.15
Choline Chloride	0.10	0.10
Wheat pollard	0.135	1.00
Calculated nutrient content (g/kg DM)		
ME (kcal/Kg)	3081.1	3152.8
Crude protein	22.04	20.09
Crude fat	7.57	8.004
Calcium	1.189	1.0440
Phosphorus	0.786	0.768
Avail. P for Poultry	0.472	0.450
Analyzed Se (mg/kg)[d]	0.085	0.099
Analyzed vitamin E (mg/kg)[e]	224.9	167.1

[a]Mineral premix provided the following per kg diet: iron 120 mg, manganese 150 mg, copper 15 mg, zinc 120 mg, iodine 1.5 mg, and cobalt 0.4 mg
[b]Vitamin premix provided the following per kg diet: Vitamin A (retinyl acetate) 10.32 mg, cholecalciferol 0.250 mg, vitamin E (DL-tocopheryl acetate) 90 mg, vitamin K 6 mg, cobalamin 0.07 mg, thiamine 7 mg, riboflavin 22 mg, folic acid 3 mg, biotin 0.04 mg, pantothenic acid 35 mg, niacin 120 mg and pyridoxine 12 mg
[c]Toxin binder contains natural hydrated sodium calcium aluminium silicates to reduce the exposure of feed to mycotoxins
[d]The Se content measured using ICP.MS.
[e]Vit E content measured using spectrophotometer

Reagent (Qiagen, Germany) and processed for storage at – 80 °C, according to the manufacturer's instructions.

Plasma immunoglobulin concentration

Blood samples were collected at days 21 and 42 in vacutainer tubes containing ethylene diamine tetra acetic acid (EDTA). The samples were centrifuged at 3000 rpm for 15 min at 4 °C, and the plasma was stored at – 80 °C until antibody analyses. The chicken immunoglobulin (IgA, IgG, and IgM) were established employing commercial kits (Chicken IgA ELISA, Immunology Consultants Laboratory, Inc. USA), (Chicken IgM ELISA, Immunology Consultants Laboratory, Inc., USA), and (CEA544Ga, Enzyme-linked Immunosorbent Assay Kit, Cloud-Clone Corp., USA), respectively, following the manufacturer's instructions.

Analysis of caecal bacteria by quantitative real-time PCR

Collection of the caecal digesta was done directly after slaughter and kept at – 20 °C before it was used for quantification of caecal microbial population. The populations of *Lactobacillus* spp., *Bifidobacteria* spp., *Enterococcus* spp., *Enterobacteria* spp., *E. coli,*. and *Salmonella* spp. were established following the procedure reported by Navidshad et al. [16]. The genomic DNA extraction from the caecal digesta was done by using QIAamp® DNA Stool Mini kits following the manufacturer's instructions. DNA concentration and purity were measured with a Nanodrop ND-1000 spectrophotometer. Standard curves created by amplifying a known amount of target bacteria DNA were formed using serial dilution of PCR products from pure cultures of the targeted bacteria. The qPCR reaction was carried out using master mix of maxima SYBR® Green qPCR Master Mixes, ROX solution (Cat. no. K0252, Thermo Scientific Fermentas, UK). The primer sequences and annealing temperature of the targeted caecal bacteria used in this study are shown in Table 2. Each reaction volume comprised 12.5 µL of SYBR Green Master Mix, 1 µL of 10 µM forward primer, 1 µL of 10 µM reverse primer, 2 µL of DNA samples and 8.5 µL of molecular H2O. The qPCR assay was carried out with the BioRad CFX96 real-time PCR system (BioRad, USA) by utilising optical grade plates as follows: the reaction conditions consisted of an initial denaturation at 94 °C for 5 min, then by 40 cycles of denaturation at 94 °C for 20 s, primer annealing at 55 °C total bacteria, 58 °C for *Lactobacilli* spp., 60 °C for *Bifidobacteria* spp., and 50 °C for *Salmonella* spp., *E. coli, Enterococcus* spp., and *Enterobacteria* spp. for 30 s respectively, and extension at 72 °C for 20 s. To verify the specificity of amplification melting curve analysis was performed following the last cycle of each amplification.

RNA isolation and real-time RT-PCR for cytokines gene expression

For RNA extraction, 30 mg of tissues was extracted using the RNeasy® Mini kit (Cat. No. 74104, Qiagen, Hilden, Germany). The concentration of the extracted RNA was examined with NanoDrop ND-1000 UV-Vis Spectrophotometer (NanoDrop Technologies, Wilmington, DE, USA) at 260/280 nm absorbance. Then I µg of extracted RNA was reversely transcribed employing the Quantitect® reverse transcription kit as per manufacturer's instructions.

Real-time PCR was carried out with the use of Bio-Rad CFX96 Touch (Bio- Rad Laboratories, Hercules, CA, USA), in 96-well optical reaction plates. The GAPDH was taken as the reference gene to normalise the targeted genes. Primers were designed according to Table 3. Real-time qPCR analyses were conducted using 25 µL PCR master mix containing 12.5 µL SYBR Green Master Mix, 1 µL forward primer, 1 µL reverse primer, 2 µL template

Table 2 The primer sequences of caecal targeting total bacteria, *Lactobacillus*, *Bifidobacteria*, *Enterococcus*, *Enterobacteriaceae*, *E.coli*, and *Salmonella*

Microorganism	Primer	Size of amplified fragments (bp)	References
Lactobacillus	F-5'-CATCCAGTGCAAACCTAAGAG-3' R-5'-GATCCGCTTGCCTTCGCA-3'	341	[42]
Enterococcus genus	F-5'-CCCTTATTGTTAGTTGCCATCATT-3' R-5'-ACTCGTTGTACTTCCCATTGT-3'	144	[9]
Bifidobacterium	F-5'- GGGTGGTAATGCCGGATG-3' R-5'- TAAGCCATGGACTTTCACACC-3'	440	[43]
Escherichia coli	F-5'-GTGTGATATCTACCCGCTTCGC-3' R-5'-AGAACGCTTTGTGGTTAATCAGGA-3'	82	[42]
Enterobacteriace	F- 5'-CAT TGACGTTACCCGCAGAAGAAGC-3' R-5'-CTCTACGAGACTCAAGCTTGC-3'	195	[42]
Total *Salmonella*	F-5'-TCGTCATTCCATTACCTACC-3' R-5'-AAACGTTGAAAAACTGAGGA-3'	119	[44]

cDNA and 8.5 µL RNase-free water. Target genes were amplified using the following thermo cycling programme: 95 °C for 10 min, 40 PCR cycles at 95 °C for 10s, 60 °C for 15 s. Efficiency of amplification was established for each primer pair by utilising the serial dilutions of cDNA. The cycle numbers at which amplified DNA samples were in excess of the computer-generated fluorescence threshold level were normalised and comparisons made to establish the relative gene expression. Higher cycle number values showed lower initial concentrations of cDNA, and hence lowered levels of mRNA expression. Each sample was run in duplicate. The quantification of PCR reactions for each primer pair was carried out by comparing the target gene with the housekeeping gene. The formulation below was used to compute the gene expression of the target gene according to the method described by Pfaffl [17]:

$$Ratio = \frac{\left(E_{target}\right)^{\Delta CT_{target}(Control-Treatment)}}{\left(E_{reference}\right)^{\Delta CT_{reference}(Control-Treatment)}}$$

The result was presented as a fold change between treatment and control group.

Table 3 Primers used for qRT-PCR

Gene	size (bp)	Sequence (5'_3')	References
IL-2	144	F- GTGGCTAACTAATCTGCTGTCCA R- CCGTAGGGCTTACAGAAAGG	[45]
IL-10	172	F- TAACATCCAACTGCTCAGCTC R- TGATGACTGGTGCTGGTCTG	[45]
IFN- γ	214	F- GAGCCATCACCAAGAAGATGA R- TAGGTCCACCGTCAGCTACA	[45]
TNF-α	–	F- GCTGTTCTATGACCGCCCAGTT R- AACAACCAGCTATGCACCCCA	[46]
GAPDH	312	F- CTGGCAAAGTCCAAGTGGTG R- AGCACCACCCTTCAGATGAG	[45]

Organ collection

Twelve birds of each treatment were slaughtered on day 42. The lymphoid organs (thymus, spleen, and bursa of Fabricius) were collected and weighed individually.

Statistical analysis

The present study followed a factorial completely randomized design (3 (Se factors) × 2 (Vit E levels)). All data obtained were subjected to the generalised linear model (GLM) procedure of SAS (SAS, 2005). Tukey HSD test was used to separate means at $p < 0.05$ significance level.

Results

Plasma immunoglobulin concentration

The effect of Se and Vit E and their combination on plasma immunoglobulins in broiler chickens is shown in Table 4. Vitamin E supplementation had no effect on plasma immunoglobulin levels except significant ($P < 0.05$) elevation which was observed at day21 IgM. On the other hand, at day21 bacterial organic Se of ADS18 showed the highest IgA level compared to SS and NS groups with no significant differences between SS and NS treatments. At day 42, both ADS18-Se and SS showed significant ($P < 0.05$) elevation in IgG level than NS group, while SS showed the highest level of IgA and IgM however the differences between SS and ADS18-Se was in-significant. The interaction between Vit E and Se was significant ($P < 0.05$) on day 42 IgM. Without Vit E supplementation there were no significant differences between SS and ADS18-Se, however both of them were higher significantly than the NS group and Vit E alone. The combination of 0.3 mg/kg ADS18-Se with 100 mg/kg Vit E showed significantly ($P < 0.05$) highest IgM level compared to Vit E alone and Vit E- SS complex.

Ceacum microbial population

The main effect of dietary Se sources and Vit E levels on ceacum microbial population of broiler chickens is shown

Table 4 Effect of dietary selenium sources and Vit E levels on antibody response in broiler chickens

Treatments		DAY 21			DAY 42		
		IgA (g/L)	IgG (g/L)	IgM (g/L)	IgA (g/L)	IgG (g/L)	IgM (g/L)
Vit E mg/kg							
0		1.135	4.239	0.837[b]	1.599	7.148	0.967
100		1.169	4.234	1.003[a]	1.524	7.279	1.038
Se sources							
NS		1.053[b]	3.695	0.875	1.357[b]	6.556[b]	0.941
SS		1.101[b]	4.439	0.966	1.645[a]	7.505[a]	1.040
ADS18-Se		1.302[a]	4.577	0.917	1.482[ab]	7.577[a]	1.027
SEM		0.039	0.179	0.032	0.074	0.181	0.020
p Values							
Vit		0.618	0.987	0.004	0.547	0.682	0.018
Se		0.019	0.105	0.378	0.011	0.028	0.042
Se*Vit		0.354	0.364	0.134	0.174	0.201	0.032
Vit E 0	NS	0.987	3.353	0.723	1.387	6.078	0.938[b]
	SS	1.153	4.690	0.888	2.033	7.690	0.999[a]
	ADS18-Se	1.263	4.675	0.899	1.378	7.676	1.036[a]
Vit E 100	NS	1.118	4.035	1.028	1.328	7.036	0.943[b]
	SS	1.048	4.187	1.045	1.659	7.321	0.940[b]
	ADS18-Se	1.342	4.479	0.936	1.588	7.479	1.017[a]
SEM		0.039	0.179	0.031	0.073	0.180	0.020

[a-b]means with different superscripts within a column-subgroup are significantly different ($P < 0.05$)
[a-b]means with different superscripts within a column of significant interaction are significantly different ($P < 0.05$)
NS no Se supplement, SS sodium selenite, ADS18-Se bacterial organic Se
Experimental unit, ($n = 12$)

in Table 5. The *Lactobacilli* spp. in the group of birds treated with ADS18-Se was significantly higher than the SS and NS treated groups. Moreover, ADS18-Se supplementation was associated with the highest *Bifidobacteria* spp., and the lowest *E.coli* and *Salmonella* spp. compared to SS and NS groups, however, the difference between ADS18-Se and SS group was insignificant.

On the other hand, dietary supplementation of Vit E had no effect on ceacum microbial population except for moderate reduction observed in *Salmonella* spp. count, which was significantly ($P < 0.05$) different compared to un-supplemented diet.

Splenic cytokines gene expression

The effect of Se and Vit E on spleen cytokines gene expression is shown in Table 6. Selenium × Vit E interactions were significant ($p < 0.0001$) for a pro-inflammatory cytokine (TNF-α, IFN-γ) and anti-inflammatory cytokine

Table 5 Main effect of dietary selenium sources and Vit E levels on ceacum microbial population of 42-day broiler chickens

Parameters	Se			Vit E		SEM	p values		
Log 10 copy no/g ceacum	NS	SS	ADS18-Se	0	100		Se	Vit	Se*Vit
Lactobacilli spp.	6.91[b]	6.98[b]	7.74[a]	7.03	7.33	0.099	0.001	0.699	0.060
Bifidobacteria spp.	7.01[b]	7.57[ab]	8.21[a]	7.40	7.65	0.163	0.029	0.489	0.145
Enterobacteria spp.	4.20	4.02	4.53	4.23	4.25	0.087	0.146	0.914	0.784
Enterococcus spp.	6.86	7.25	6.88	7.08	6.76	0.081	0.128	0.118	0.240
E.coli	4.56[a]	4.33[ab]	4.21[b]	4.44	4.34	0.049	0.012	0.315	0.787
Salmonella spp.	3.41[a]	3.04[ab]	2.80[b]	3.38[a]	2.84[b]	0.105	0.031	0.006	0.126

[a-b]Means with different superscripts within a row-subgroup are significantly different ($P < 0.05$). NS no Se supplement, SS sodium selenite, ADS18-Se bacterial organic Se. Experimental unit, ($n = 12$)

Table 6 Effects of dietary selenium sources and vitamin E levels on cytokines gene expression of 42-day broiler chickens

Items		TNF-	IFN-γ	IL-2	IL-10
Vit E mg/kg					
0		0.879	0.786	2.019	2.066
100		1.100	0.808	3.019	4.609
Se sources					
NS		0.854	0.911	1.524	2.829
SS		1.134	0.798	3.029	3.633
ADS18-Se		0.981	0.682	3.006	3.551
SEM		0.226	0.169	0.259	0.296
P values					
Vit		0.0048	0.6935	<.0001	<.0001
Se		0.0133	0.0117	<.0001	<.0006
Se*Vit		<.0001	<.0001	<.0001	<.0001
Vit E 0	NS	1.000[a]	1.000[a]	1.000[c]	1.000[c]
	SS	0.992[a]	0.875[b]	1.203[b]	2.796[b]
	ADS18-Se	0.644[b]	0.483[c]	2.756[a]	2.402[b]
Vit E 100	NS	0.708[b]	0.822[b]	1.048[c]	4.658[a]
	SS	0.975[a]	0.720[b]	3.655[a]	4.470[a]
	ADS18-Se	0.918[a]	0.882[b]	2.257[b]	4.699[a]
SEM		0.061	0.042	0.258	0.294

[a-b]Means with different superscripts within a row-subgroup are significantly different ($P < 0.05$)
[a-c]means with different superscripts within a column are significantly different ($P < 0.05$)
NS no Se supplement, SS sodium selenite, ADS18-Se bacterial organic Se. Experimental unit, ($n = 12$)

(IL-2, IL-10). Without Vit E supplementation, Dietary Se of ADS18 down-regulated the TNF-α and IFN-γ significantly compared to SS and NS groups, and up-regulated the IL-2 and IL-10 significantly compared to other treatments, however, on IL-10 the effect of SS was higher compared to ADS18-Se. On the other hand, combination of either SS or ADS18-Se with Vit E had no significant effect on IFN-γ and IL-10 compared to Vit E alone, while Vit E alone showed the significantly lowest TNF-α compared to the Se combinations. Moreover, both Se combinations up-regulated IL-2 significantly compared to Vit E alone, but the SS combination was significantly higher than ADS18-Se.

Furthermore, it is clear that the combination of both sources of Se with the Vit E showed no better regulation compared to using each source alone, except for significant up-regulation observed on IL-10 of both sources, and up-regulation of 1 L-2 observed on SS.

Body weight, feed intake and lymphoid organ weights

The effects of vitamin E, Se sources, and their different combinations on the body weight, feed intake and lymphoid organ weights are shown in Table 7. The

final body weight was improved significantly ($P < 0.05$) when the diet was supplemented with Vit E compared to un-supplemented diet, Moreover, both SS and ADS18-Se showed high final body weight compared to NS group. The ADFI showed that dietary Vit E lowered ADFI significantly compared to un-supplemented diet, Moreover Se supplementation in the form of SS or ADS18-Se showed significant reduction in ADFI compared to NS diet.

All dietary Se sources and Vit E supplementation had no significant effect on lymphoid organ weights. Moreover, there were no synergistic effects between Se and Vit E on lymphoid organ weights.

Discussion

Immune system is a main factor that influences the animal's health and performance. It is well known that Se and Vit E can act synergistically and affect biological processes mainly, antioxidant and immunity [3]. Dietary Vit E and Se combination improved the humoral immunity and provided better immunity response through their role on free radical elimination and oxidative stress stability of the immune cells [8] Generally, the results of this study indicated that there are synergistic effects between Vit E and Se on plasma immunoglobulin, which appeared just in plasma IgM level Table 4. Combination of Vit E with bacterial organic Se of ADS18 significantly increased plasma IgM concentration in broiler chickens compared with the chicks fed SS- Vit E complex or Vit E alone. This result was consistent with the finding that Vit E and Se combination improved the humoral immunity and provided better immunity response [8, 11], when a dietary vitamin E (0, 125 and 250 mg/kg), selenium (Se, 0, 0.5 and 1 mg/kg), and their different combinations on humoral immunity was examined by intravenous injection of 7% sheep red blood cell (SRBC) followed by evaluation of serum for antibody titers in primary and secondary responses. Vitamin E and Se showed interactive effects on antiSRBC titers. Dietary vitamin E and Se alone also resulted in improvement of primary and secondary antibody responses [11]. On the other hand, Supplementation of 200 mg vitamin E/kg and 0·2 mg selenium/kg resulted in a significantly higher antibody titres, that associated with an increased serum concentration of total immunoglobulins and circulatory immune complexes [8]. Moreover, combined Vit E and Se, significantly increased serum IgG and IgM levels in mice after their exposure to sodium azide [9] .

Dietary supplementation of Vit E in broiler chicken improved primary and secondary antibody responses after heat stress challenge [18]. According to Habibian et al. [11], supplementation of Vit E at both 125 and 250 mg/kg levels showed no effect on IgM level in broiler chickens. Furthermore, Vit E supplementation had no significant effect on immunoglobulin levels of IgA, IgM, and IgG in the serum of duck [19]. This partially agreed with this

Table 7 Main effect means of dietary selenium sources and vitamin E levels on body weight, feed intake and lymphoid organ weight of 42-day broiler chickens

Items (g)	Se			Vit E		SEM	P values		
	NS	SS	ADS18-Se	0	100		Se	Vit	Se* Vit
Initial BW	41.9	42.1	43.3	43.2	42.5	0.28	0.325	0.135	0.543
Final BW	2747.7[b]	2858.3[a]	2900.8[a]	2799.7[b]	2871.4[a]	21.79	0.004	0.048	0.565
Average DFI	98.34[a]	92.67 [b]	90.89[b]	99.71[a]	94.23[b]	1.21	≤.0001	0.001	0.061
Lymphoid organ weight (% of BW)									
Thymus	0.204	0.169	0.209	0.205	0.178	0.014	0.483	0.367	0.272
Bursa	0.064	0.059	0.057	0.053	0.067	0.006	0.873	0.218	0.152
Spleen	0.123	0.137	0.114	0.115	0.138	0.010	0.755	0.365	0.788

[a-b] Means with different superscripts within a row-subgroup are significantly different (P < 0.05)
NS no Se supplement, SS sodium selenite, ADS18-Se, bacterial organic Se
BW body weight, DFI daily feed intake per pen (n = 6)

study's finding that there was no significant effect observed in IgA and IgG levels due to Vit E supplementation, however IgM level was significantly increased at day 21, but at day 42 the effect was significantly interactive with Se factor.

On the other hand, Khan et al. [20], demonstrated that dietary Se (inorganic Se) could improve immunity and significantly enhance the synthesis of IgA and IgG in broilers. This was clearly observed in this study, that Se supplementation of both inorganic and bacterial organic sources improved the bird's immunity via IgA, IgG, and IgM elevation at day 42, but at day 21 bacterial organic Se showed significantly highest IgG level compared to SS and NS groups Table 5. However, our study concern about the different Se sources mainly the bacterial organic Se as unusual source of Se. This could be explained by the role of Se in protection and thus activation of B-lymphocytes cells which is the source of immunoglobulin [21]. Moreover, Se could increase the interleukin 2 receptors on the surface of lymphocytes [22].

The regulation of gut microbiota can be achieved via dietary supplements which have the ability to stimulate the growth of beneficial bacteria, or selectively can suppress the activity and growth of pathogenic bacteria. Trace elements as a diet component may affect the diversity of intestinal microbiota [23]. A study conducted by Molan et al. [24], revealed that the addition of sodium selenite or sodium selenate alone in the concentration of (1, 2, 3, 4, and 5 μg/ml) for each source, or their combination with China green tea to MRS culture of *Lactobacillus rhamnosus* and *Bifidobacterium breve*, enhanced their growth significantly compared to the control MRS. Oral supplementation of Se- china tea extract significantly (P < 0.05) increased the count of both *Lactobacillus* spp. and *Bifidobacterium* spp. in rat's ceacum compared to tea extract without Se [25]. Moreover, bacterial culture of *Lactobacillus casei rhamnosus* showed improved

cell viability when Se and cadmium (Cd) were added to the culture compared to the culture contained in the Cd alone [26]. These studies supported the finding of the current study that Se supplementation enhances the population of ceacum *Lactobacillus* spp. and *Bifidobacterium* spp. compared to the basal diet, but the Se sourced from ADS18 showed better count than SS treatment.

Furthermore, the current study showed that Se supplementation of inorganic and bacterial organic Se reduced the ceacum numbers of *E-coli* and *Salmonella* spp., but the difference was significant just between ADS18-Se and NS groups. In the same manner, feeding of probiotics or Se-enriched probiotics to piglets was associated with higher *Lactobacillus* spp. count and lower *E-coli* compared to the basal diet and sodium selenite diet [27]. Selenium-enriched probiotics also decreased *E-coli* via undefined antimicrobial metabolites [28]. In contrast, dietary Se-yeast in chickens showed no effect on the caecal microbiota or *Campylobacter jejuni* colonisation [29]. Intestinal microbiota, are probably sensitive to some trace elements such as Se, which is important for normal function for some bacteria, however, at the same time is considered a toxic element to other bacteria. Therefore, changes in dietary Se which acts as an antioxidant may modulate the diversity of intestinal microbiota via oxidative stress suppression and providing a better medium for the growth of beneficial bacteria. Lactic acids and *Bifidobacterium* spp. are able to incorporate Se from the growth medium to their cells [26, 30], which may enhance their growth and activity. Moreover, lactic acid bacteria have a role in inhibiting the colonization of pathogenic microorganisms through their secreted hydrogen peroxide, acids, and other antimicrobial substances. Published data on the effect of Vit E on caecum microorganisms are scant, thus, the reduction in *Salmonella* spp. count in the present study due to Vit E supplementation remain unclear.

Cytokines are small protein messengers released by the host as immune responses to infection, inflammation, and trauma. Some cytokines are anti-inflammatory and others are pro-inflammatory, and this also plays a role in the up-regulation of inflammatory reactions [31]. TNF-α, IFN-γ, and IL2 are pro-inflammatory cytokines that are produced by activated monocytes, macrophages, T cells, and natural killer cells. Adequate Se supplementation may enhance the immunity and decrease the host susceptibility to diseases [32]. Infected Se- deficient mice were associated with significant increases in the expression of cytokines IL-6, TNF-α, IFN-γ IL-18, and IL-10 in the liver, while Se adequate mice showed over-expression in the liver IL-10 [33]. However, in the present study, there was significant interaction between Se and Vit E on all examined splenic anti-inflammatory and pro-inflammatory cytokines expression, dietary Se of both ADS18 and SS down-regulated the IFN-γ and up-regulated IL-2 and IL-10 significantly compared to NS group, while ADS18 showed significant down-regulation of TNF-α level compared to both SS and NS groups. The down-regulation of pro-inflammatory cytokines observed in this study was due to IL-10 elevation, which is a known potent anti-inflammatory cytokine and deactivator of pro-inflammatory cytokine synthesis, macrophage, and monocyte [31]. However, the IL-2 up-regulation in this study was unexpected but according to Yang et al. [34], IL-2, is also required for the growth, proliferation, and differentiation of T cells, and the spleen sight is highly enriched with T cells, B cells, and monocytes.

On the other hand, Vit E supplementation down-regulated the pro-inflammatory cytokines expression in chickens receiving lipopolysaccharide [35]. The present study indicated that combination of either SS or ADS18-Se with Vit E had no significant effect on IFN- γ and IL-10 compared to Vit E alone, while Vit E alone showed the significantly lowest TNF-αcompared to both Se combinations. To the best of the researcher's knowledge, there is no report about the effect of Se and Vit E combination on splenic cytokines expression, however, previous studies indicated that dietary Vit E could lower pro-inflammatory cytokine expression through the NF-κB pathway alteration [36]. On the other hand, dietary Se-regulated inflammatory cytokines via NF-κB and MAPK signaling pathways [37]. Therefore, it is clear that, Se can induce immune response more than Vit E, through activation of anti-inflammatory cytokines and suppression of pro-inflammatory cytokines. The balance between anti-inflammatory and pro-inflammatory cytokines determines the severity of the disease.

In the current study, there was improvement in the final body weight and ADFI due to Vit E supplementation, and due to dietary Se either in bacterial organic or inorganic form. This was proved by the finding that supplementation of organic selenium and Vit E in the layer diet was efficient for improving performance [38]. Supplementation of 200 mg/kg of Vit E in broiler diet improved weight gain and feed intake compared to the basal diet [39]. In contrast, dietary Vit E and Se had no effect on the body weight of layer hens [40], and different Vit E levels showed no significant changes in the broiler performance [41]. On the other hand, present study showed that both Se and Vit E supplementation had no significant effect on the lymphoid organ weights (thymus, bursa, and spleen) in broiler chickens. These findings are consistent with previous results of [18] who revealed that Vit E supplementation could not affect the lymphoid organ. Moreover, Habibian et al. [11] indicated that dietary Se had no positive effect on the lymphoid organ weights under heat stress, however, the dietary inclusion of Vit E showed improvement of the relative weights of lymphoid organs. Along the same lines of the findings of this study, no synergestic effect between Se and Vit E were observed for relative lymphoid organ weights in the study conducted by Habibian et al. [11], however, Swain et al. [10] reported that dietary Se and Vit E had a synergestic effect on the lymphoid organ weights in broiler chickens under normal environmental conditions.The reason for this difference is not clear.

Conclusion

In conclusion, the present study showed that dietary supplementation of bacterial organic Se of ADS18 in broiler chickens increased the ceacum beneficial bacteria, and support the immune system more than SS. The synergistic effect of Se and Vit E was apparent on the plasma IgM levels and splenic cytokines gene expression. The inclusion of 100 mg/kg Vit E with 0.3 mg/kg ADS18-Se, effectively could support the immune system through regulation of some cytokines expression and immunoglobulin levels more than using ADS18-Se alone, while there was no difference between using SS alone or combined with Vit E.

Abbreviations

ADS18: Stenotrophomonas maltophilia; IFNγ: Interferon gamma; IgA: Immunoglobulin A; IgG: Immunoglobulin G; IgM: Immunoglobulin M; IL-10: Interleukin 10; IL-2: Interleukin-2; Se: Selenium; SS: Sodium selenite; TNFα: tumor necrosis factor alpha; Vit E: Vitamin E

Funding

This study was financed by the Fundamental Research Grant Scheme (FRGS 5524272) granted by Malaysian Ministry of Higher Education. A.M.D. was a recipient of scholarship from the Ministry of Higher Education and Scientific Research of Sudan and University of Khartoum, Sudan.

Authors' contributions

A.M.D. analysed and interpreted data regarding birds performance and carried out laboratory analysis. M.F.J was a major contributor in the part of gene expression and qPCR. A.M.D., T.C.L, A.Q.S and A.A.S participated in the whole design of the study and performed the statistical analysis and contributed to the preparation of the manuscript. All authors read and approved the final manuscript.

Consent for publication
"Not applicable"

Competing interests
The authors declare that they have no competing interests.

Author details
[1]Department of Animal Science, Faculty of Agriculture, Universiti Putra Malaysia, 43400 Serdang, Selangor, Malaysia. [2]Department of Animal Nutrition, Faculty of Animal Production, University of Khartoum, Khartoum, Sudan. [3]Institute of Tropical Agriculture, Universiti Putra Malaysia, 43400 Serdang, Selangor, Malaysia.

References
1. Meydani SN, Chung H, Han SN. Effect of selenium and vitamin E status on host defense and resistance to infection. In: Micronutrient Deficiencies in the First Months of Life, vol. 52. Basel: Karger Publishers; 2003. p. 165–80.
2. Hernken R., Harmon R., Trammel S. Selenium of dairy cattle: a role for organic selenium. In: Jacques TPL and KA, editor. Biotechnol. Feed Ind. Loughborough, LEC, UK,: proc. Alltech 14th Ann. Symp. Nottingham: Nottingham University press; 1998. p. 797–803.
3. Liu Q, Lanari MC, Schaefer DM. A review of dietary vitamin E supplementation for improvement of beef quality. J Anim Sci. 1995;73:3131–40.
4. Hoffmann PR, Berry MJ. The influence of selenium on immune responses. Mol Nutr Food Res. 2008;52(11):1273–80.
5. Bellinger FP, Raman AV, Reeves MA, Berry MJ. Regulation and function of selenoproteins in human disease. Biochem J. 2009;422(1):11–22.
6. Köhrle J, Brigelius-Flohé R, Böck A, Gärtner R, Meyer O, Flohé L. Selenium in biology: facts and medical perspectives. Biol Chem. 2000;381(9–10):849–64.
7. Arthur JR, McKenzie RC, Beckett GJ. Selenium in the immune system. J Nutr. 2003;133(5):1457S–9S.
8. Singh H, Sodhi S, Kaur R. Effects of dietary supplements of selenium, vitamin E or combinations of the two on antibody responses of broilers. Br Poult Sci. 2006;47:714–9.
9. El-Shenawy NS, AL-Harbi MS, Hamza RZ. Effect of vitamin E and selenium separately and in combination on biochemical, immunological and histological changes induced by sodium azide in male mice. Exp Toxicol Pathol. 2015;67:65–76.
10. Swain BK, Johri TS, Majumdar S. Effect of supplementation of vitamin E, selenium and their different combinations on the performance and immune response of broilers. Br Poult Sci. 2000;41:287–92.
11. Habibian M, Ghazi S, Moeini MM, Abdolmohammadi A. Effects of dietary selenium and vitamin E on immune response and biological blood parameters of broilers reared under thermoneutral or heat stress conditions. Int J Biometeorol. 2014;58:741–52.
12. Suzuki KT. Metabolomics of selenium: se metabolites based on speciation studies. J Health Sci. 2005;51(2):107–14.
13. Burk RF, Hill KE, Motley AK. Selenoprotein metabolism and function: evidence for more than one function for Selenoprotein P, 2. J Nutr. 2003;133(5):1517S–20S.
14. Surai PF. Natural antioxidants in avian nutrition and Reproduction. Nottingham: Nottingham University Press; 2002.
15. Dalia AM, Loh TC, Sazili AQ, Jahromi MF, Samsudin AA. The effect of dietary bacterial organic selenium on growth performance, antioxidant capacity, and Selenoproteins gene expression in broiler chickens. BMC Vet Res. 2017;13:254.
16. Navidshad B, Liang JB, Jahromi MF. Correlation coefficients between different methods of expressing bacterial quantification using real time PCR. Int J Mol Sci. 2012;13:2119–32.
17. Pfaffl MW. A new mathematical model for relative quantification in real-time RT-PCR. Nucleic Acids Res. 2001;29:e45.
18. Niu Z, Liu F, Yan Q, Li W. Effects of different levels of vitamin E on growth performance and immune responses of broilers under heat stress. Poult Sci. 2009;88(10):2101–7. 13
19. He J, Zhang KY, Chen DW, Ding XM, Feng GD, Ao X. Effects of vitamin E and selenium yeast on growth performance and immune function in ducks fed maize naturally contaminated with aflatoxin B1. Livest Sci. 2013;152:200–7.
20. Khan MZI, Akter SH, Islam MN, Karim MR, Islam MR, Kon Y. The effect of selenium and vitamin e on the lymphocytes and immunoglobulin-containing plasma cells in the lymphoid organ and mucosa-associated lymphatic tissues of broiler chickens. J Vet Med Ser C Anat Histol Embryol. 2008;37:52–9.
21. Combs G, Combs S Jr. The role of selenium in nutrition. In: Academic Press, Inc; 1986.
22. Roy M, Kiremidjian-Schumacher L, Wishe HI, Cohen MW, Stotzky G. Effect of selenium on the expression of high affinity interleukin 2 receptors. Proc Soc Exp Biol Med. 1992:36–43.
23. Kasaikina MV, Kravtsova MA, Lee BC, Seravalli J, Peterson DA, Walter J, et al. Dietary selenium affects host selenoproteome expression by influencing the gut microbiota. FASEB J. 2011;25:2492–9.
24. Molan AL, Flanagan J, Wei W, Moughan PJ. Selenium-containing green tea has higher antioxidant and prebiotic activities than regular green tea. Food Chem. 2009;114:829–35.
25. Molan AL. Antioxidant and prebiotic activities of selenium-containing green tea. Nutrients. 2013;29:476–7.
26. Araúz ILC, Afton S, Wrobel K, Caruso JA, Corona JFG, Wrobel K. Study on the protective role of selenium against cadmium toxicity in lactic acid bacteria: an advanced application of ICP-MS. J Hazard Mater. 2008;153:1157–64.
27. Lv CH, Wang T, Regmi N, Chen X, Huang K, Liao SF. Effects of dietary supplementation of selenium-enriched probiotics on production performance and intestinal microbiota of weanling piglets raised under high ambient temperature. J Anim Physiol Anim Nutr. 2015;99:1161–71.
28. Yang J, Huang K, Qin S, Wu X, Zhao Z, Chen F. Antibacterial action of selenium-enriched probiotics against pathogenic Escherichia coli. Dig Dis Sci. 2009;54:246–54.
29. Thibodeau A, Letellier A, Yergeau É, Larrivière-Gauthier G, Fravalo P. Lack of evidence that selenium-yeast improves chicken health and modulates the caecal microbiota in the context of colonization by Campylobacter jejuni. Front Microbiol. 2017;8:1–9.
30. Zhang B, Zhou K, Zhang J, Chen Q, Liu G, Shang N, et al. Accumulation and species distribution of selenium in se-enriched bacterial cells of the Bifidobacterium animalis 01. Food Chem. 2009;115:727–34.
31. Dinarello CA. Proinflammatory cytokines. Chest. 2000;118:503–8.
32. Tsuji PA, Carlson BA, Anderson CB, Seifried HE, Hatfield DL, Howard MT. Dietary selenium levels affect selenoprotein expression and support the interferon-γ and IL-6 immune response pathways in mice. Nutrients. 2015;7:6529–49.
33. Wang C, Wang H, Luo J, Hu Y, Wei L, Duan M, et al. Selenium deficiency impairs host innate immune response and induces susceptibility to Listeria monocytogenes infection. BMC Immunol. 2009;10:55.
34. Yang J, Liu L, Sheikhahmadi A, Wang Y, Li C, Jiao H, et al. Effects of corticosterone and dietary energy on immune function of broiler chickens. PLoS One. 2015;10:1–14.
35. Leshchinsky TV, Klasing KC. Profile of chicken cytokines induced by lipopolysaccharide is modulated by dietary alpha-tocopheryl acetate. Poult Sci. 2003;82:1266–73.
36. Sen CK, Packer L. Antioxidant and redox regulation of gene transcription. FASEB J. 1996;10:709–20.
37. Zhang W, Zhang R, Wang T, Jiang H, Guo M, Zhou E, et al. Selenium inhibits LPS-induced pro-inflammatory gene expression by modulating MAPK and NF-κB signaling pathways in mouse mammary epithelial cells in primary culture. Inflammation. 2014;37:478–85.
38. Ziaei N, Pour EE. The effects of different levels of vitamin-E and organic selenium on performance and immune response of laying hens. Afr J Biotechnol. 2013;12(24)
39. Maini S, Rastogi SK, Korde JP, Madan AK, Shukla SK. Evaluation of oxidative stress and its amelioration through certain antioxidants in broilers during summer. J Poult Sci. 2007;44(3):339–47.
40. Zanini SF, Torres CAA, Bragagnolo N, Turatti JM, Silva MG, Zanini MS. Effect of oil sources and vitamin E levels in the diet on the composition of fatty acids in rooster thigh and chest meat. J Sci Food Agric. 2004;84(7):672–82.

41. Albuquerque D, Lopes JB, Ferraz MS, Ribeiro MN, Silva SR, Costa E, Lima DC, Ferreira JD, Gomes PE, Lopes JC. Vitamin E and organic selenium for broilers from 22 to 42 days old: performance and carcass traits. An Acad Bras Cienc. 2017;89(2):1259–68.

42. Jahromi MF, Altaher YW, Shokryazdan P, Ebrahimi R, Ebrahimi M, Idrus Z, et al. Dietary supplementation of a mixture of lactobacillus strains enhances performance of broiler chickens raised under heat stress conditions. Int J Biometeorol. 2016;60:1099–110.

43. Bartosch S, Fite A, Macfarlane GT, Mcmurdo MET. Characterization of bacterial communities in feces from healthy elderly volunteers and hospitalized elderly patients by using real-time PCR and effects of antibiotic treatment on the fecal microbiota. Appl Environ Microbiol. 2004;70:3575–81.

44. Nam H-M, Srinivasan V, Gillespie BE, Murinda SE, Oliver SP. Application of SYBR green real-time PCR assay for specific detection of *Salmonella* spp. in dairy farm environmental samples. Int J Food Microbiol. 2005;102:161–71.

45. Rasoli M, Yeap SK, Tan SW, Moeini H, Ideris A, Bejo MH, et al. Alteration in lymphocyte responses, cytokine and chemokine profiles in chickens infected with genotype VII and VIII velogenic Newcastle disease virus. Comp Immunol Microbiol Infect Dis. 2014;37:11–21.

46. Dai M, Wu S, Feng M, Feng S, Sun C, Bai D, et al. Recombinant chicken interferon-alpha inhibits the replication of exogenous avian leukosis virus (ALV) in DF-1 cells. Mol Immunol. 2016;76:62–9.

16

Modulation of ovine SBD-1 expression by *Saccharomyces cerevisiae* in ovine ruminal epithelial cells

Xin Jin[1,2†] , Man Zhang[1,2†], Xue-min Zhu[1,2,3], Yan-ru Fan[1,2], Chen-guang Du[1,2,4], Hua-er Bao[1,2], Siri-guleng Xu[1,2], Qiao-zhen Tian[1,2], Yun-he Wang[1,2] and Yin-feng Yang[1,2*]

Abstract

Background: The ovine rumen is involved in host defense responses and acts as the immune interface with the environment. The ruminal mucosal epithelium plays an important role in innate immunity and secretes antimicrobial innate immune molecules that have bactericidal activity against a variety of pathogens. Defensins are cationic peptides that are produced by the mucosal epithelia and have broad-spectrum antimicrobial activity. Sheep β-defensin-1 (SBD-1) is one of the most important antibacterial peptides in the rumen. The expression of SBD-1 is regulated by the probiotic, *Saccharomyces cerevisiae* (S.c); however, the regulatory mechanism has not yet been elucidated. In the current study, the effects of S.c on the expression and secretion of SBD-1 in ovine ruminal epithelial cells were investigated using quantitative real-time PCR (qPCR) and enzyme-linked immunosorbent assay (ELISA). In addition, specific inhibitors were used to block the nuclear factor kappa-light-chain enhancer of activated B cells (NF-κB), p38, JNK, and ERK1/2 signalling pathways separately or simultaneously, to determine the regulatory mechanism(s) governing S.c-induced SBD-1 upregulation.

Results: Incubation with S.c induced release of SBD-1 by ovine ruminal epithelial cells, with SBD-1 expression peaking after 12 h of incubation. The highest SBD-1 expression levels were achieved after treatment with 5.2 × 10^7 CFU·mL^{−1} S.c. Treatment with S.c resulted in significantly increased NF-κB, p38, JNK, ERK1/2, TLR2, and MyD88 mRNA expression. Whereas inhibition of mitogen-activated protein kinases (MAPKs) and NF-κB gene expression led to a decrease in SBD-1 expression.

Conclusions: S.c was induced SBD-1 expression and the S.c-induced up-regulation of SBD-1 expression may be related to TLR2 and MyD88 in ovine ruminal epithelial cells. This is likely simultaneously regulated by the MAPKs and NF-κB pathways with the p38 axis of the MAPKs pathway acting as the primary regulator. Thus, the pathways regulating S.c-induced SBD-1 expression may be related to TLR2-MyD88-NF-κB/MAPKs, with the TLR2-MyD88-p38 component of the TLR2-MyD88-MAPKs signalling acting as the main pathway.

Keywords: Sheep, Ruminal epithelium, *Saccharomyces cerevisiae*, SBD-1, Modulation, Signalling pathway

* Correspondence: nmyangyinfeng@imau.edu.cn
†Equal contributors
[1]Veterinary Medicine College of Inner Mongolia Agricultural University, Hohhot 010018, People's Republic of China
[2]Key Laboratory of Clinical Diagnosis and Treatment Technology in Animal Disease, Ministry of Agriculture, Hohhot 010018, People's Republic of China
Full list of author information is available at the end of the article

Background

Defensins, a group of broad-spectrum antimicrobial agents secreted by epithelial cells in response to microbial infection and stimulation from the main components of microbial pathogens, have recently garnered a lot of attention. Defensins are small-molecular-weight peptides, generally consisting of 29–42 amino acids, which play an important role in both the innate and adaptive immune systems of vertebrates [1–3]. In contrast, pathogen defense in invertebrates and plants occurs exclusively via mechanisms involved in innate immunity [4, 5].

Defensins have a lethal effect on both gram-negative and gram-positive bacteria, as well as on viruses and fungi [6–8]. Defensins are divided into 3 main classes, based on different structural characteristics: α-, β-, and θ-defensins. To date, α- and θ-defensins have only been identified in mammals [6, 9]. The expression of α-defensin genes has been observed in humans [10], mice [11], rhesus macaques [12], rats [13], rabbits [14], guinea pigs [15], hamsters [16], and horses [17]. The α-defensins have also been identified in opossum [18], elephant, and hedgehog tenrec genomes in silico [19], but are absent from cattle [20] and dog genomes [21]. The θ-defensins have only been identified in the rhesus macaque (*Macaca mulatta*) and olive baboon (*Papio anubis*) [22]. The β-Defensins have been found in various vertebrates, including cows [23], humans [24], mice [25], birds [26], reptiles [27], and fish [28]. Thus far, only beta defensin-1 (BD-1) and beta defensin-2 (BD-2) have been identified in sheep [29]. In adult sheep, SBD-2 expression was found to be confined to the tongue, ileum, and colon, while SBD-1 expression was identified in the entire digestive tract (from the tongue to the colon), with highest expression located in the rumen [30, 31]. This suggests that β-defensins constitute an important component of ovine rumen innate immunity.

Animal feed producers have used specific strains of *S.c* as feed supplements, based on claims that these products can improve feed intake [32, 33], weight gain [34], fiber digestion [35, 36], and reduce the need for antibiotic use. It has also been reported that live yeast can stabilize the rumen pH [37, 38]. In addition to the nutritional value of yeast, there is evidence that yeast probiotics and components, such as zymosan, can increase the production of the host defense peptide, cathelicidin, and the cytokine, IL-1β, in the intestinal epithelial cell line RTgutGC, at the mRNA and protein levels [39]. In addition, whole yeast (*S.c*), β-glucan and laminaran have been used as immunostimulants in farmed Nile tilapia. The β-glucans have been used in farmed Nile tilapia under stressful, immune-depressive conditions, in order to increase resistance to disease [40]. Therefore, it is possible that dietary supplementation with yeast probiotics and/or their components may improve ovine innate immunity in animals that are vulnerable to disease.

Nonetheless, there is a paucity of information concerning the role and regulation of SBD-1 gene expression in the sheep rumen; particularly whether *S.c* can modulate SBD-1 expression. In this study, the expression of SBD-1 was investigated in ovine ruminal epithelial cells treated with *S.c* using qPCR and ELISA assays. In addition, the effect of the p38, ERK1/2, JNK, and NF-κB– pathways on SBD-1 expression in ruminal epithelial cell culture was examined. The results indicated that *S.c* provides a stimulus that may regulate defensins by MAPKs and NF-κB pathways.

Methods

Reagents

The NF-κB inhibitor, PDTC, the ERK1/2 inhibitor, PD98059, the p38 inhibitor, SB202190, and the JNK inhibitor, SP600125, were purchased from Sigma Chem. Co. (Munich, Germany). All other chemicals used were of analytical grade and obtained from commercial sources.

Fungal strains and culture conditions

The *S.c* used in this study was purchased from the Chinese microbial strain network (code: CGMCC 2. 161). The yeast strains were inoculated in 100 mL malt extract medium and incubated for 48 h at 28 °C in an orbital shaker (180 rpm).

Ovine ruminal epithelial cells and culture conditions

Ten adult Mongolian sheep (5 ewes and 5 rams, aged 10–15 months) were obtained from Inner Mongolia Agricultural University (IMAU) Experimental Animal Center. None of the sheep had clinical signs of parasitic or infectious disease. The sheep were euthanized with an overdose of the proprietary euthanasia solution Euthasol (pentobarbital sodium 100 mg/kg and phenytoin sodium 10 mg/kg) and the rumens were harvested. Rumen epithelial cells were obtained from each of the 10 sheep and were tested separately. This study was approved by the Institutional Animal Care and Use Committee of the IMAU (License No. SYXK, Inner Mongolia, 2014–0008) with adherence to IMAU guidelines.

After euthanasia, the rumen tissue (25 cm^2) was immediately extracted, flushed with physiological saline, and placed in ice-cold phosphate buffered saline (PBS; Sigma-Aldrich) supplemented with 5% penicillin/streptomycin (Sigma). The ruminal epithelial cells were cultured as previously described [41, 42]. All procedures were performed under sterile conditions. The tissue was washed several times with PBS and the mucosa was removed from the underlying epithelium and washed 3 times in PBS supplemented with 1 mg/mL penicillin, 500 μg/mL streptomycin, 100 μg/mL gentamicin, and 50 μg/mL amphotericin. Seven digestions of the ruminal muco-sal tissue were performed with 0.25% pancreatin (Sigma) incubated at 37 °C for 45, 40, 30, 20, 15, 8, and 3 min; the digestion products were then observed under a microscope. A large number of small cells were observed after the third digestion that were pre-dominantly oval or round in shape, had smooth edges, and high refractive indexes. Ruminal tissue was removed and the cell pellet was resuspended in DMEM containing 20% fetal bovine serum (FBS, ap-proximately 20 mL) to stop enzymatic digestion and then concentrated by centrifugation at 1000 rpm for 6 min. The cell pellet was again resuspended in DMEM, agitated by pipetting up and down using a movette pipette 3–5 times, and cultured at 37 °C and 5% CO_2 in DMEM/F12 supplemented with 20% heat-inactivated FBS, 200 µg/mL penicillin, 100 µg/mL streptomycin, 50 µg/mL gentamicin, 5 µg/mL ampho-tericin, 2 µg/mL insulin-protein- selenium additive, and 2 µg/mL β-mercaptoethanol. The cells remained attached to the cell culture plate for more than 96 h and the medium was replaced every 2 d. Once the number of primary cells grew to more than 85% confluence, the cells were passaged into 12-well flat-bottom culture plates.

Induction tests

After reaching 80–90% confluence, the ovine ruminal epithelial cells were washed 3 times with PBS containing 1% penicillin/streptomycin and then passaged into 12-well flat-bottom culture plates containing 1 mL DMEM/ F12 medium, without FBS or antibiotics, and were incu-bated at 37 °C and 5% CO_2 for a 24 h starvation treat-ment. Following the starvation treatment, the cells were washed 3 times with PBS and placed into 900 µL DMEM/F12 without FBS or antibiotics. The cells were then randomly divided into 6 groups: 5 S.c-treated groups and 1 control group. The treatment groups were exposed to a range of concentrations (5.2×10^8, 5.2×10^7, 5.2×10^6, 5.2×10^5, 5.2×10^4 CFU·mL^{-1}) of S.c (100 µL) at 37 °C and 5% CO_2 for 2 h; control group cells were cultured in DMEM/F12 medium without S.c. After 2 h of stimulation, the medium was discarded and the cells were washed 3 times with PBS containing 5% amphotericin and incubated for 2, 4, 8, 12, or 24 h in DMEM/F12 with antibiotics. Finally, total RNA was extracted from the cells following induction for 2, 4, 8, 12, or 24 h.

Inhibition tests

The NF-κB, p38, JNK, and ERK1/2 pathways were blocked using specific inhibitors: PDTC (50 µM) for NF-κB, SB202190 (20 µM) for p38, SP600125 (20 µM) for JNK, and PD98059 (20 µM) for ERK1/2. The cells were treated with the inhibitor for 1 h and the 4 different treatment groups were then stimulated with S.c (S.c + PDTC, S.c + PD98059, S.c + SB202190, or S.c + SP600125). Cells treated with inhibitors (PDTC, PD98059, SB202190, SP600125), but not S.c, were the negative controls. Cells treated with S.c, but not inhibitors were the positive con-trols and untreated cells were the blank controls.

Primers

Primers used to detect the expression of target genes (SBD-1, TLR2, MyD88, NF-κB, p38, JNK, ERK1/2) in ovine ruminal epithelial cells treated with S.c are shown in Table 1. The reference gene (β-actin) in the current study was used as a reference gene in a similar previ-ous study [43, 44]. Stable expression of this gene was validated using PCR and Western blot. All primers (Table 1) were designed and synthesized by Sangon Biotech (Shanghai, China).

RNA isolation

After reaching 85–95% confluence in 12-well flat-bottom plates (~ 450,000 cells per well), the epithelial cells were washed with PBS. Total cellular RNA was ex-tracted using RNA Fast2000 (Fastgene, China), in ac-cordance with the manufacturer's instructions. The total RNA concentration and purity were analysed by measur-ing the absorbance at 260 and 280 nm using a Synergy H4 Hybrid microplate reader (BioTek Inc., Winooski, VT, USA). Only samples with an OD 260/280 ratio be-tween 1.8 and 2.0 were included in subsequent studies.

Table 1 Primer sequences for qPCR

Gene names	GenBank accession	Fragment size (bp)	Primer pair sequences (5`-3`)
SBD-1	U75250	206	F: GGCTCCATCACCTGCTCCTC
			R: CGTCTTCGCCTTCTGTTACTTCTT
β-actin	U39357	208	F: GTCACCAACTGGGACGACA
			R: AGGCGTACAGGGACAGCA
TLR2	DQ890157.1	190	F: GTGTCCGCCGTGTGCTGTGC
			R: AGTAGGAATCCCGCTCGCTGTAGG
MyD88	GQ221044.1	203	F: AGGTGCCGTCGGATGGTGGTGGTT
			R: TGGTGGCAGGGGTTAGTGTAGTCA
NF-κB	XM_012119628.1	95	F: CACCTTCTCCCAGCCCTTTG
			R: TGCCACCTCCTCCTCCAG
p38	NM_001142894.1	74	F: CGTTCAGTTCCTTATCTACCAG
			R: GCTCACAGTCTTCATTCACAG
JNK	XM_004002020.3	113	F: ATGACTGCAAAGATGGAAACGA
			R: ATGCTCTGCTTCAGAATCTTGG
ERK1/2	XM_012157699.1	90	F: GCGCTACACCAATCTCTCGT
			R: ATGGCGACTCGGACTTTGTT

cDNA synthesis

RNA was reverse transcribed into cDNA using the PrimerScript RT reagent Kit with gDNA Eraser (TaKaRa, Japan) via a thermal cycler (GeneAmp PCR System 9700, Thermo Fisher Scientific Inc., Massachusetts, USA). To remove genomic DNA, a total of 500 ng of RNA from each sample was first incubated at 42 °C for 2 min in the presence of 0.5 μL of RNase-Free dH$_2$O, 1.0 μL of gDNA Eraser, and 2.0 μL of 5× gDNA Eraser Buffer. Next, reverse- transcription (RT) was conducted in a total reaction volume of 20 μL, containing 10 μL of extracted DNA template, 4.0 μL of RNase-Free dH$_2$O, 4.0 μL of 5× Prime Script Buffer 2 (for qPCR), and 1.0 μL of Prime Script RT Enzyme Mix I. The thermal profile consisted of 37 °C for 15 min, 85 °C for 5 s, and the synthesized cDNA stored at − 20 °C. The absence of contaminating gDNA was confirmed by the absence of product in control tubes (no RT), which included all components of the cDNA synthesis reaction, except Prime Script RT Enzyme Mix I.

qPCR

Following reverse transcription, the cDNA samples were analysed by qPCR using the VIIATM7 Real-Time PCR System. Each 20 μL reaction was used for qPCR analysis in PCR strip tubes (PCR-0208-C, Axygen) and consisted of 10 μL of SYBR Premix Ex Taq (2×, Perfect Real Time, TaKaRa), 0.8 μL of each gene-specific primer (10 μM), 2.0 μL of the cDNA template, and 6.4 μL of ddH$_2$O, which was used to normalize the fluorescent reporter signal between the reactions. The reaction conditions were as follows: 95 °C (30 s); 45 cycles of 95 °C (5 s); 60 °C (34 s). Each condition was followed by a 46-step melt-curve analysis (95 °C for 5 s, 60 °C for 30 s, and 95 °C for 15 s). All PCR reactions were performed in triplicate and primer specificity was confirmed by melting (dissociation) curve analysis (Fig. 1). Gene-specific amplification efficiencies for primer were also measured. Quantification of relative expression of the target gene was performed using the $2^{-\Delta\Delta Ct}$ method and QuantStudio™ Real-Time PCR software.

SBD-1 ELISA

Cell culture supernatants were collected to determine the secretion of SBD-1 by ovine ruminal epithelial cells upon induction with different concentrations of *S.c* (5.2 × 10^8, 5.2 × 10^7, 5.2 × 10^6, 5.2 × 10^5, 5.2 × 10^4 CFU·mL^{-1}) for 2, 4, 8, 12, or 24 h. The SBD-1 protein was quantified in the cell culture supernatants from ovine ruminal epithelial cells using the Ovine defensin β1 (DEFβ1) ELISA kit (Wuhan Xinqidi Biological Technology, China) according to the supplier's protocol.

Statistical analysis

All experiments were performed in triplicate and were repeated at least 3 times. The data are presented as the mean ± SD of 3 independent experiments. A 1-way analysis of variance (ANOVA) was used to compare the differences between the control and treatment groups using IBM SPSS Statistics 20.0 (SPSS Institute Inc.). The Duncan's multiple range test was used to assess the differences after verifying normality and homogeneity of variance. *P* values of less than 0.05 were considered to be statistically significant.

Results

S.c induced SBD-1 mRNA expression in ovine ruminal epithelial cells

In the current study, results of qPCR indicated that *S.c* promoted SBD-1 mRNA transcription in a time- and dose-dependent manner (Fig. 2a). When the concentration of *S.c* was constant, the induction of SBD-1 was shown to be time-dependent. The maximal amount of SBD-1 mRNA was expressed after 12 h of incubation and decreased markedly after 24 h of incubation. When the incubation time was constant, the expression of SBD-1 mRNA was highest when cells were stimulated with 5.2 × 10^7 CFU·mL^{-1} *S.c*, and was significantly higher than compared with cells stimulated with other *S.c* concentrations and compared to the control group (*P* < 0.01). Thus, the expression of SBD-1 was highest after incubation with 5.2 × 10^7 CFU·mL^{-1} *S.c* for 12 h.

S.c induced SBD-1 protein expression

The ELISA results demonstrated that the expression of SBD-1 at the protein level was consistent with that observed at the mRNA level (Fig. 2b). After the ovine ruminal epithelial cells were induced with various concentrations of *S.c* for different incubation periods, the SBD-1 protein expression in the co-culture supernatants was significantly higher compared to the control cells (*P* < 0.01). In short, the highest SBD-1 expression levels were achieved after a 12 h incubation with 5.2 × 10^7 CFU·mL^{-1} *S.c*, which suggesting that these are the optimal *S.c* concentration and incubation time for SBD-1 induction. Therefore, an *S.c* concentration of 5.2 × 10^7 CFU·mL^{-1} and an incubation time of 12 h was used to investigate the signalling pathways involved in the *S.c*-induced up-regulation of SBD-1 expression.

mRNA expression levels of putative factors involved in *S.c*-induced up-regulation of SBD-1 in ruminal epithelial cells

To investigate the possible roles of TLR2, MyD88, p38, ERK1/2, JNK, and NF-κB activation in *S.c*-induced SBD-1 expression, ovine ruminal epithelial cells were stimulated

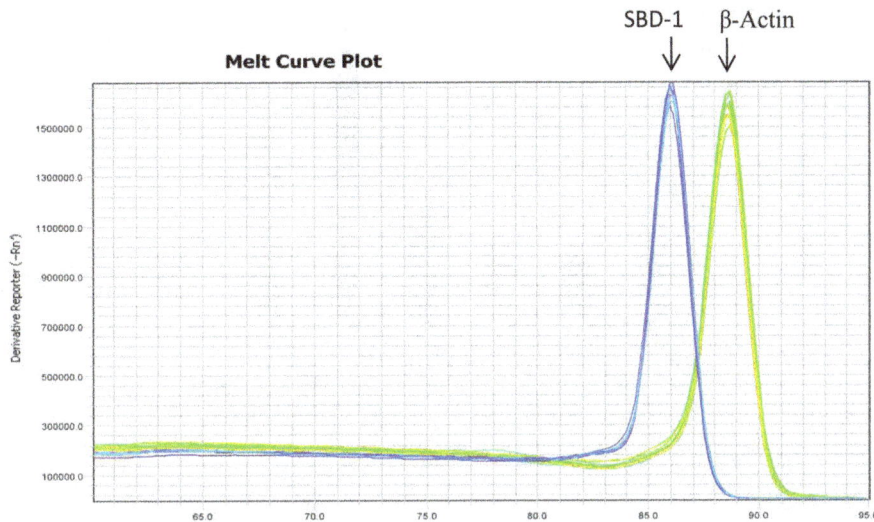

Fig. 1 qPCR melt peak curve for SBD-1 and β-Actin genes. Primers are valid for qPCR as demonstrated by a single peak observed in each dissociation curve using SYBR Green II

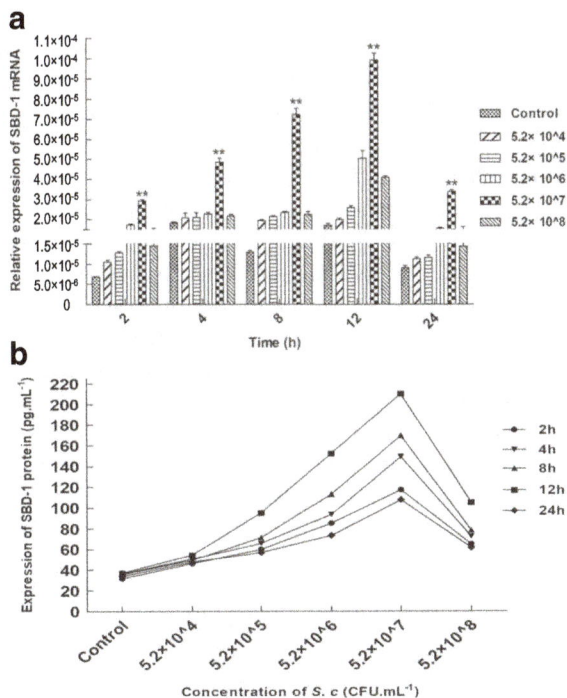

Fig. 2 S.c induces SBD-1 mRNA and protein expression. **a** Ovine ruminal epithelial cells treated with S.c (5.2×10^8, 5.2×10^7, 5.2×10^6, 5.2×10^5, 5.2×10^4 CFU·mL^{-1}) for 2, 4, 8, 12, or 24 h compared to untreated controls. qPCR analysis showed that S.c induces SBD-1 mRNA expression in a time- and concentration-dependent manner. **b** Ruminal epithelial cells treated with S.c (5.2×10^8, 5.2×10^7, 5.2×10^6, 5.2×10^5, 5.2×10^4 CFU·mL^{-1}) for 2, 4, 8, 12, or 24 h compared to untreated controls. ELISA showed that expression of SBD-1 protein was consistent with that observed for SBD-1 mRNA. All experiments were repeated at least 3 times. $*P < 0.05$, $**P < 0.01$ vs. the control group

with S.c and mRNA expression of the above factors was examined. As shown in Fig. 3, S.c treatment resulted in significantly increased NF-κB, p38, JNK, ERK1/2, TLR2, and MyD88 mRNA expression compared to the untreated cells ($P < 0.05$). The increased expression of these molecules suggests a putative role for these factors in S.c-mediated SBD-1 upregulation in ovine ruminal epithelial cells.

MAPKs and NF-κB pathways were essential for S.c-induced up-regulation of SBD-1 expression

The inhibition tests demonstrated that MAPKs and NF-κB pathways are essential for S.c-induced up-regulation of SBD-1 expression (Fig. 4a). S.c significantly up-regulated the expression of SBD-1 mRNA ($P < 0.01$) in the positive control compared to the blank control group. Treatment with the specific NF-κB inhibitor, PDTC, significantly inhibited the expression of SBD-1 mRNA ($P < 0.01$) in the treatment groups compared to the positive control group. Furthermore, treatment with the specific inhibitors PD98059, SB202190, or SP600125 (MAPKs pathway inhibitors) also significantly inhibited the up-regulation of SBD-1 by S.c ($P < 0.01$). No significant difference was observed between the negative control group and the blank control group ($P > 0.05$). These results indicate that S.c can induce the up-regulation of SBD-1 expression through the NF-κB and MAPKs pathways. The 4 inhibitors decreased SBD-1 mRNA to different degrees with SB202190 having the biggest inhibitory effect. The effect of the 4 inhibitors was as follows: SB202190 > PDTC > SP600125 > PD98059. The effect of SB202190 was significantly higher than PDTC ($P < 0.01$), however the effect of PDTC was not significantly different compared to SP600125 or PD98059 ($P > 0.05$). These results suggest that the NF-κB and MAPKs pathways

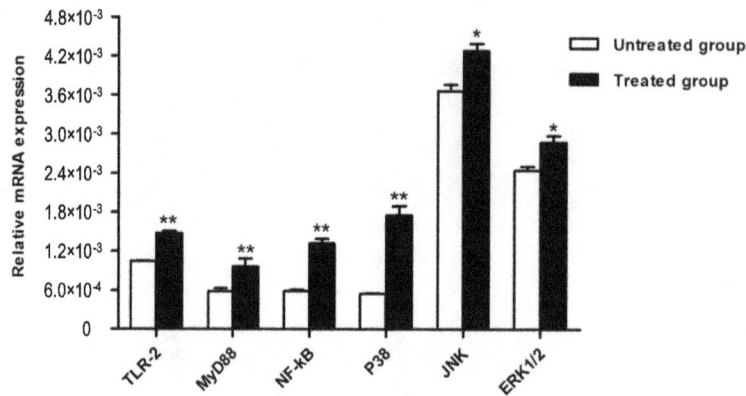

Fig. 3 *S.c* stimulates expression of TLR2, MyD88, NF-kB, p38, JNK, and ERK1/2 mRNA as measured with qPCR. *$P < 0.05$, **$P < 0.01$ vs. the untreated group

mediate the *S.c*-induced up-regulation of SBD-1 expression and that p38 in the MAPKs pathway may constitute a key signalling axis.

To further investigate the potential interaction between the NF-κB, p38, JNK, and ERK1/2 pathways, the 4 inhibitors were applied to the cells in combination. Groups of ovine ruminal epithelial cells were treated with various combinations of the inhibitors and then stimulated with *S.c* as follows: *S.c* + SB202190 + PDTC, *S.c* + SB202190 + SP600125, *S.c* + SB202190 + PD98059, *S.c* + PDTC+SP600125, *S.c* + PDTC+PD98059, *S.c* + SP60 0125 + PD98059, *S.c* + SB202190 + PDTC+SP600125, *S.c* + SB202190 + PDTC+PD98059, *S.c* + SB202190 + SP6001 25 + PD98059, or *S.c* + PDTC+SP600125 + PD98059. Cells treated with *S.c* alone served as a positive control group and cells not treated served as a blank control group (Fig. 4b). *S.c* significantly up-regulated SBD-1 expression ($P < 0.01$) in the positive control compared to the blank control group. In addition, when cells were treated with various combinations of the inhibitors, the *S.c*-mediated induction of SBD-1 mRNA was significantly reduced ($P < 0.01$) in treated groups compared to the positive control group. SB202190, the specific inhibitor of p38, had the most pronounced inhibitory effect.

Discussion

Defensins are normal antibacterial peptides that act as important components of innate immunity in many organisms. In recent years, the role of probiotics in the regulation of β-defensin expression in the gastrointestinal tract of mammals has garnered a lot of attention. The relationship between probiotics and the expression of β-defensin genes in the gastrointestinal tracts of mammals has largely been investigated in Caco-2 human intestinal epithelial cells, in which inducible defensin expression by *Lactobacillus* and probiotic *Escherichia coli* was identified [45, 46]. However, few studies have been done on the relationship between fungi (such as *S.c*) and the defensin expression.

At present, the broadly accepted view is that probiotics can induce the expression of antimicrobial peptides in mammalian intestinal epithelial cells. In studying human intestinal epithelial cells (Caco-2), Wehkamp et al. [47] and Schlee et al. [46] found that the interactions between *Lactobacillus* and other probiotics and epithelial cells can increase the defensin expression and improve the body's natural immune functions. However, these studies focused on the expression of antimicrobial peptides in human colon cancer epithelial cells and not in normal intestinal epithelial cells. Clearly, there are some differences in the basic structure, metabolism and function between cancer epithelial cells and normal epithelial cells, thus the understanding of these processes in normal cells is limited. Gastrointestinal tract antimicrobial peptides are mainly derived from epithelial cells, but can also be derived from intestinal mucosal immune cells [48]. Moreover, the role of probiotics in the body is affected by many factors, including gastric intestinal pH value, digestive enzymes, and bile. These factors can affect the viability of probiotic bacteria and the integrity of cell wall components. Therefore, to avoid interference from these complex variables and the impact of intestinal symbiotic bacteria, the effect of the probiotic *S.c* on the expression of the SBD-1 gene was investigated in normal sheep rumen epithelial cells.

SBD-1 mRNA levels were detected to elucidate the relationship between the probiotic concentration, the induction time, and the defensin expression. The results suggest that *S.c*-induced SBD-1 gene expression in sheep ruminal epithelial cells is dose- and time-dependent and that the effect on SBD-1 gene expression decreased when the *S.c* concentration was too low or too high. The SBD-1 mRNA levels were highest after the rumen epithelial cells were induced for 12 h at an *S.c* concentration of 5.2×10^7 CFU·mL^{-1}. In 2008, Schlee et al. [46]

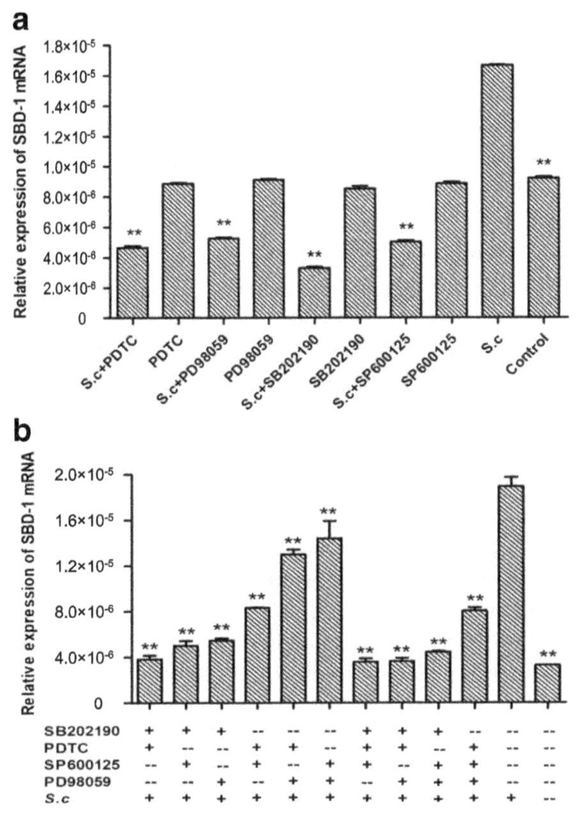

Fig. 4 The role of MAPKs and NF-κB in *S.c*-induced SBD-1 mRNA expression. **a** Effect of different signalling pathway inhibitors on SBD-1 mRNA expression induced by *S.c*. Ruminal epithelial cells were cultured with *S.c* (5.2×10^7 CFU·mL^{-1}), with or without NF-κB inhibitor (PDTC), ERK 1/2 inhibitor (PD98059), p38 inhibitor (SB203580) or JNK inhibitor (SP600125) for 12 h. Total RNA was isolated, reverse-transcribed to cDNA, and the expression of SBD-1 mRNA was quantified with qPCR using specific primers for SBD-1 and β-Actin. **b** Effect of a combination of different inhibitors on *S.c*-induced SBD-1 mRNA expression. Ruminal epithelial cells were cultured with *S.c* (5.2×10^7 CFU·mL^{-1}), with or without NF-κB inhibitor (PDTC), ERK 1/2 inhibitor (PD98059), p38 inhibitor (SB203580), and JNK inhibitor (SP600125) for 12 h. Total RNA was isolated, reverse-transcribed to cDNA, and SBD-1 mRNA expression was measured using qPCR and specific primers for SBD-1 and β-Actin. All experiments were repeated at least 3 times. *$P < 0.05$, **$P < 0.01$ vs. positive controls

found that stimulation of Caco-2 cells with different probiotic lactic acid bacteria induced the expression of human β-defensin-2 (HBD-2) and that there was a dose- and time-dependent relationship between the bacterial concentration and the defensin expression. The expression of HBD-2 increased with the increasing dosage of different probiotics and reached a peak level after incubation for 6 h. In 2012, Guanhong Li and colleagues [49] determined that the expression level of HBD-2 mRNA peaked after the cultured chicken small intestinal epithelial cells were induced by *Lactobacillus rhamnosus LGA* at a concentration of 2×10^6 CFU·mL^{-1} for 12 h. In 2014, Gácser et al. [50] showed that *Candida* spp. could

induce the expression of HBD-2 in Caco-2 cells, with *Candida albicans* inducing the highest expression levels. Similarly, α-defensin (human neutrophil peptides, HNP 1–3) secretion was significantly increased in human whole blood after exposure to *Candida* yeast cells with *C. albicans* producing the greatest effect. Although there were differences in the concentration of bacteria and the incubation time, which resulted in the highest levels of the antimicrobial peptides, these differences may be species-specific and dependent on the particular stimulating components.

In the current study, ELISA was used to investigate SBD-1 expression at the protein level. The results showed that the expression of SBD-1 at the protein level was consistent with that observed at the mRNA level. Therefore, the *S.c*-stimulated expression of SBD-1 in ruminal epithelial cells was significantly higher than in the control group at both the RNA and protein levels, suggesting that SBD-1 expression is transcriptionally regulated. However, SBD-1 gene expression levels were not consistent at the mRNA and protein levels after the ruminal epithelial cells were cultured with 5. 2×10^7 CFU·mL^{-1} *S.c* for 2 or 24 h. This suggests that the expression of SBD-1 protein in ruminal epithelial cells may also be regulated post-transcriptionally, in addition to being regulated at the transcriptional level. The specific regulatory mechanisms require further investigation.

The results of this study indicate that the probiotic *S.c* can induce the expression of the SBD-1 gene in sheep rumen epithelial cells. If this also occurs in vivo, it may be of physiological significance as SBD-1 up-regulation may provide immunostimulatory effects. Thus, if the probiotic *S.c* can increase the ruminal innate immune function by up-regulating the expression of SBD-1 gene in ruminal epithelial cells in sheep, this may confer an immune benefit to the animal. The secretion of SBD-1 was confirmed by ELISA in in vitro studies using sheep ruminal epithelial cells. If this also occurs in vivo, SBD-1 may have extracellular biological functions. In addition, antimicrobial peptides secreted by ruminal epithelial cells may have a multitude of immunomodulatory effects as intercellular signalling molecules.

It is well-established that TLRs act as natural immune recognition receptors for the initial detection of microbes and serve as important bridges to activate the adaptive immune response [51]. It has been reported that probiotics are mainly recognized by TLRs in the intestin, and are involved in producing a prebiotic immune effect via the TLRs-mediated NF-κB signalling pathway. This interaction plays a crucial role in the maintenance of intestinal microbial and mucosal immune homeostasis [52]. Several studies have also confirmed that the peptidoglycan and lipoteichoic acid on the cell walls of beneficial bacteria can recognize the TLRs in epithelial cells and activate the downstream NF-κB signalling pathway [53, 54]. There is also evidence that the yeast, zymosan, activates TLR2/TLR6 heterodimers, whereas *S.c-* and *C. albicans-* derived mannan seems to be detected by TLR4 [55]. Glyc101 is a β-glucan isolated from *S.c,* Glyc101-induced immunomodulatory effector molecule production has been observed to be mediated via TLR-2 and NF-κB activation [56]. Based on this knowledge, the possible signal transduction mechanisms governing *S.c*-induced up-regulation of SBD-1 expression in ovine ruminal epithelial cells were investigated. It was found that the up-regulation of SBD-1 gene expression by *S.c* can affect the expression of TLR2 and MyD88 mRNA. This suggests that SBD-1 gene expression induced by *S.c* may be mediated by TLR2- and MyD88-dependent pathways. SBD-1, as an immune signalling molecule, can regulate the rumen mucosal immune response, thereby enhancing the animal's immune system.

Recent studies have confirmed that the NF-κB pathway mediates the expression of some antimicrobial peptides in the intestines of mammals, including humans [57]. However, the expression of defensins is not only regulated by the NF-κB pathway, but also by MAPKs pathways. The expression of HBD-2 in oral mucosa epithelial cells can be induced by *Fusobacterium nucleatum* via the p38 and JNK components of the MAPKs signal transduction pathways [58]. Studies have also shown that the induction of defensin expression is co-mediated by the NF-κB and MAPKs pathways. Zhu et al. [59] reported that the release of mBD-14 by mouse osteoblasts was mediated by the activation of p38 MAPK and NF-κB in response to *S. aureus*-secreted bacterial exoproducts. Jia et al. [60] also confirmed that *Lactobacillus rhamnosus MLG_A*, and its cell wall component, peptidoglycan, induced AvBD9 gene expression in chicken intestinal epithelial cells and that this was mediated by the TLR2-NF-κB/AP-1 signalling pathway, where TLR2-NF-κB constituted the main signalling axis. Results of this study showed that *S.c* up-regulated NF-κB and MAPKs signalling pathway molecules (NF-κB, p38, JNK and ERK1/2) at the mRNA level. Four specific inhibitors were used to elucidate the signalling pathways involved in *S.c*-induced up-regulation of SBD-1 expression and the results demonstrated a pronounced inhibition of SBD-1 mRNA levels following treatment with any of the 4 inhibitors, either alone or in combination, prior to *S.c* stimulation. Furthermore, SB202190, a well-characterised chemical inhibitor of p38 [61], was the most effective inhibitor of SBD-1, suggesting that while the NF-κB and MAPKs pathways may mediate the SBD-1 expression induced by *S.c,* the p38 axis may act as the main signalling mechanism. Therefore, signalling pathways regulating

defensin expression induced by probiotics are likely not identical. This may be due to differences in the stimulating components of the specific species, but the explicit reasons require in-depth, follow-up study. At the same time, the results of this study showed that the 4 inhibitors could hinder the expression of SBD-1 only when the ruminal epithelial cells were stimulated by *S.c.* It may be that the expression of SBD-1 induced by *S.c* may occur through TLR2 membrane receptor ligation with the effective stimulating factor(s) of *S.c,* subsequent signalling to the kinase complex by the adapter protein MyD88, activating the NF-κB and MAPKs signalling pathways, resulting in the transcription of the SBD-1 gene by a variety of other coordinating proteins.

Conclusion

In conclusion, *S.c* can increase the expression of SBD-1 in sheep ruminal epithelial cells. The SBD-1 expression levels were highest when the rumen epithelial cells were induced with *S.c* for 12 h at a concentration of 5.2×10^7 CFU·mL^{-1}. The regulatory mechanisms controlling *S.c*-mediated up-regulation of SBD-1 expression may function through the activation of the TLR2 and MyD88-dependent pathway and the downstream MAPKs and NF-κB pathways. Thus, this work suggests that the pathways involved in *S.c*-induced SBD-1 expression may be related to TLR2-MyD88-NF-κB/MAPKs signalling and that the TLR2-MyD88-p38 axis of the TLR2-MyD88-MAPKs signalling may act as the main pathway.

Abbreviations
ELISA: enzyme-linked immunosorbent assay; MAPKs: mitogen-activated protein kinases; MyD88: myeloid differentiation factor 88; NF-κB: nuclear factor kappa-light-chain-enhancer of activated B cells; qPCR: quantitative real-time PCR; S.c: *Saccharomyces cerevisiae*; SBD-1: sheep β-defensin-1; TLR2: Toll-like receptor 2

Acknowledgments
We thank Accdon for their assistance in editing our article and for language revision. We thank Prof. Gui-fang Cao for providing us with laboratory space for the experiments.

Funding
This study was supported by the National Natural Science Foundation of China (Grant No. 31160491, 31560682), and they provided suggestions about the study design.

Authors' contributions
XJ designed the experiments, extracted RNA and prepared cDNA, performed qPCR experiments, performed statistical analysis, and prepared the manuscript and figures; MZ performed ELISA, statistical analysis, and prepared the manuscript and figures; YY and CD designed the experiments and revised the manuscript; XZ, YF, and HB designed the experiments, conducted qPCR, and prepared figures; SX and QT performed cell culture, RNA extraction, and cDNA preparation; YW conducted statistical analysis. All authors read and approved the final manuscript.

Consent for publication

Not applicable.

Competing interests

The authors declare that they have no competing interests.

Author details

[1]Veterinary Medicine College of Inner Mongolia Agricultural University, Hohhot 010018, People's Republic of China. [2]Key Laboratory of Clinical Diagnosis and Treatment Technology in Animal Disease, Ministry of Agriculture, Hohhot 010018, People's Republic of China. [3]College of Animal Science and Technology, Henan University of Science and Technology, Luoyang 471000, People's Republic of China. [4]Vocational and Technical College of Inner Mongolia Agricultural University, Baotou 014109, People's Republic of China.

References

1. Tohidnezhad M, Varoga D, Podschun R, Wruck CJ, Seekamp, Brandenburg LO, et al. Thrombocytes are effectors of the innate immune system releasing human beta defensin-3. Injury 2011;42(7):682–686.
2. Diamond G, Beckloff N, Ryan LK. Host defense peptides in the oral cavity and the lung: similarities and differences. J Dent Res. 2008;87(10):915–27.
3. Rehaume LM, Hancock RE. Neutrophil-derived defensins as modulators of innate immune function. Crit Rev Immunol. 2008;28(3):185–200.
4. Wu J, Jin X, Zhao Y, Dong Q, Jiang H, Ma Q. Evolution of the defensin-like gene family in grass genomes. J Genet. 2016;95(1):53–62.
5. Li M, Zhu L, Zhou CY, Sun S, Fan YJ, Zhuang ZM. Molecular characterization and expression of a novel big defensin (Sb-BDef1) from ark shell, Scapharca broughtonii. Fish Shellfish Immunol. 2012;33(5):1167–73.
6. Ganz T. Defensins: antimicrobial peptides of innate immunity. Nat Rev Immunol. 2003;3(9):710–20.
7. Ganz T, Selsted ME, Defensins LRI. Eur J Haematol. 1990;44(1):1–8.
8. Ganz T, Defensins LRI. Curr Opin Immunol. 1994;6(4):584–9.
9. Yang D, Biragyn A, Hoover DM, Lubkowski J, Oppenheim JJ. Multiple roles of antimicrobial defensins, cathelicidins, and eosinophil-derived neurotoxin in host defense. Annu Rev Immunol. 2004;22:181–215.
10. Lough D, Dai H, Yang M, Reichensperger J, Cox L, Harrison C, et al. Stimulation of the follicular bulge LGR5+ and LGR6+ stem cells with the gut-derived humanalpha defensin 5 results in decreased bacterial presence, enhanced wound healing, and hair growth from tissues devoid of adnexal structures. Plast Reconstr Surg. 2013;132(5):1159–71.
11. Eisenhauer PB, Harwig SSL, Cryptdins LRI. Antimicrobial defensins of the murine small intestine. Infect Immun. 1992;60(9):3556–65.
12. Tang YQ, Yuan J, Miller CJ, Isolation SME. Characterization, cDNA cloning, and antimicrobial properties of two distinct subfamilies of α-defensins from rhesus macaque leukocytes. Infect Immun. 1999;67(11):6139–44.
13. Yount NY, Wang MS, Yuan J, Banaiee N, Ouellette AJ, Selsted ME. Rat neutrophil defensins. Precursor structures and expression during neutrophilic myelopoiesis. J Immunol. 1995;55(9):4476–84.
14. Sinha S, Cheshenko N, Lehrer RI, Herold BC. NP-1, a rabbit α-defensin, prevents the entry and intercellular spread of herpes simplex virus type 2. Antimicrob Agents Chemother. 2003;47(2):494–500.
15. Selsted ME, Purification HSS. Primary structure, and antimicrobial activities of a Guinea pig neutrophil defensin. Infect Immun. 1987;55(9):2281–6.
16. Mak P, Wójcik K, Thogersen IB, Dubin A. Isolation antimicrobial activities, and primary structures of hamster neutrophil defensins. Infect Immun. 1996; 64(11):4444–9.
17. Bruhn O, Regenhard P, Michalek M, Paul S, Gelhaus C, Jung S, et al. A novel horse alpha-defensin: gene transcription, recombinant expression and characterization of the structure and function. Biochem J. 2007;407(2):267–76.
18. Belov K, Sanderson CE, Deakin JE, Wong ES, Assange D, McColl KA, et al. Characterization of the opossum immune genome provides insights into the evolution of the mammalian immune system. Genome Res. 2007;17(7): 982–91.
19. Lynn DJ, Bradley DG. Discovery of alpha-defensins in basal mammals. Dev Comp Immunol. 2007;31(10):963–7.
20. Fjell CD, Jenssen H, Fries P, Aich P, Griebel P, Hilpert K, et al. Identification of novel host defense peptides and the absence of alpha-defensins in the bovine genome. Proteins. 2008;73(2):420–30.
21. Patil A, Hughes AL, Zhang G. Rapid evolution and diversification of mammalian alpha-defensins as revealed by comparative analysis of rodent and primate genes. Physiol Genomics. 2004;20(1):1–11.
22. Nguyen TX, Cole AM, Lehrer RI. Evolution of primate theta-defensins: a serpentine path to a sweet tooth. Peptides. 2003;24(11):1647–54.
23. Diamond G, Zasloff M, Eck H, Brasseur M, Maloy WL, Bevins CL. Tracheal antimicrobial peptide, a cysteine-rich peptide from mammalian tracheal mucosa: peptide isolation and cloning of a cDNA. Proc Natl Acad Sci U S A. 1991;88(9):3952–6.
24. Bensch KW, Raida M, Magert HJ, Schulz-Knappe P, Forssmann WG. hBD-1: a novel beta-defensin from human plasma. FEBS Lett. 1995;368(2):331–5.
25. Huttner KM, Kozak CA, Bevins CL. The mouse genome encodes a single homolog of the antimicrobial peptide human beta-defensin 1. FEBS Lett. 1997;413(1):45–9.
26. Evans EW, Beach GG, Wunderlich J, Harmon BG. Isolation of antimicrobial peptides from avian heterophils. J Leukoc Biol. 1994;56(5):661–5.
27. Rádis-Baptista G, Oguiura N, Hayashi MA, Camargo ME, Grego KF, Oliveira EB, et al. Nucleotide sequence of crotamine isoform precursors from a single south American rattlesnake (Crotalus durissus terrificus). Toxicon. 1999;37(7):973–84.
28. Zou J, Mercier C, Koussounadis A, Secombes C. Discovery of multiple beta-defensin like homologues in teleost fish. Mol Immunol. 2007;44(4):638–47.
29. Monteleone G, Calascibetta D, Scaturro M, Galluzzo P, Palmeri M, Riggio V, et al. Polymorphisms of β-defensin genes in Valle del Belice dairy sheep. Mol Biol Rep. 2011;38(8):5405–12.
30. Huttner KM, Brezinski-Caliguri DJ, Mahoney MM, Diamond G. Antimicrobial peptide expression is developmentally regulated in the ovine gastrointestinal tract. J Nutr. 1998;128(2 Suppl):297S–9S.
31. Li Y, Yang YF. Research Progress of Polymorphism and Expression of Defensins in vivo of Livestock. China Animal Husbandry & Veterinary Medicine. 2013; 40(3):160–168.
32. Williams PE, Tait CA, Innes GM, Newbold CJ. Effects of the inclusion of yeast culture (Saccharomyces cerevisiae plus growth medium) in the diet of dairy cows on milk yield and forage degradation and fermentation patterns in the rumen of steers. J Anim Sci. 1991;69(7):3016–26.
33. Robinson PH, Garrett JE. Effect of yeast culture (Saccharomyces cerevisiae) on adaptation of cows to postpartum diets and on lactational performance. J Anim Sci. 1999;77(4):988–99.
34. Salama AAK, Caja G, Garín D, Albanell E, Such X, Casals R. Effects of adding a mixture of malate and yeast culture (Saccharomyces cerevisiae) on milk production of Murciano-Granadina dairy goats. Anim Res. 2002;51(4):295–303.
35. Wohlt JE, Corcione TT, Zajac PK. Effect of yeast on feed intake and performance of cows fed diets based on corn silage during early lactation. J Dairy Sci. 1998; 81(5):1345–52.
36. Kamel HEM, Sekine J, El-Waziry AM, Yacout MHM. Effect of Saccharomyces cerevisiae on the synchronization of organic matter and nitrogen degradation kinetics and microbial nitrogen synthesis in sheep fed berseem hay (Trifolium alexandrinum). Small Ruminant Res. 2004;52(3):211–6.
37. Doreau M, Jouany JP. Effect of a Saccharomyces cerevisiae culture on nutrient digestion in lactating dairy cows. J Dairy Sci. 1998;81(12):3214–21.
38. Jouany JP, Mathieu F, Senaud J, Bohatier J, Bertin G, Mercier M. The effect of Saccharomyces cerevisiae and aspergillus oryzae on the digestion of the cell wall fraction of a mixed diet in defaunated and refaunated sheep rumen. Reprod Nutr Dev. 1998;38(4):401–16.
39. Schmitt P, Wacyk J, Morales-Lange B, Rojas V, Guzmán F, Dixon B, et al. Immunomodulatory effect of cathelicidins in response to a β-glucan in intestinal epithelial cells from rainbow trout. Dev Comp Immunol. 2015; 51(1):160–9.
40. El-Boshy ME, El-Ashram AM, Abdelhamid FM, Gadalla HA. Immunomodulatory effect of dietary Saccharomyces cerevisiae, beta-glucan and laminaran in mercuric chloride treated Nile tilapia (Oreochromis niloticus) and experimentally infected with Aeromonas hydrophila. Fish Shellfish Immunol. 2010;28(5–6):802–8.
41. Klotz JL, Baldwin RL 6th, Gillis RC, Heitmann RN. Refinements in primary rumen epithelial cell incubation techniques. J Dairy Sci 2001;84(1):183–193.
42. Sun ZH, Zhang QL, He ZX, Han XF, Tan ZL, Zhang HP, et al. Research on

primary culture method for ruminal epithelial and jejunum epithelial cells of goats. Chinese Journal of Animal Nutrition. 2010;22(3):602–10.

43. Wen S, Cao G, Bao T, Cheng L, Li H, Du C, et al. Modulation of ovine SBD-1 expression by 17 beta-estradiol in ovine oviduct epithelial cells. BMC Vet Res. 2012;8:143.

44. Li Q, Bao F, Zhi D, Liu M, Yan Q, Zheng X, et al. Lipopolysaccharide induces SBD-1 expression via the p38 MAPK signalling pathway in ovine oviduct epithelial cells. Lipids Health Dis. 2016;15(1):127.

45. Schlee M, Wehkamp J, Altenhoefer A, Oelschlaeger TA, Stange EF, Fellermann K. Induction of human beta-defensin 2 by the probiotic Escherichia coli Nissle 1917 is mediated through flagellin. Infect Immun. 2007;75(5):2399–407.

46. Schlee M, Harder J, Köten B, Stange EF, Wehkamp J, Fellermann K. Probiotic lactobacilli and VSL#3 induce enterocyte beta-defensin 2. Clin Exp Immunol. 2008;151(3):528–35.

47. Wehkamp J, Harder J, Wehkamp K, Wehkamp-von Meissner B, Schlee M, Enders C, et al. NF-kappaB-and AP-1-mediated induction of human beta defensin-2 in intestinal epithelial cells by Escherichia coli Nissle 1917: a novel effect of a probiotic bacterium. Infect Immun. 2004;72(10):5750–8.

48. Cunliffe RN, Mahida YR. Expression and regulation of antimicrobial peptides in the gastrointestinal tract. J Leukoc Biol. 2004;75(1):49–58.

49. Li GH, Hong ZM, Jia YJ, Yi ZH, Qu MR, Liu SG. Effect of lactobacillus rhamnosus LGA on β-defensin-9 expression in cultured chicken small intestine epithelial cells. Acta Veterinaria et Zootechnica Sinica. 2012;43(4):634–41.

50. Gácser A, Tiszlavicz Z, Németh T, Seprényi G, Mándi Y. Induction of human defensins by intestinal Caco-2 cells after interactions with opportunistic Candida species. Microbes Infect. 2014;16(1):80–5.

51. Wells JM, Rossi O, Meijerink M, van Baarlen P. Epithelial crosstalk at the microbiota-mucosal interface. Proc Natl Acad Sci U S A. 2011;108(Suppl 1): 4607–14.

52. Rakoff-Nahoum S, Paglino J, Eslami-Varzaneh F, Edberg S, Medzhitov R. Recognition of commensal microflora by toll-like receptors is required for intestinal homeostasis. Cell. 2004;118(2):229–41.

53. Vinderola G, Mater C, Perdigon G. Role of intestinal epithelial celles in immune effects mediated by gram-positive probiotic bacteria: involvement of toll-like receptors. Clin Diagn Lab Immunol. 2005;12(9):1075–84.

54. Galdeano CM, De Moreno De LeBlanc A, Vinderola G, Bonet ME, Perdigón G. Proposed model: mechanisms of immunomodulation induced by probiotic bacteria. Clin Vaccine Immunol. 2007;14(5):485–92.

55. Roeder A, Kirschning CJ, Rupec RA, Schaller M, Weindl G, Korting HC. Toll-like receptors as key mediators in innate antifungal immunity. Med Mycol. 2004;42(6):485–98.

56. Roy S, Dickerson R, Khanna S, Collard E, Gnyawali U, Gordillo GM, et al. Particulate β-glucan induces TNF-α production in wound macrophages via a redox-sensitive NF-κB-dependent pathway. Wound Repair Regen. 2011; 19(3):411–9.

57. Kaiser V, Diamond G. Expression of mammalian defensin genes. J Leukoc Biol. 2000;68(6):779–84.

58. Krisanaprakornkit S, Kimball JR, Dale BA. Regulation of human-defensin-2 in gingival epithelial cells: the involvement of mitogen-activated portein kinase pahtways, but not the NF-kappa B tnanscription factor family. J Immunol. 2002;168(1):316–24.

59. Zhu C, Qin H, Cheng T, Tan HL, Guo YY, Shi SF, et al. Staphylococcus aureus supernatant induces the release of mouse β-defensin-14 from osteoblasts via the p38 MAPK and NF-κB pathways. Int J Mol Med. 2013;31(6):1484–94.

60. Jia YJ. Effects of lactobacillus rhamnosus on β-defensin 9 expression and its signal transduction pathway in chicken small intestinal epithelial cells. Nanchang: Jiangxi Agricultural University; 2012.

61. Nassar K, Tura A, Lüke J, Lüke M, Grisanti S, Grisanti S. A p38 MAPK inhibitor improves outcome after glaucoma filtration surgery. J Glaucoma. 2015;24(2): 165–78.

17

Cutaneous lupus erythematosus in dogs

Thierry Olivry[1,2]* (iD), Keith E. Linder[2,3] and Frane Banovic[4]

Abstract

Since the first description of discoid lupus erythematosus (LE) in two dogs in 1979, the spectrum of canine cutaneous lupus erythematosus (CLE) variants has expanded markedly.

In this review, we first propose an adaptation of the Gilliam-Sontheimer classification of CLE for dogs. We then review the signalment, clinical signs, laboratory and histopathology and treatment outcome of the currently recognized variants of canine CLE, which are vesicular CLE, exfoliative CLE, mucocutaneous LE and facial or generalized discoid LE. We end with a short description of the rare cutaneous manifestations of systemic LE in dogs.

Canine CLE variants are heterogeneous, some of them mirror their human counterparts while others appear—thus far—unique to the dog. As most CLE subtypes seem to have a good prognosis after diagnosis, veterinarians are encouraged to become familiar with the spectrum of often-characteristic and unique clinical signs that would permit an early diagnosis and the rapid implementation of an effective treatment.

Keywords: Auto-immune skin diseases, Auto-immunity, Canine, Dermatology, Lupus, Skin

Background

In 1979, Griffin and colleagues were the first to report a skin disease of dogs that resembled discoid lupus erythematosus (DLE), one of the variants of cutaneous lupus erythematosus (CLE) of humans [1]. Within the ensuing two decades, new information was limited to a large case series of canine DLE [2–4] and a catalog of skin lesions present in dogs with systemic lupus erythematosus (SLE) [5]. It was only around the turn of the millennium that other cutaneous variants of canine LE were characterized, notably type I bullous systemic LE, as well as exfoliative and vesicular CLE [6–8]. Finally, a third wave of descriptions of canine CLE subsets occurred more recently with the publication of case series of mucocutaneous LE and generalized DLE in dogs [9, 10].

In this paper, we first propose a classification of canine CLE variants, which is derived from the princepst modern nosology of the corresponding human diseases. This first section will be followed by a series of monographs reviewing relevant information published to date on the various canine CLE subsets.

Classification of cutaneous lupus erythematosus
Classification in humans

In 1997, Gilliam-Sontheimer proposed a nosology that is the modern foundation of the classification of cutaneous manifestations of LE in humans [11]. This system separates skin lesions associated with LE into two groups. Those that have microscopic skin lesions specific for lupus (i.e. a lymphocyte-rich interface dermatitis with basal keratinocyte apoptosis) are named *"LE-specific skin diseases"* (or CLE sensu stricto) while those that do not share such a histopathologic pattern are grouped under the denomination *"LE-nonspecific skin diseases"* [11, 12].

In this classification, LE-specific skin diseases (CLE) are further subdivided into three major subcategories based on the lesional morphology and the average duration of individual skin lesions; these are named acute cutaneous LE (ACLE), subacute cutaneous LE (SCLE) and chronic cutaneous LE (CCLE) (Fig. 1a). Lupus erythematosus-nonspecific skin lesions encompass those associated with the underlying autoimmune disease, but that are not specific for LE itself, since the same lesions can be seen also in other diseases. Examples of LE-nonspecific skin lesions are those due to vasculitis, cryoglobulinemias, or vesicobullous lesions associated with basement-membrane autoantibodies (i.e. bullous SLE).

* Correspondence: tolivry@ncsu.edu
[1]Department of Clinical Sciences, College of Veterinary Medicine, North Carolina State University, Raleigh, NC 27606, USA
[2]Comparative Medicine Institute, North Carolina State University, Raleigh, NC, USA

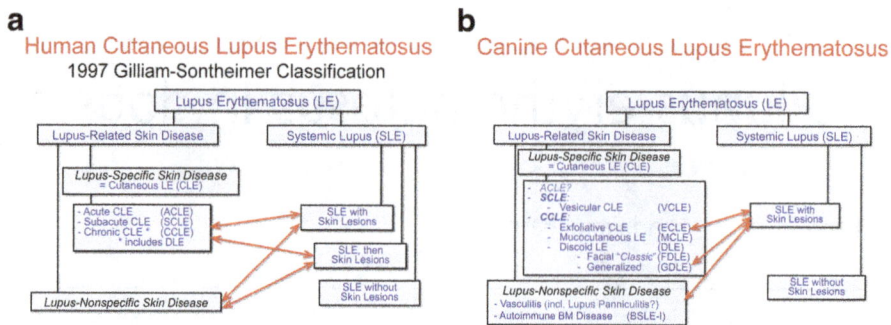

Fig. 1 Classification of skin manifestations of lupus erythematosus in humans and dogs. **a** Gilliam-Sontheimer classification of human cutaneous lupus erythematosus variants; **b**: proposed classification of canine cutaneous lupus erythematosus variants

Importantly, human patients with SLE might exhibit cutaneous lesions that can be either specific or nonspecific (SLE with or without CLE). Conversely, LE-specific skin lesions can be present with or without systemic involvement (CLE with or without SLE) (Fig. 1a).

A simplified version of this classification has been reported recently [13]. A recent review summarizes the salient clinical and diagnostic features of human CLE variants [14].

Proposed classification in dogs

It seems logical to use the same logic to classify the cutaneous manifestations of LE in dogs as that first developed by Gilliam and Sontheimer (Fig. 1b). Herein, we also suggest to separate LE-specific skin diseases (CLE *sensu stricto*) from those that are lupus-non-specific. Among CLEs, a canine homologue of ACLE of humans has not yet been reported. In contrast, vesicular cutaneous LE (VCLE) is the only identified canine CLE variant that is an equivalent to human SCLE. Exfoliative cutaneous LE (ECLE), localized (facial) or generalized discoid LE (DLE) and mucocutaneous LE (MCLE) are the currently recognized subtypes of canine CCLE.

At this time, we would also regroup under the umbrella of LE-nonspecific skin diseases the various skin lesions that are seen not only in the context of SLE, but also outside of this syndrome. Examples are vasculitis and the type I-bullous SLE associated with collagen VII autoantibodies (i.e. an epidermolysis bullosa acquisita occurring in the context of SLE); one case of putative "lupus panniculitis" was mentioned in a case series of cutaneous manifestations of SLE in dogs [5].

Lupus-specific skin diseases

The salient features of lupus-systemic skin diseases in dogs are summarized in Table 1.

Subacute cutaneous lupus erythematosus

Vesicular cutaneous lupus erythematosus

Historical perspective

First recognized in the late 1960's, "*hidradenitis suppurativa*" was a unique skin disease described in Collies, Shetland sheepdogs and their crosses [15, 16]. Since the early 1980's, the disease mentioned above was suspected to represent, in fact, bullous pemphigoid [17, 18] or erythema multiforme in these breeds [19, 20]. In 1995, an "*idiopathic ulcerative dermatosis of Collies and Shetland sheepdogs*" was individualized as a separate entity that was initially linked to juvenile dermatomyositis, also seen in these breeds [21]. In 2001, Jackson and Olivry separated this ulcerative dermatosis from dermatomyositis based on clinical and histological grounds, and the denomination of VCLE was then coined [8]. In 2004, the same authors reported the detection of circulating anti-Ro autoantibodies in dogs with VCLE [22], and they highlighted the similarity of this canine disease with human SCLE.

Incidence and prevalence

At this time, there is insufficient information on canine VCLE to appropriately assess the incidence and prevalence of this disease in dogs. However, this entity has been diagnosed in several countries and continents over the last five decades.

Signalment

The clinical characteristics of canine VCLE can be inferred from six reports including 25 dogs [23–28]. Among these cases, there were 11 Shetland sheepdogs and their crosses (44%), seven (rough) collies (28%) and seven pure- or cross-bred border collies (28%). The female-to-male ratio was 0.9 and the age of onset varied between 2.0 and 11. 0 years of age (median 5.5 years). That VCLE has been recognized almost entirely in collie-related breeds suggests the existence of a strong genetic predisposition, but the genetics of this disease have not yet been elucidated.

Clinical signs

Dogs with VCLE present with erythema and flaccid vesicles that slough to leave erosions and ulcers; these predominate on glabrous skin of the abdomen, axillae, groin and medial thighs [8, 23–28]. Skin lesions exhibit a unique sharp-edged annular, polycyclic or serpiginous pattern (Fig. 2a-d). There is accompanying

Table 1 Comparative characteristics of cutaneous lupus erythematosus variants in dogs

| | SCLE | CCLE | | | |
	VCLE	ECLE	MCLE	FDLE	GDLE
Most commonly affected breeds	Shetland sheepdogs, rough collies and border collies	German shorthaired pointers and Magyar viszlas	German shepherd dogs	German shepherd dogs	Chinese crested dogs
Ages of onset: median (range)	5.5 (2.0–11.0)	0.7 (0.2–3.5)	6.0 (3.0–13.0)	7.0 (1.0–12.0)	9.0 (5.0–12.0)
female-to-male ratios	0.9	1.4	1.8	0.7	1.0
Most common skin lesions	figurate erythema, flaccid vesicles and erosions	erythema, scaling, follicular casts, alopecia and occasional scarring	erosions, ulcers with or without peripheral hyperpigmentation	dyspigmentation, erythema, erosions, ulcers, scaling crusting,	dyspigmentation, erythema, erosions, ulcers, scaling, crusting
Most common lesion distribution	abdomen, axillae, medial thighs, concave pinnae and perimucosal areas	trunk, muzzle, pinnae and abdomen	genital, perigenital, anal, perianal, periocular and perilabial areas	nasal planum and dorsal muzzle	trunk, lateral legs and abdomen
Systemic signs	typically not seen	lymphadenomegaly, arthralgia, and reproductive defects	typically not seen	typically not seen	typically not seen
Most relevant clinical mimics	erythema multiforme	sebaceous adenitis	mucocutaneous pyoderma, mucous membrane pemphigoid and erythema multiforme variants	mucocutaneous pyoderma, epitheliotropic cell lymphoma and uveodermatological syndrome	hyperkeratotic erythema multiforme and generalized ischemic dermatopathies

Disease name abbreviations are listed at the end of this paper

ulceration of mucocutaneous junctions (Fig. 2e,f), concave pinnae and oral cavity in some patients, but these nonventral lesions are usually minor in extent and severity [8, 23–28]. The secondary bacterial colonization of erosive/ ulcerative lesions is common. Altogether, these lesions resemble those of the vesicular variant of human SCLE. Pruritus manifestations are usually absent, except, perhaps, for a licking of eroded lesions [23–28].

In eight of 11 (73%) dogs with VCLE, clinical signs were reported to first arise in the summer [23]. In three cases where this information was available, lesions recurred during summer months [23]. Systemic signs are typically not seen in dogs with VCLE, though one dog was reported with weakness and lethargy with associated electromyographic changes interpreted as myositis [24]. There are normally no relevant hematology and clinical biochemistry changes.

The main dermatosis with clinical signs mimicking VCLE is erythema multiforme and its variants.

Histopathology

In canine VCLE, a lymphocyte cell-rich interface dermatitis is associated with prominent basal keratinocyte vacuolation, apoptosis and loss, which is often sufficient to cause intrabasal clefts and epidermal vesiculation, typical of the disease (Fig. 3a-c) [8]. Basal cell apoptosis is reported to be as high as 16 apoptotic basal cells per 1 mm of epidermis utilizing immunohistochemical detection methods [23]. Hair follicle infundibula have a similar lymphocytic interface and mural

folliculitis [8]. Pigment dispersal to dermal macrophages (pigmentary incontinence) is often not a feature or is very mild, likely due to breed coat coloration and the tendency for lesions to occur in poorly- or non-pigmented skin. The thickening of the basement membrane zone and superficial dermal fibrosis are uncommon, which is attributable to the subacute nature of the disease, but they can occur in persistent lesions (Fig. 3d). Cell-rich lesions dominate biopsies but very mild lymphocytic dermal infiltrates or even cell-poor areas of lesions can occur that lack a subepidermal, band-like (lichenoid), dermal infiltrate of lymphocytes (Fig. 3c) [8]. Cell-poor areas of lesions can lead to confusion with juvenile dermatomyositis, which is seen often in the same breeds [8]. Dermatomyositis presents with lesions of ischemic dermatopathy (i.e. cell-poor interface dermatitis and ischemic follicular atrophy), but cell-poor VCLE lesions have more lymphocyte exocytosis into the basal epidermal layer, with lymphocytic satellitosis of apoptotic basal keratinocytes. If the intrabasal level of epidermal clefts is not recognized (Fig. 3b), then vesiculation can be confused with subepidermal autoimmune blistering skin diseases such as mucous membrane pemphigoid (MMP), bullous pemphigoid (BP) and epidermolysis bullosa acquisita (EBA). The prominence of basal apoptosis and intrabasal epidermal vesiculation, when present, supports the histological diagnosis of VCLE over that of other variants of CCLE, but this distinction is difficult for more chronic lesions and is best done clinically, as for all forms of canine

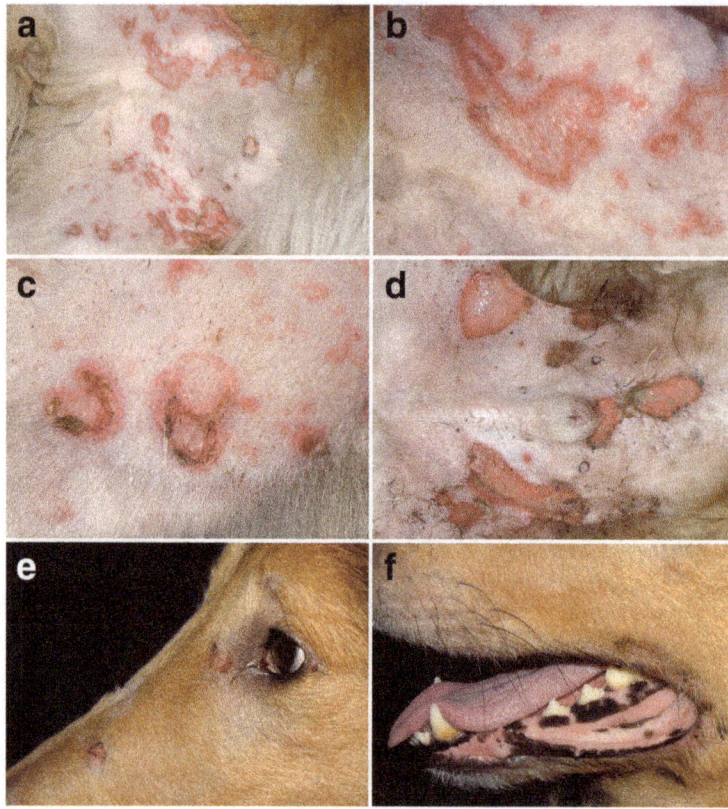

Fig. 2 Clinical characteristics of canine vesicular cutaneous lupus erythematosus. **a**, **b**, **c**: erythematous macules progress to annular-to-polycyclic lesions with central flaccid vesiculation and peripheral erythema; skin lesions predominate on the ventral abdomen, medial thighs and axillae. **d**: with chronicity, ulceration can become more prominent. **e**, **f**: erosions at mucocutaneous junctions can be seen in some dogs

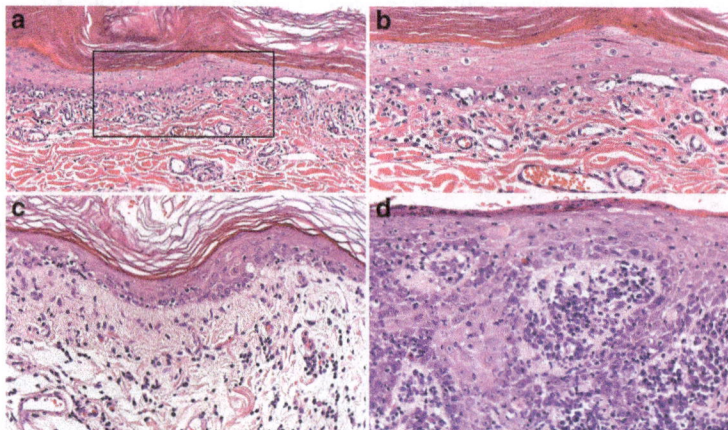

Fig. 3 Histopathology of canine vesicular cutaneous lupus erythematosus. **a**: cell-rich, lymphocytic interface dermatitis is present. Marked basal keratinocyte apoptosis has caused a secondary cleft (vesiculation) through the epidermal basal cell layer, which is typical of the disease. 100X (**b**): inset box from image "a", lymphocytes infiltrate the basal layer and are associated with basal cell vacuolation, apoptosis, loss and disorganization at the cleft margin. 200X (**c**): dermal lymphocytic inflammation can be mild, lacking a clear subepidermal band-like (lichenoid) pattern, but lymphocytes are still observed in the basal epidermal layer in association with basal cell loss. 200X (**d**): chronic lesions can develop epidermal hyperplasia, a prominent dermal infiltrate of lymphocytes and plasma cells and thickening of the basement membrane zone. 200X

CLE. Occasionally superficial epidermal apoptosis with lymphocytic satellitosis might erroneously suggest the diagnosis of erythema multiforme and its morphologically related conditions [29]. Neutrophilic inflammation is common in lesions that progress to ulcers and support the development of secondary bacterial infection.

Immunohistochemistry

In one of the two largest case series [22], detailed information on mononuclear cell immunophenotyping was reported. T-lymphocytes expressing CD3 were found in epidermal sections of all 11 dogs examined. In two of these dogs with VCLE, the phenotype of skin-infiltrating leukocytes was similar: approximately 25 to 50% of epidermal leukocytes were T-lymphocytes expressing the alpha-beta T-cell receptor, CD3 and CD8; less commonly, epitheliotropic lymphocytes expressed CD4. The other epithelial leukocytes were identified as CD1-positive Langerhans cells. In the superficial dermis, infiltrating cells consisted of an approximately equal population of alpha-beta T-lymphocytes expressing CD4 or CD8-alpha and CD1-positive dermal dendritic cells. Rare CD21-positive B-lymphocytes were detected in the superficial dermis. In contrast, gamma-delta T-cells were not identified in either the epidermis or dermis. Basal keratinocytes expressed high levels of ICAM-1 and low levels of class II major histocompatibility complex molecules signifying their activated state. In this study, apoptotic keratinocytes were observed in the basal epidermis of seven of the 12 dogs evaluated (58%) [22].

Immunopathology

Direct immunofluorescence Direct immunofluorescence revealed the presence of IgG at the basement membrane zone in 7/14 (50%) dogs with VCLE [22]. The deposition of IgG around blood vessels was observed in 13/14 dogs (93%). Finally, cytoplasmic basal keratinocyte IgG was detected in 6/14 subjects (43%); the deposition of activated complement was not seen [22].

Indirect immunofluorescence Indirect immunofluorescence did not reveal anti-basement membrane circulating IgG autoantibodies in the serum of five dogs with VCLE [22]. Similarly circulating antinuclear IgG autoantibodies were not detected in the serum of any of 11 dogs with VCLE using human Hep2 cells as a substrate [22].

Immunoblotting and ELISA Using Hep2 cell extracts, immunoblotting permitted the detection of autoantibodies against soluble nuclear antigens in 9/11 tested sera (82%) [22]. When an ELISA was performed with purified human soluble nuclear antigens, the serum from 8/11 dogs with VCLE (73%) was found to have IgG autoantibodies that bound to these antigens. Antibodies were found to target

Ro/SSA (45% of dogs), La/SSB (45%), Sm/RNP (45%), Scl70 (36%), Jo-1 (36%) and Sm-SnRNP (18%) [22]. Overall, and as seen in humans with SCLE, most dogs with VCLE (6/11; 55%) were found to have IgG antibodies that targeted Ro/SSA and/or La/SSB antigens [22].

Treatment and outcome

As VCLE is induced and/or worsened by UV light, sun avoidance should be implemented immediately after a diagnosis is made. The first case series provided detailed information on the post-treatment outcome in 11 dogs with VCLE [23]. In six of these dogs (55%), clinical signs resolved with the oral administration of prednisone at low immunosuppressive dosages (2 mg/kg/day), which were tapered according to treatment response. In three dogs (27%), azathioprine (at about 2 mg/kg/day) was added to the treatment regimen due to the insufficient reduction of lesions with glucocorticoids. Finally, the response to pentoxifylline (initially prescribed due to the then erroneous inclusion of VCLE in the dermatomyositis spectrum) was reported as poor in four dogs (36%). In this case study of 11 dogs, one (9%) died of unknown cause, and three (27%) were euthanized at the owner's request due to poor response to treatment. In the remaining seven dogs (64%), a complete or sub-complete remission of signs was achieved with glucocorticoids alone or in combination with azathioprine [23]. Lesions have also been shown to respond to the immunosuppressant mycophenolate mofetil in one rough collie with VCLE, as the introduction of this drug led to the complete remission of skin lesions after the discontinuation of oral glucocorticoids [27].

More recently, the benefit of calcineurin inhibitors, which had been previously reported in two dogs with VCLE [24, 26], was confirmed in 11 additional patients [28]. In all dogs, treatment was initiated with sun avoidance, oral glucocorticoids and oral ciclosporin at a median dosage of 5.5 mg/kg/day. A complete remission of skin lesions occurred in 8/11 dogs (73%) within one to two months of starting treatment. In two dogs (18%), lesion remission was achieved by increasing the dose of ciclosporin and adding topical 0.1% tacrolimus ointment. While relapses of clinical signs were common when the dosage of ciclosporin was lowered, the long-term remission of signs was possible with calcineurin inhibitors, either alone or in combination. These observations suggest that calcineurin inhibitors might be the drug category of choice to treat canine VCLE.

Chronic cutaneous lupus erythematosus
Exfoliative cutaneous lupus erythematosus
Historical perspective
In 1992, Ihrke, Gross and Walder described a scaly dermatosis in young German shorthaired pointers (GSHP). Because microscopic lesions resembled those seen in subjects with lupus, the disease was named "*hereditary lupoid*

dermatosis" [30]. One brief case report [31], one series of five cases [32] and a book chapter [33] constituted the early descriptions of this rare disease.

In 1999, we reviewed the histopathological and immunological characteristics of eight dogs with this disease, and proposed the name exfoliative cutaneous lupus erythematosus (ECLE) [7]. Clinical, histopathological and immunological data from 25 dogs with ECLE were later collated and described in more detail [34].

Incidence and prevalence
At this time, there is insufficient information on canine ECLE to appropriately assess the incidence and prevalence of this disease in dogs. It appears to have a worldwide distribution.

Signalment
This variant of CCLE is predominantly seen in GSHPs [34]. A large pedigree analysis of 235 purebred GSHPs and experimental mating studies established that this disease was transmitted on an autosomal recessive manner [35]. A single nucleotide polymorphism on the CFA 18 chromosome was found to perfectly segregate with the trait in 267 dogs [35]. Interestingly, ECLE has been diagnosed also in several Magyar viszlas living in western Europe [36, 37]; this observation is noteworthy, as viszlas share a common ancestry with GSHPs [37].

Adding the cases from the largest case series [34] to those of the genome-wide association study [35] yielded 45 GSHPs already reported with ECLE: there were 26 females and 19 males with a female-to-male ratio of 1.4. The first clinical signs usually occurred in juveniles or young adult dogs with a median age of onset of 8 months (range: 7 weeks to 3.5 years) [32, 34].

Clinical signs
In the largest clinical case series of ECLE in GSHPs [34], the most prominent skin lesions were scaling and alopecia, which affected 25 (100%) and 19 (76%) of the reported dogs, respectively (Fig. 4a,b). Follicular casts were noted in one third of patients (Fig. 4a,b). Recently seen GSHPs with ECLE were found to also exhibit irregular and polycyclic patches and plaques with dyspigmentation and some scarring (personal observations; Fig. 4c,f). In this form of canine CCLE, skin lesions typically affect the muzzle, pinnae and dorsal trunk and then progress to involve the limbs, sternum and ventral abdomen. Generalized skin lesions are found in most dogs, while crusting, with or without an underlying ulceration, was recorded in one fourth of patients in the largest series of GSHPs [34]. In one dog of that report, ulcers were so extensive that they resulted in bacterial septicemia. Mild pruritus was recorded in one third of GSHPs with ECLE [34].

Overall, skin lesions of ECLE in viszla dogs are nearly identical to those seen in GSHPs with the same disease (Fig.

5a-d). Furthermore, in some viszlas, the alopecic lesions are circumscribed and resemble those of the so-called "*sebaceous adenitis of viszlas*" (Fig, 5a,d). This observation, as well as the presence of typical histological changes of CLE in these dogs, raises the suspicion that some of the viszlas reported with sebaceous adenitis might have had, in fact, ECLE. In fact, in both GSHPs and Magyar viszlas, (granulomatous) sebaceous adenitis is the perfect mimic for ECLE.

A generalized peripheral lymphadenomegaly was reported in one-third of GSHPs with ECLE [34]; lymph node enlargement was also described in other reports [31, 32, 38]. Many GSHPs with ECLE eventually develop signs suggestive of arthralgia, which manifests as a stiff gait, lameness or an arched back [34, 38, 39] In one report, all six dogs were infertile, with azoospermia and irregular or arrested cycles in females [38].

Laboratory evaluation
While rare GSHPs with ECLE have mild anemia, fluctuating thrombocytopenia is seen more commonly in these dogs [34, 38]; serum biochemistry and urinalysis usually do not exhibit consistent changes, except for hyperglobulinemia seen occasionally [34, 38].

Fine needle aspirate material from enlarged peripheral lymph nodes was submitted for cytological evaluation in one GSHP with lymphadenomegaly, and it revealed lymphoid hyperplasia. Spinal radiographs, myelogram and cerebrospinal fluid analysis and stifle and hock joint aspirates were performed in dogs suffering from intermittent arthralgia, but they failed to identify any underlying abnormality [34].

Histopathology
The largest compilation of dogs with ECLE confirms previous information regarding the histopathology of this disease [34]. In this study, microscopic examination revealed a cell-rich interface dermatitis (Fig. 6a,b) characterized by moderate to marked dermal lymphocyte infiltrate that tended to be multifocal, rather than always organized into a subepidermal band. Typical of cell-rich interface lesions, the apoptosis of basal keratinocytes was accompanied by moderate to marked lymphocytic exocytosis in the lower epidermis (Fig. 6b). In addition, biopsies of most dogs had mild lymphocytic exocytosis and keratinocyte apoptosis in the upper epidermis. Diffuse orthokeratotic hyperkeratosis was a notable feature of most biopsies and was usually moderate (Fig. 6b).

In the study by Bryden and colleagues, a lymphocytic interface mural folliculitis was also present in the infundibulum in all dogs, for which biopsy sections captured the infundibula of follicles, and it extended to inferior follicular segments in 92% of dogs [34] (Fig. 6c,d). Sebaceous glands were also affected. A periglandular lymphocytic infiltrate was present in 63% of dogs, sebaceous glands were absent in 50% of all biopsy sections evaluated, and 16% of dogs lacked sebaceous glands in all biopsies (Fig. 6c) [34].

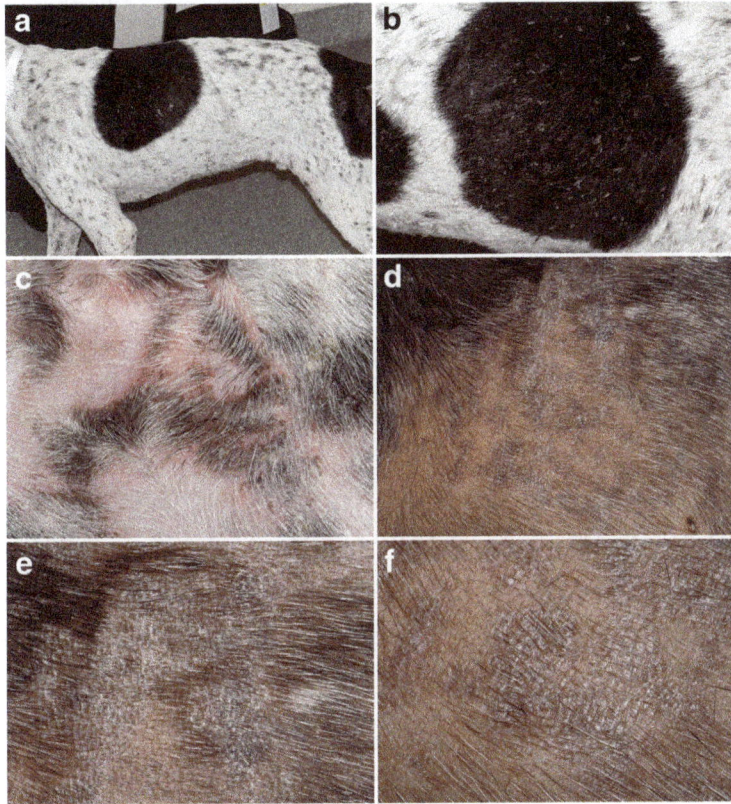

Fig. 4 Clinical characteristics of canine exfoliative cutaneous lupus erythematosus in German shorthaired pointers. **a**, **b**: poor hair coat, scaling and follicular casts are visible from a distance. **c**, **d**, **e**, **f**: irregular plaques with hyperpigmentation and scaling can be seen on closer examination - (**d-f**) courtesy of Petra Bizikova, NC State University

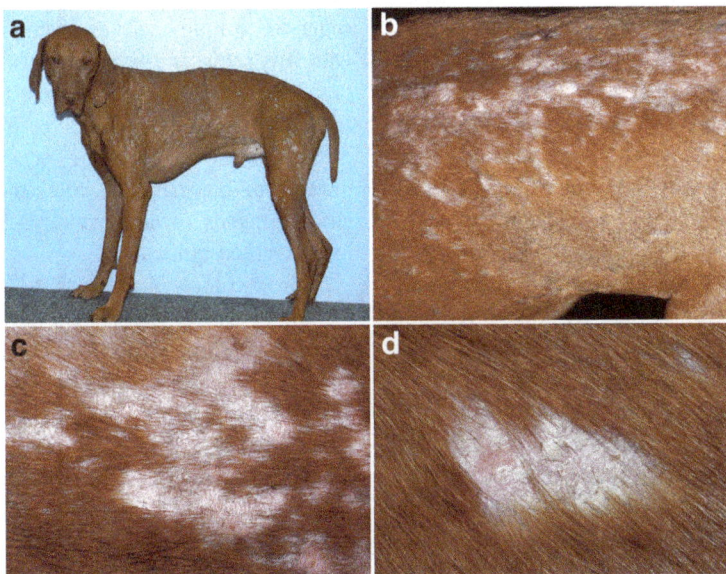

Fig. 5 Clinical characteristics of canine exfoliative cutaneous lupus erythematosus in Magyar viszlas. **a**, **b**: multifocal, often coalescing, patches of alopecia are noted from afar. **c**, **d**: atrophic scars and follicular casts and large scales develop in alopecic areas - courtesy of Émilie Vidémont, University of Lyon, France

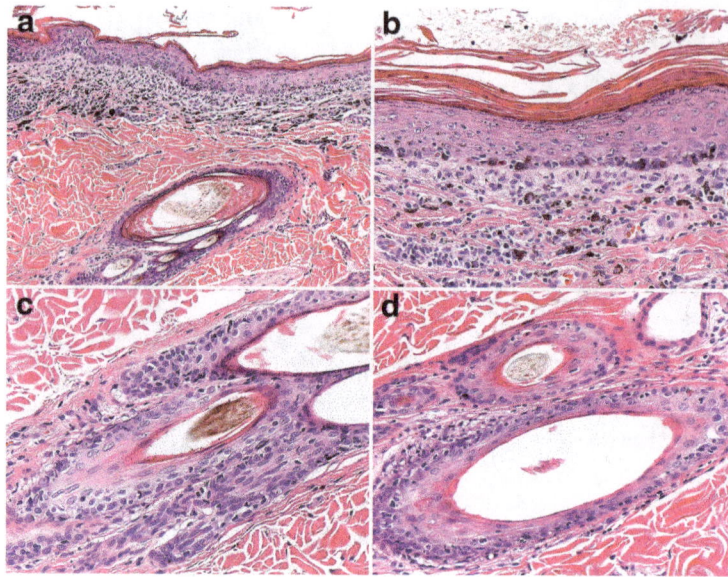

Fig. 6 Histopathology of canine exfoliative cutaneous lupus erythematosus. **a**: cell-rich, lymphocytic interface dermatitis is present with a distinct band-like (lichenoid) dermal infiltrate of lymphocytes, plasma cells and a few histiocytes. 100X (**b**): in an area of well-developed interface dermatitis, laminated, orthokeratotic hyperkeratosis (exfoliation) is present, which is typical of the disease. 200X. **c**: lymphocytic interface folliculitis and mural folliculitis involve the infundibulum (upper-right) as well as the isthmus and inferior segments (lower-left) of hair follicles. Sebaceous glands are absent in this biopsy, as is reported in some cases. 200X (**d**): lymphocytic interface folliculitis and mural folliculitis are present in the external root sheath of anagen hair follicles. Telogen hair follicles can also be affected (not shown). 200X

These latter features can lead to confusion with (primary) sebaceous adenitis. Additionally, a lymphocytic apocrine gland infiltrate was observed in 46% of dogs [34].

Immunopathology

Direct immunofluorescence In one study [34], direct immunofluorescence testing performed on paraffin-embedded sections revealed the presence of in situ deposition of IgG, IgM, IgA and C3 in the epidermal basement membrane of 100%, 47%, 11% and 5% of GSHPs, respectively. The multifocal or continuous fine deposition of IgG was recorded in 61%, 35% and 77% of skin biopsy sections, respectively. Interestingly, the follicular basement membrane deposition of IgG was found in 41% of tested biopsies.

Indirect immunofluorescence Indirect immunofluorescence testing on sections of normal canine haired and salt-split-skin revealed the existence of circulating anti-follicular IgG antibodies in the serum of 57% of tested GSHPs with ECLE [34]. In addition, anti-sebaceous gland IgG antibodies were also detected in these dogs. Circulating anti-epidermal basement membrane antibodies were not observed, however. In three studies, antinuclear antibody serology usually remained below positive thresholds in GSHPs with ECLE [32, 34, 38].

Immunohistochemistry Immunohistochemical staining confirmed the predominance of CD3-bearing T lymphocytes

in the lower epidermis, superficial dermis, in the infundibulum of hair follicles and around sweat glands [34]. These CD3-positive T lymphocytes infiltrated sebaceous glands and their associated ducts in samples collected from two dogs.

Treatment and outcome The review of published reports has yielded inconsistent information on the treatment and outcome of this disease. The early descriptions of ECLE suggested some benefit of dietary changes, supplementation with fatty acids, anti-seborrheic shampoos, antibiotics and/or oral retinoids [31, 32] The most recent case series [34, 38] reported the limited efficacy of immune-modulating drugs prescribed either as single or combination therapy (e.g. tetracycline-niacinamide combinations, doxycycline, oral glucocorticoids, azathioprine, ciclosporin, leflunomide, or hydroxychloroquine).

Hydroxychloroquine, an first-line antimalarial drug used in human CCLE, appeared to slow down the clinical progression in some dogs with ECLE; in contrast, high-dose ciclosporin reportedly was not able to halt lesion worsening [38]. As the response to immunomodulators is heterogeneous in human CCLE variants [40], the use of high-dose oral glucocorticoids and adjunctive immunosuppressive regimens need to be investigated on an individual patient basis [34, 38, 39].

Taking into account all GSHPs with ECLE for which a long-term outcome has been reported [31, 32, 34, 38, 39], over half of dogs are eventually euthanized for their lack of disease response to therapy. This makes this CLE variant the most challenging to treat among all those of canine CCLE.

Mucocutaneous lupus erythematosus

Historical perspective In the mid 1990's, two German shepherd dogs (one in France and one in Québec, Canada) were described as having a genital-predominant DLE [41, 42]. In 1998, we proposed the disease name of MCLE for dogs with perimucosal ulcerative lesions and microscopic characteristics of CLE (Olivry T: British Veterinary Dermatology Study Group, York, 1998). Additional cases with identical phenotypes were later published with the diagnoses of MCLE [43], DLE [44], or, more recently, perianal/perivulvar LE [45]. Finally, we reported a large series of 21 additional dogs with MCLE was reported in 2015 [9] and a single case report from Chile was later published in 2017 [46].

Incidence and prevalence There are no available data to estimate the incidence of prevalence of MCLE in dogs.

Signalment Collating the signalment of all published cases of canine MCLE yielded pertinent information. Of the 36 dogs [9, 41–46], there were 17 German shepherd dogs and their crosses (47%); adding the two Belgian shepherds [43] leads to about half of the dogs with MCLE belonging to breeds related to German shepherds. Altogether, females appear nearly twice over-represented with a female-to-male ratio of 1.8; there was an equal representation of intact and neutered individuals. Interestingly, this female-to-male ratio increases to 3.8 if we only collate data from German/Belgian shepherds and their crosses. In all, the age of onset of skin lesions of MCLE varied between 3 to 13 years (median and means: 6 years). Most dogs for which this information was available (17/28; 61%) began exhibiting noticeable mucocutaneous lesions in mid-adulthood (i.e. between 4 and 8 years of age).

Odds ratios for breed, sex or age predispositions for the development of MCLE cannot be estimated, as dogs come from multiple continents (North and South America, Japan, Europe), and a reference population therefore is not available.

Clinical signs The owners of dogs with MCLE often report perimucosal ulcerative skin lesions with vocalization suggesting pain why defecating or urinating.

At the time of presentation to the veterinarian, lesions have been reported to occur most commonly on or around the anus (24/36; 67%) (Fig. 7a) or on the genitalia or perigenital region (17/36; 47%) (Fig. 7b,c) [9, 41–46]. Similar lesions can also be seen, but less commonly, abutting the lips, but they usually do not cross into the mucosa itself (10 dogs; 28%) (Fig. 7e,f). More rarely, lesions have

been noted around the eyes (6 dogs; 17%) (Fig. 7d) and nasal planum (4 dogs; 11%); oral lesion are rarest (3 dogs; 9%) [9, 41–46]. In the largest case series, most dogs had two or more areas affected, and the lesions were usually symmetrically distributed [9].

The characteristic lesions of MCLE are erosions and ulcers (Fig. 7a-f), but the latter do not tend to heal with scarring [9, 41–46], an important difference with the lesions of facial and generalized DLE. Crusts are present when lesions extend into haired skin. Hyperpigmentation can be seen often around ulcerative lesions or at the site of previous ones, thus leaving a figurate or reticulated pattern [9, 41–46]. Pruritus is normally absent or mild, but pain is described when defecating and urinating or when touching the lesions; systemic signs have not been reported [9, 41–46].

The most relevant clinical differential diagnoses of MCLE are mucocutaneous pyoderma (MCP), MMP and EM variants.

Histopathology In the largest case series, and per inclusion criteria, skin biopsies contained a cell-rich lymphocytic interface dermatitis with basal keratinocyte damage (i.e. basal cell apoptosis, loss and/or hydropic degeneration) [9] (Fig. 8a-c). This pattern was often patchy, or in limited areas, sometimes only being observed at close proximity to an ulcer margin. Interface dermatitis commonly extended to the infundibula of hair follicles (Fig. 8d), while inferior segments of hair follicles are sometimes also involved (Fig. 8e). Basement membrane thickening was found to be multifocal, patchy to diffuse (Fig. 8c). Pigmentary incontinence varied from mild to marked. Plasma cells were present in all cases (Fig. 8b,c), mixed with lymphocytes and were often numerous in subepidermal, perivascular, periadnexal and in dermal areas below erosions and ulcers. Erosions and ulcers were common but granulation tissue was limited and fibrosis (scarring) was not seen. Occasional suprabasal keratinocyte apoptosis was noted in half of the cases, but suprabasal lymphocytic satellitosis, when present, was always mild. Nonetheless, superficial keratinocyte cell death can lead to confusion with EM and morphologically related conditions. Not surprisingly, for a perimucosal ulcerative disease, lesions of concurrent bacterial infection were common, including neutrophilic crusting, pustules, perifolliculitis and folliculitis, as well as presence of bacteria in surface exudates. Such infection will complicate the histological diagnosis and the successful treatment of pyoderma is warranted prior to biopsy.

Immunopathology In dogs in whom this information was reported, direct IF almost always revealed a positive IgG lupus band test (LBT) [9, 44]. Positive LBTs were sometimes also uncovered for IgA, IgM and C3. Positive ANA titers were rarely found, however.

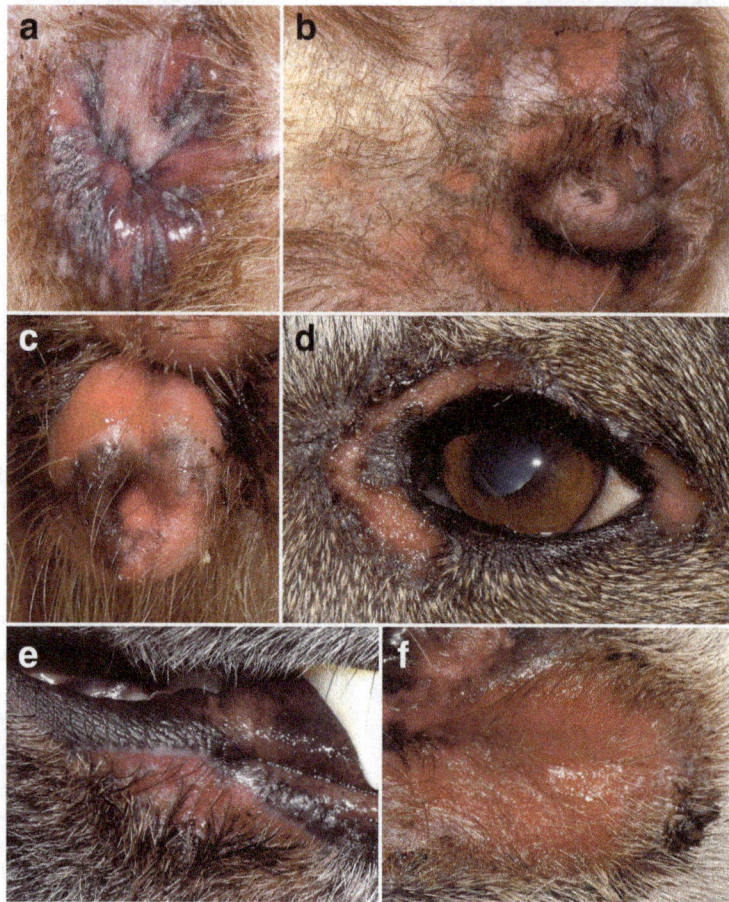

Fig. 7 Clinical characteristics of canine mucocutaneous lupus erythematosus. **a**: anal erosions with peripheral hyperpigmentation in a German shepherd dog; (**b**): multifocal perigenital erosions with peripheral hyperpigmentation are often seen in female German shepherd bitches; (**c**): erosions on the lateral sides of the vulva in a German shepherd bitch (courtesy of Pablo Del Mestre, Mar Del Plata Argentina); (**d**): periocular erosions in a German shepherd – these lesions were bilateral (courtesy of Petra Bizikova, NC State University, Raleigh; (**e**): erosion abutting the lip in the same German shepherd dog as in (**a**); (**f**): same dog as in (**b**) – large perilabial erosion; this lesion was also symmetric

Treatment and outcome The skin lesions of canine MCLE appear to respond best to immunosuppressive dosages of oral glucocorticoids [9, 41–46]. The complete remission of signs is generally obtained within one month of treatment induction [9]. A combination of a tetracycline antibiotic, with or without niacinamide, appears beneficial either alone or as adjunctive combination in some dogs [9, 41, 45]. In most patients, the tapering of oral glucocorticoids leads to the prompt relapse of skin lesions, which will undergo remission once the dosage is re-escalated again. The usefulness of adding additional immunosuppressive drugs (e.g. azathioprine, ciclosporin, mycophenolate mofetil etc.) to permit the reduction of oral glucocorticoid doses needs further investigations.

Discoid lupus erythematosus

Historical perspective Among the several variants of human chronic CLE (e.g. discoid LE [DLE], verrucous (hyperkeratotic) LE, chilblain LE, lupus tumidus and lupus profundus), DLE represents the most common form: it is divided into a localized variant where skin lesions are confined to the head and neck, and a generalized form, in which skin lesions also occur below the neck [47].

In 1979, Griffin and colleagues reported clinical, histopathological and immunological characteristics of two dogs with localized facial lesions that were diagnosed as being affected with the canine counterpart of human DLE [1]. In these two dogs, the nasal-predominant dermatitis was associated with microscopic focal interface dermatitis, basement membrane thickening and a superficial lymphocytic and plasmacytic dermatitis. Since then, there were three large case series describing dogs with nasal skin-predominant DLE lesions [2–4], two of them including some of the same cases [2, 4]. The then-proposed terminology resulted in the widespread acceptance of "*canine DLE*" being equated mainly to facial localized lesions. In the 2010s, we began reporting dogs with a more widespread phenotype that

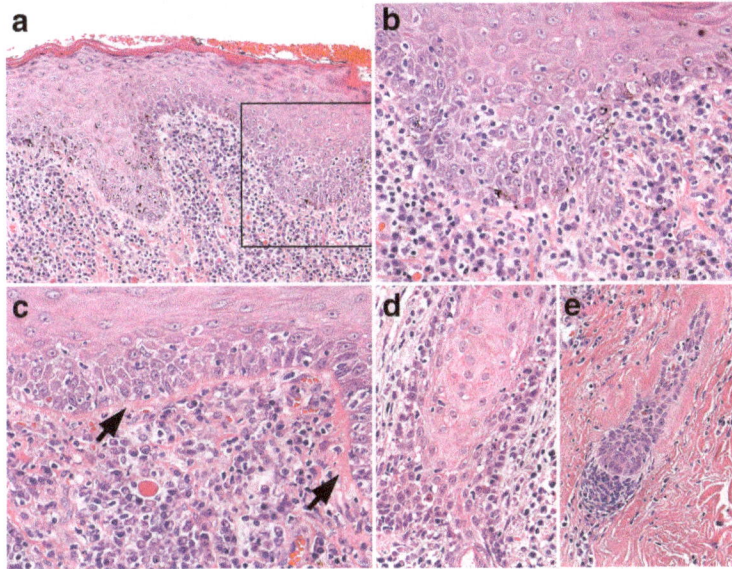

Fig. 8 Histopathology of canine mucocutaneous lupus erythematosus. **a**: cell-rich, lymphocytic interface dermatitis is present with numerous plasma cells, including Mott cells, which is common with inflammation in perimucosal skin and is exacerbated by secondary bacterial infection. 100X (**b**): inset box from image "a", lymphocytes infiltrate the basal and suprabasal layers of the epidermis in association with multifocal basal cell apoptosis. 400X (**c**): basement membrane thickening (arrows) is present and is usually patchy and multifocal. 400X (**d**): lymphocytic interface folliculitis and mural folliculitis involve the infundibulum and extend to the isthmus (not shown) of a hair follicle. 400X (**e**): lymphocytic mural folliculitis of the inferior hair follicle (external root sheath), with apoptosis and follicular atrophy. 200X

resembled that of the generalized variant of human DLE [48–50]; this was followed with the publication of a case series of ten dogs with generalized DLE (GDLE) [10], this article encompassing the three cases already published by the NC State Dermatology group [48–50].

Signalment The four largest series of dogs with the "classic" localized facial-predominant DLE (FDLE) allows the analysis of a cohort of 104 dogs [3, 4, 45, 51]. Among these cases, there were 32 German shepherd dogs and their crosses (31%). The age of onset of FDLE skin lesions varied between 1 and 12 years of age (median: 7 years); while the female-to-male ratio was 0.7, there was an equal representation of intact and neutered individuals.

A retrospective study recently evaluated the historical and outcome information in ten dogs with GDLE [10]. Amongst these dogs, there were two Chinese crested dogs and two Labrador retrievers; there was one each of the following pure breeds: miniature pinscher, Leonberger, Shih-Tzu and toy poodle. The age of onset of GDLE skin lesions varied between 5 and 12 years of age (median 9 years). The female-to-male ratio was 1.0 and all dogs were castrated. Interestingly—and surprisingly—German shepherd dogs, a breed predisposed to develop several forms of LE, such as SLE, localized FDLE and MCLE, did not seem affected by GDLE. This discrepancy may be explained by the German shepherd breed not being predisposed to this disease, by the small size of the reported cohort or by a possible clinical

misdiagnosis of GDLE as one of the" *idiopathic lichenoid dermatoses*" as they were diagnosed in the 1980's solely based on the histopathological identification of a "lichenoid tissue reaction" in dogs [52].

Incidence and prevalence At this time, there is no usable information to determine the frequency of occurrence of FDLE and GDLE in dogs.

Clinical signs The classic skin lesions of human DLE usually consist of early erythematous and variably scaly macules or papules that slowly evolve into a coin-shaped (i.e. discoid) , plaques with adherent scales, follicular plugging (i.e. comedones) and peripheral hyperpigmentation presumed to occur secondarily to inflammation [47]. These discoid plaques can coalesce and develop central scarring and depigmentation [47]. Atypical presentations of GDLE have been reported in patients of differing ethnic groups; the morphological appearance of lesions in these patients varies from hyperpigmented macules to hyperkeratotic, hyperpigmented plaques with an erythematous border [53].

The early skin lesions in canine FDLE consist of erythema, depigmentation and scaling that progress into erosions and ulcerations with atrophy and loss of the architecture of the nasal planum (Fig. 9a-f); crusting may be present if the epithelial integrity is damaged [3, 4]. Skin lesions usually affect the nasal planum (Fig. 9a-f) and might even involve the nares (Fig. 9c,d,f); several dogs exhibit additional skin lesions on the dorso-proximal

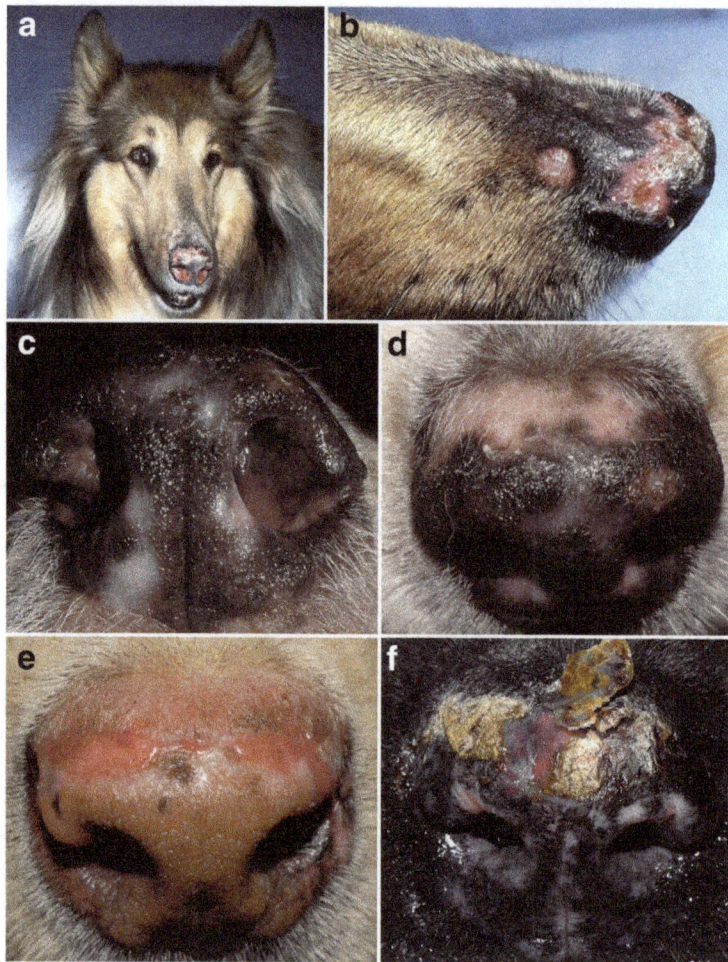

Fig. 9 clinical characteristics of canine facial discoid lupus erythematosus. **a**, **b**: erythematous, depigmented, ulcerated, crusted and scarred nasal lesions of FDLE in a rough collie; a discoid lesion is visible in the proximal dorsal muzzle; (**c**, **d**): during the chronic phase of FDLE, depigmentation and scarring without inflammation are present; (**e**): erosions leading to scars in a Labrador with active FDLE; (**f**) depigmentation, scarring and crusting in a dog with FDLE. The presence of prominent inflammation often heralds a secondary bacterial colonization, like in the so-called MCP (courtesy of Petra Bizikova, NC State University, Raleigh)

muzzle (Fig. 9a,b), lips, periorbital skin and pinnae [3, 4]. Squamous cell carcinoma was reported to develop from chronic DLE nasal lesions in dogs [54], as in humans [55]. Pruritus has been reported to be variable in dogs with FDLE [3, 4].

Clinicians should remember that cutaneous (epitheliotropic) T-cell lymphomas can have localized lesions that affect the nose and could mimic those of FDLE. Other differential diagnosis for depigmentation and inflammation on the nasal planum are MCP and the uveodermatological syndrome, which resembles the Vogt-Koyanagi-Harada syndrome of humans. One should keep in mind that the "so-called MCP" is a poorly described disease that, if it were to even exist as a primary disease, is likely to occur secondarily to other diseases such as FDLE, MMP and MCLE and other nasal-targeting auto-immune and immune-mediated diseases.

Dogs with GDLE present with generalized or multifocal, annular (discoid) to polycyclic plaques with dyspigmentation, an erythematous margin, adherent scaling, follicular plugging and central alopecia; these predominate on the neck, dorsum and lateral thorax (Fig. 10a,f) [10]. In many of these dogs, the plaques evolved into ulcerations healing with a central atrophic or hypertrophic scar and dyspigmentation (depigmentation and hyperpigmentation) (Fig. 10a,f). Four of ten of the reported dogs (40%) had mucocutaneous regions involved with plaques usually appearing on or around the genitalia. An unusual pattern of reticulated (net-like) hyperpigmentation was visible on the ventral abdomen and lateral thorax in two of these cases, a feature also seen in other CCLE variants such as MCLE [9]. In the largest series of cases, systemic signs were not reported; pruritus and pain at the site of lesions were observed in four (40%) and three of ten dogs (30%), respectively [10]. There are only two

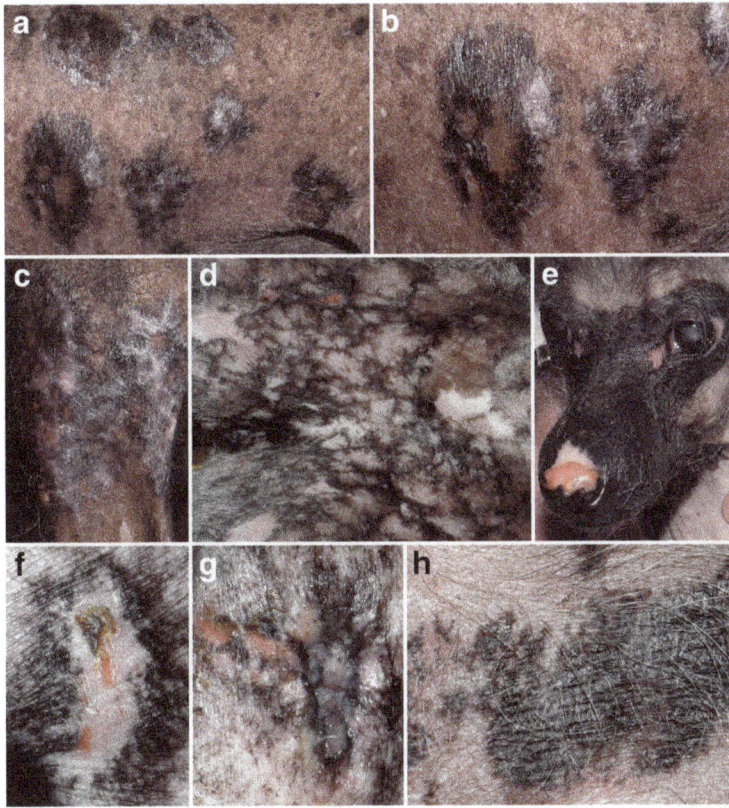

Fig. 10 Clinical characteristics of canine generalized discoid lupus erythematosus. **a, b**: disc-shaped, annular and polycyclic plaques with hyperpigmentation, focal depigmentation and scarring on the thorax of a Chinese crested dog with GDLE; (**c**): large irregular plaque with dyspigmentation, scarring and erythema on the lateral knee of the same dog as in (**a, b**); **d**: reticulated depigmentation with occasional plaques and focal ulceration on the abdomen; (**e**): unusual "mask-like" bilateral and symmetric hyperpigmentation and dorsal proximal ulceration and scarring in another Chinese crested dog with GDLE; (**f**): same dog as in (**e**) – classic disc-shaped dyspigmented plaque with scarring and focal ulceration and crusting; (**g**): same dog as in (**e**) – anal and perianal dyspigmentation and scarring with focal ulceration; (**h**): large polycyclic hyperpigmented and scaly plaque on the abdomen of a crossbred dog with GDLE

canine skin diseases that could closely mimic GDLE: generalized (and often vaccine-induced) ischemic dermatopathies and the very rare hyperkeratotic EM (a.k.a. "old dog" EM).

Laboratory evaluation In humans affected with the generalized variant of GDLE, a positive ANA titer is frequently found, and it represents a risk factor for development of SLE within five years after the initial diagnosis of skin lesions [56]. So far, out of the 104 dogs with classic FDLE included in the four largest series of cases, there were no reports of progression to SLE [3, 4, 45, 51]. Seven dogs with GDLE had a low positive ANA serum titer, but a progression with acquisition of additional criteria for SLE was not seen in any dog within the median follow up of 2.5 years (ranging 0.5 to 6 years) in the published series [10]. To our knowledge, the progression of a DLE variant to "clinical" SLE has been reported only in one dog [57].

Histopathology The histology of DLE in dogs is similar to that of humans and is characterized by a lichenoid cell-rich,

lymphocytic interface dermatitis reaction pattern with basal keratinocyte vacuolar degeneration, apoptosis, loss of basal cells and basement membrane thickening [1, 10].

In canine FDLE, the interface reaction (vacuolar degeneration, apoptosis and loss of basal cells) is often subtle or mild in biopsy samples (Fig. 11a-c) [1, 10]. Only small areas might exhibit an active interface reaction and these lesions are easily missed, as nasal planum biopsies tend to be few and small. Interface changes can involve the follicular infundibula (Fig. 11d), when lesions extend off of the nasal planum; however, folliculitis has not been specifically investigated in canine FDLE. Pigmentary incontinence occurs secondarily to the interface reaction (Fig. 11a,b) but it is not specific to this type of injury and it can be found, persistent, in the nasal planum of dogs without concurrent nasal dermatitis [58, 59] Thickening of the basement membrane zone is patchy or multifocal but is not specific, as it occurs with other chronic inflammatory disorders of the nasal planum, such as leishmaniosis, where geographically relevant [60]. Superficial dermal fibrosis can be absent or range from mild-to-marked. Secondary bacterial

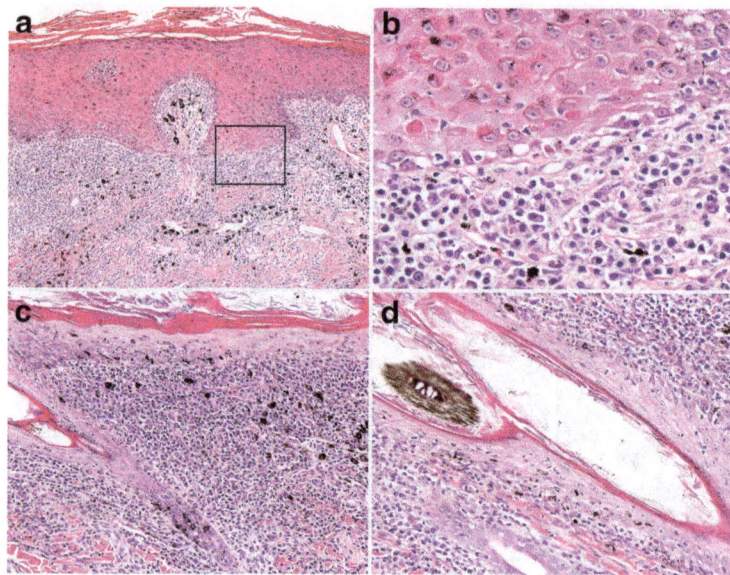

Fig. 11 Histopathology of facial canine discoid lupus erythematosus. **a**: in a biopsy from the nasal planum, cell-rich, lymphocytic interface dermatitis is present with a prominent band-like (lichenoid) dermal infiltrate of lymphocytes and plasma cells. Pigmentary incontinence is moderate. 100× (**b**): inset box from image "a", a short epidermal segment with well-developed interface change, where lymphocytes infiltrate predominantly the basal layer in conjunction with basal cell vacuolation, apoptosis, and loss. 400X (**c**): a similar interface reaction pattern affects the epidermis of haired skin in the dorsal nasal area. 200X (**d**): lymphocytic interface folliculitis and mural folliculitis of the hair follicle infundibulum. 200X

colonization is common in FDLE and often complicates the histological diagnosis. These issues are compounded by the fact that, historically, the diagnosis of nasal-predominant "*canine DLE*" was given to dogs when microscopic examination of nasal planum skin biopsy specimens revealed a superficial dermal "*band-like*" pattern of inflammation rich in lymphocytes and plasma cells (a so-called "*lichenoid infiltrate*"), without any emphasis on the presence of an interface reaction. In fact, it is now believed that such "*lichenoid*" lymphocyte and plasma cell rich inflammation is a nonspecific inflammatory pattern seen in and near mucosae or related tissues (oral cavity, nasal planum, eyelids, genitalia, etc.). In a retrospective histological study of nasal dermatitis in dogs, a cell-rich lichenoid infiltrate was common, but only a small subset of subjects with nasal lesions exhibited the interface dermatitis associated with CLE [61].

In canine GDLE, in contrast to FDLE, the interface reaction is usually well developed, when an adequate number of biopsies are examined from the active margins of lesions (Fig. 12a,b) [10]. The epidermis may be atrophic or mildly hyperplastic (Fig. 12a,b) as a consequence of regional variation in severity of the interface reaction. Pigmentary incontinence can be pronounced, especially at the margins of lesions, where the interface reaction extends into zones of secondary hyperpigmentation induced by chronic inflammation (Fig. 12a-d). In chronic lesions, dermal fibrosis occasionally displaces the cell-rich inflammatory infiltrate from the superficial dermis (Fig. 12c,d). Cell-poor zones of lesion occasionally occur but often individual lymphocytes

can be found in the basal layer of the epidermis in good numbers, with satellitosis of apoptotic basal keratinocytes. In GDLE, superficial epidermal apoptosis occurs, with or without lymphocytic satellitosis, which can erroneously suggest the diagnosis of erythema multiforme or morphologically related conditions. However, the collection of multiple biopsies reveals apoptosis to be most prominent in the basal epidermal layer in cases of GDLE.

In the recent case series of canine GDLE [10], alopecia occurred in nearly all patients; lymphocytic interface folliculitis involved the infundibulum and extended into the isthmus. A lymphocytic mural folliculitis was also common, but it was usually milder and involved the infundibulum, isthmus and inferior hair follicle segments, typically sparing the bulbs. This mural pattern mirrors that of human DLE, where it is also called a panfollicular pattern; it is usually minimally severe, but such a pattern is insufficiently described [62]. Sebaceous gland atrophy occurred in GDLE cases, where it was mostly mild and partial in biopsies but sometimes it was complete [10]. It should be noted that diagnostic biopsies typically focus on epidermal changes at the margins of skin lesions where hair follicle and sebaceous gland changes might not be fully developed.

Immunopathology A linear deposition of IgG and IgM at the dermo-epidermal basement membrane zone (i.e. a positive LBT) of lesional skin was found in 90% of dogs with GDLE, and this proportion is similar to what is seen

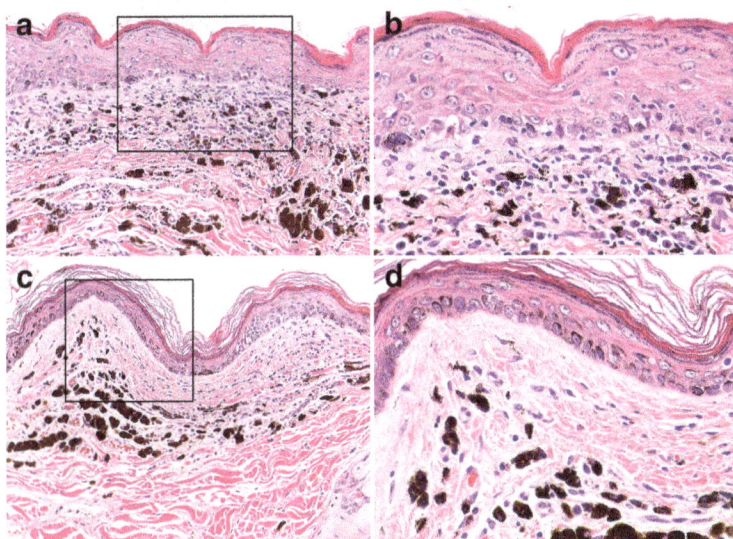

Fig. 12 Histopathology of generalized canine discoid lupus erythematosus (**a**): in a skin biopsy from the trunk, a cell-rich lymphocytic interface dermatitis is present with prominent pigmentary incontinence. While epidermal atrophy (not shown) is classically seen in areas of prominent interface change, epidermal hyperplasia (shown here) can occur in chronic smoldering areas of lesions. 200X (**b**): inset box from image "a", lymphocytes infiltrate predominately the basal layer in conjunction with basal cell vacuolation, apoptosis, and loss. 400X (**c**): some chronic lesions develop mild subepidermal fibrosis with a paucity of inflammation, while retaining pigmentary incontinence. 100X (**d**): inset box from image "c", higher magnification image shows mild subepidermal fibrosis, few inflammatory cells and prominent pigmentary incontinence. 400X

in human DLE lesions [10]. Interestingly, the most commonly detected immunoreactant deposited in one series of dogs with classic FDLE was C3 (90–100%), while IgG and IgM were revealed in 40–70% of cases, respectively [4]. In contrast, in the second case series, a positive LBT showed immunoglobulins (all classes together) and activated complement (C3) in 85–90% of 22 cases [3]. These variable results between canine localized and generalized DLE could be related to differences in tissue fixation techniques (frozen vs. formalin), antigen retrieval methods and/or immunofluorescence staining protocols that were performed 30 years apart. To investigate the value of performing DIF in canine CLE diagnostic work-up, further studies regarding the sensitivity and specificity of a positive LBT for the diagnosis of CLE variants are warranted.

Treatment and outcome Besides the obvious need for photoprotection (sun avoidance), the 2017 update of the Cochrane systematic review of interventions for human DLE reported evidence for the benefit of a potent topical glucocorticoid and the oral drugs hydroxychloroquine and acitretin (a retinoid) [63] Furthermore, there was insufficient evidence for the efficacy of other interventions, such as topical calcineurin inhibitors (e.g. tacrolimus), [63].

Since 1992, antibiotics of the tetracycline family, with or without concurrent niacinamide (a.k.a. nicotinamide), have been suggested to be helpful for the treatment of canine immune-mediated skin diseases including FDLE. An initial report by White and colleagues showed that 14/20 (70%) dogs with FDLE had a good-to-excellent response

using a tetracycline-niacinamide combination [64]; a recent retrospective study revealed a similar positive response rate in dogs with FDLE [45]. While tetracycline-niacinamide therapy is considered to be safe, tetracycline is no longer available commercially in many countries. Although tetracycline and doxycycline were shown to be relatively similar in their effectiveness to treat the so-called canine lupoid onychodystrophy, a poorly-understood onychitis [65], therapeutic equipotency data for other canine auto-immune and immune-mediated diseases, such as DLE are unavailable; additional studies are necessary to confirm the effectiveness of substituting doxycycline or minocycline for the tetracycline used beforehand to treat dogs with CLE.

Topical tacrolimus ointment has been used successfully for the topical treatment of canine FDLE. At first, Griffies and colleagues evaluated the use of 0.1% tacrolimus ointment applied topically to the lesional (facial) skin of ten dogs with DLE, most of these dogs receiving topical tacrolimus as an adjunctive therapy to oral glucocorticoids [66]. There was a positive response in eight dogs (80%), three of them having had an excellent improvement in skin lesions [66]. Recently, Messinger and colleagues conducted a randomized, double-blinded, placebo-controlled crossover study to evaluate the efficacy of a lower concentration of tacrolimus ointment (0.03%) in 19 dogs with FDLE [51]. Tacrolimus ointment, applied twice daily as monotherapy for up to 10 weeks, appeared safe and effective. A noticeable clinical improvement was seen in 13/18 (72%) of the dogs, whereas only three dogs receiving the placebo had lesions that improved. To summarize, limited outcome data suggest that topical tacrolimus ointment and/or a niacinamide-cyclin combination therapy should be considered as potentially effective therapeutic options for canine FDLE.

Skin lesions of canine GDLE appear to respond to a wide range of treatments but half of the patients experienced relapses upon the tapering of drug dosages. In a recent report [10], a remarkable improvement or a complete remission in GDLE skin lesions followed treatment with oral ciclosporin (mean 4.8 mg/kg once daily) along with a short course of glucocorticoids at treatment onset. Furthermore, oral hydroxychloroquine, in conjunction with topical 0.1% tacrolimus ointment application, helped induce and maintain remission of skin lesions in two dogs with GDLE [10].

Lupus nonspecific skin diseases
In the Gilliam-Sontheimer CLE classification, lupus-nonspecific skin diseases are those that are not only present in the context of SLE, but also in other diseases; they do not have histopathology typical of CLE, however [11].

Cutaneous lesions associated with systemic lupus erythematosus
There is only scant information of skin lesions that occur during canine SLE. In the largest compilations of dogs with SLE, skin lesions were described in 33% [5] to 60% [67] of dogs, while oral ulcers were reported in 4 to 11% of cases, respectively [5, 67] Of note is that the first paper regrouped data from all cases published beforehand [5], while, in the other [67], skin lesions were not described in detail. In the first paper [5], Scott also reported characteristics on 26 new cases. In these cases, scaling (86% of the 14 dogs with dermatitis), mucocutaneous ulcerations (50%) and footpad ulcers and/or hyperkeratosis (42%) were most commonly seen [5]; two of 14 dogs (14%) exhibited lesions reportedly consistent with "lupus panniculitis" [5].

The microscopic lesions reported in 18 of these new cases were most commonly an interface dermatitis with variable inflammation [5]. While vasculitis was reported in only one case, the images of cell-poor interface dermatitis might represent sequelae of a lupus-associated vasculitis, a lupus-nonspecific skin disease; a lymphocytic septal panniculitis was observed in two dogs.

There is a clear need for more detailed descriptions of skin lesions associated with canine SLE. Future reports should also attempt to classify these lesions in the context of the human and canine CLE subsets described above.

Bullous systemic lupus erythematosus
In 1999, we reported a case that clinically resembled type I bullous SLE of humans (BSLE-I) [6]. In this four-year-old male castrated bichon frisé, erosions and crusts were present on the right elbow, axilla, thorax, pinna and labial commissures, and ulcers were also discovered on the footpad. Skin biopsies revealed subepidermal vesiculation and immunological testing uncovered skin-fixed and circulating IgG auto-antibodies that targeted type VII collagen in the epidermal basement membrane. As this dog also exhibited an intermittent fever, oral ulcers, a persistent proteinuria, a Coombs' positive hemolytic anemia, a thrombocytopenia, a suspected pleuritis and hepatitis and elevated serum anti-nuclear autoantibodies, he was diagnosed has having concurrent SLE. The development of skin lesions associated with collagen VII auto-antibodies is normally typical of the disease epidermolysis bullosa acquisita, but, in the context of SLE, the diagnosis should change to type I bullous SLE [68]; as such, BSLE-I is a lupus-nonspecific skin disease.

Conclusions
The number of canine CLE variants has increased since the princeps description of FDLE in dogs, nearly 40 years ago [1]. The accumulation of reports has led to the identification of predisposed breeds in many subsets and to a genetic linkage in the case of ECLE [35]. The recognition of additional subtypes of CCLE has revealed the overlap in some common skin lesions, which resemble those of human DLE, (i.e. polymorphic plaques with dyspigmentation, scarring and scaling). The new frontiers of canine CLE investigations will be to characterize and report atypical and crossover CLE variants—which are anecdotally mentioned being seen by colleagues—so that to add to the expanding phenotypic spectrum of canine CLE. Clinician-scientists are also urged to begin delving into the pathogenesis of CLE in dogs, to elucidate the genetic predisposition of the breed-specific variants (e.g. VCLE in collie breeds), the flare factors and the mechanisms of lesion formation. Finally, the usefulness of oral antimalarials for treatment of canine CLE variants should be investigated further.

Abbreviations
ACLE: acute cutaneous lupus erythematosus; BP: bullous pemphigoid; BSLE-I: type-I bullous systemic lupus erythematosus; CCLE: chronic cutaneous lupus erythematosus; CLE: cutaneous lupus erythematosus; DLE: discoid lupus erythematosus; EBA: epidermolysis bullosa acquisita; ECLE: exfoliative cutaneous lupus erythematosus; EM: erythema multiforme; FDLE: facial discoid lupus erythematosus; GDLE: generalized discoid lupus erythematosus; GSHP: German shorthaired pointer; LBT: lupus band test; MCLE: mucocutaneous lupus erythematosus; MMP: mucous membrane pemphigoid; SCLE: subacute cutaneous lupus erythematosus; SLE: systemic lupus erythematosus; VCLE: vesicular cutaneous lupus erythematosus

Acknowledgements
we appreciate the BMC Veterinary Research editorship for the waiving of the page charges for this collection of articles. Ms Joanna Barton and Mr. Nathan Whitehurst from NC State University are thanked for their continuous and excellent histology laboratory support.

Funding
none.

Authors' contributions

TO designed the concept of this article and the adaptation of the CLE classification; all authors contributed to the writing and figure generation and they approved the submitted version.

Consent for publication

not applicable.

Competing interests

The authors declare that they have no competing interests.

Author details

[1]Department of Clinical Sciences, College of Veterinary Medicine, North Carolina State University, Raleigh, NC 27606, USA. [2]Comparative Medicine Institute, North Carolina State University, Raleigh, NC, USA. [3]Department of Population Health and Pathobiology, College of Veterinary Medicine, North Carolina State University, Raleigh, NC, USA. [4]Department of Small Animal Medicine and Surgery, College of Veterinary Medicine, University of Georgia, Athens, GA, USA.

References

1. Griffin CE, Stannard AA, Ihrke PJ, Ardans AA, Cello RM, Bjorling DR. Canine discoid lupus erythematosus. Vet Immunol Immunopathol. 1979;1:79–87.
2. Scott DW, Walton DK, Manning TO, Smith CA, Lewis RM. Canine lupus erythematosus. II. Discoid lupus erythematosus. J Amer Hosp Assoc. 1983;19:481–8.
3. Olivry T, Alhaidari Z, Carlotti DN, Guaguère E, Régnier A, Hubert B, Magnol JP, Oksman F. Le lupus érythémateux discoïde du chien: A propos de 22 observations (discoid lupus erythematosus in the dog: 22 cases). Prat Med Chir Anim Comp. 1987;22:205–14.
4. Scott DW, Walton DK, Slater MR, Smith CA, Lewis RM. Immune-mediated dermatoses in domestic animals: ten years after - part II. Comp Cont Ed Pract Vet. 1987;9:539–51.
5. Scott DW, Walton DK. Canine lupus erythematosus. I. Systemic lupus erythematosus. J Am Anim Hosp Assoc. 1983;19:462–79.
6. Olivry T, Savary KCM, Murphy KM, Dunston SM, Chen M. Bullous systemic lupus erythematosus (type I) in a dog. Vet Rec. 1999;145:165–9.
7. Olivry T, Luther PB, Dunston SM, Moore PF. Interface dermatitis and sebaceous adenitis in exfoliative cutaneous lupus erythematosus ("lupoid dermatosis") of German short-haired pointers. In: Proceedings of the Annual Members' Meeting of the American Academy of Veterinary Dermatology & American College of Veterinary Dermatology. Maui, HI: American Academy of Veterinary Dermatology & American College of Veterinary Dermatology; 1999. p. 41–2.
8. Jackson HA, Olivry T. Ulcerative dermatosis of the Shetland sheepdog and rough colllie dog may represent a novel vesicular variant of cutaneous lupus erythematosus. Vet Dermatol. 2001;12:19–28.
9. Olivry T, Rossi MA, Banovic F, Linder KE. Mucocutaneous lupus erythematosus in dogs (21 cases). Vet Dermatol. 2015;26:256–e55.
10. Banovic F, Linder KE, Uri M, Rossi MA, Olivry T. Clinical and microscopic features of generalized discoid lupus erythematosus in dogs (10 cases). Vet Dermatol. 2016;27:488–e131.
11. Sontheimer RD. The lexicon of cutaneous lupus erythematosus - a review and personal perspective on the nomenclature and classification of the cutaneous manifestations of lupus erythematosus. Lupus. 1997;6:84–95.
12. David-Bajar KM, Davis BM. Pathology, immunopathology, and immunohistochemistry in cutaneous lupus erythematosus. Lupus. 1997;6: 145–57.
13. Tsuchida T. Classification of lupus erythematosus based upon Japanese patients. Autoimmun Rev. 2009;8:453–5.
14. Ziemer M, Milkova L, Kunz M. Lupus erythematosus. Part II: clinical picture, diagnosis and treatment. J Dtsch Dermatol Ges. 2014;12:285,301; quiz 302.
15. Schwartzman RM, Maguire HG. Staphylococcal apocrine gland infections in the dog (canine hidradenitis suppurativa). Br Vet J. 1969;125:121–6.
16. Reedy LM, Mallett R, Freeman RG. Hidradenitis suppurativa in a female Shetland sheep dog. Vet Med Small Anim Clin. 1973;68:1262.
17. White SD, Ihrke PJ, Stannard AA. Bullous pemphigoid in a dog: treatment with six-mercaptopurine. J Am Vet Med Assoc. 1984;185:683–6.
18. Scott D, Manning T, Lewis R. Linear IgA dermatoses in the dog: bullous pemphigoid, discoid lupus erythematosus and a subcorneal pustular dermatitis. Cornell Vet. 1982;72:394–402.
19. Scott DW, Miller WH. Jr., Goldschmidt MH: erythema multiforme in the dog. J Am Anim Hosp Assoc. 1983;19:454–9.
20. Itoh T, Nibe K, Kojimoto A, Mikawa M, Mikawa K, Uchida K, Shii H. Erythema multiforme possibly triggered by food substances in a dog. J Vet Med Sci. 2006;68:869–71.
21. Ihrke PJ, Gross TL. Ulcerative dermatosis of Shetland sheepdogs and collies. In: Bonagura JD, editor. Kirk's current veterinary therapy XII (small animal practice). Philadelphia: W.B. Saunders Co; 1995. p. 639–40.
22. Jackson HA, Olivry T, Berget F, Dunston SM, Bonnefont C, Chabanne L. Immunopathology of vesicular cutaneous lupus erythematosus in the rough collie and Shetland sheepdog: a canine homologue of subacute cutaneous lupus erythematosus in humans. Vet Dermatol. 2004;15:230–9.
23. Jackson HA. Eleven cases of vesicular cutaneous lupus erythematosus in Shetland sheepdogs and rough collies: clinical management and prognosis. Vet Dermatol. 2004;15:37–41.
24. Font A, Bardagi M, Mascort J, Fondevila D. Treatment with oral cyclosporin a of a case of vesicular cutaneous lupus erythematosus in a rough collie. Vet Dermatol. 2006;17:440–2.
25. Gibson IR, Barnes J. Vesicular cutaneous lupus erythematosus in a border collie in New Zealand. N Z Vet J. 2011;59:153–4. (abstract)
26. Lehner GM, Linek M. A case of vesicular cutaneous lupus erythematosus in a border collie successfully treated with topical tacrolimus and nicotinamide-tetracycline. Vet Dermatol. 2013;24(639,41):e159–60.
27. Manzuc PJ, Koch SN, Benzoin L, Grandinetti J. Mycophenolate mofetil in the therapy of vesicular cutaneous lupus erythematosus: a case report. Vet Dermatol. 2016;27(Suppl. 1):87. (abstract)
28. Banovic F, Robson D, Linek M, Olivry T. Therapeutic effectiveness of calcineurin inhibitors in canine vesicular cutaneous lupus erythematosus. Vet Dermatol. 2017;28 in press
29. Banovic F, Dunston S, Linder KE, Rakich P, Olivry T. Apoptosis as a mechanism for keratinocyte death in canine toxic epidermal necrolysis. Vet Pathol. 2017;54:249–53.
30. Gross TL, Ihrke PJ, Walder EJ. Hereditary lupoid dermatosis of the German shorthaired pointer. In: Anonymous, editor. *Veterinary dermatopathology: a macroscopic and microscopic evaluation of canine and feline skin diseases*. St Louis, MO: Mosby year book; 1992. p. 26–8.
31. Theaker AJ, Rest JR. Lupoid dermatosis in a German short-haired pointer. Vet Rec. 1992;(21):495.
32. Vroom MW, Theaker MJ, Rest JR, White SD. Lupoid dermatosis in 5 German short-haired pointers. Vet Dermatol. 1995;6:93–8.
33. White SD, Gross TL. Hereditary lupoid dermatosis of the German short-haired pointer. In: Kirk RW, Bonagura JD, editors. Current veterinary therapy small animal practice. Volume XII; XII. Philadelphia: W.B. Saunders Co; 1995. p. 605–6.
34. Bryden SL, Olivry T, White SD, Dunston SD, Burrows AK. Clinical, histopathological and immunological characteristics of exfoliative cutaneous lupus erythematosus in 25 German shorthaired pointers. Vet Dermatol. 2005;16:239–52.
35. Wang P, Zangerl B, Werner P, Mauldin EA, Casal ML. Familial cutaneous lupus erythematosus (CLE) in the German shorthaired pointer maps to CFA18, a canine orthologue to human CLE. Immunogenetics. 2011;63:197–207.
36. Vidémont E, Pin D. Sebaceous adenitis or chronic cutaneous lupus erythematosus in a Viszla? (in French). Proceedings of the Proceedings of the Annual Congress of the GEDAC. Toulouse, France: 2010.
37. Dutoit C: Adénite sébacée granulomateuse du Vizsla: adénite ou lupus érythémateux? (granulomatous sebaceous adenitis in Vizslas: adenitis or lupus erythematosus?). Dr-Vet Thesis, Université Claude-Bernard Lyon I, Vetagro Sup Campus Vétérinaire de Lyon; 2011.
38. Mauldin EA, Morris DO, Brown DC, Casal ML. Exfoliative cutaneous lupus erythematosus in German shorthaired pointer dogs: disease development, progression and evaluation of three immunomodulatory drugs (ciclosporin, hydroxychloroquine, and adalimumab) in a controlled environment. Vet Dermatol. 2010;21:373–82.

39. Werner A. All in the family: chronic dermatitis & German shorthaired pointers. Clin Brief. 2015;(November):18–22.

40. Nutan F, Ortega-Loayza AG. Cutaneous lupus: a brief review of old and new medical therapeutic options. J Investig Dermatol Symp Proc. 2017;18:S64–8.

41. Poirier N. Discoid lupus erythematosus. Can Vet J. 1995;36:493.

42. Bensignor E, Carlotti DN, Pin D. Recto N°38 (perivulvar discoid lupus erythematosus). Prat Med Chir Anim Comp. 1997;32:323–4.

43. Schrauwen E, Junius G, Swinnen C, Maenhout I. Dyschezia in dogs with discrete erosive anal disease and histological lesions suggestive of mucocutaneous lupus erythematosus. Vet Rec. 2004;154:752–4.

44. Gerhauser I, Strothmann-Luerssen A, Baumgartner W. A case of interface perianal dermatitis in a dog: is this an unusual manifestation of lupus erythematosus? Vet Pathol. 2006;43:761–4.

45. Adolph ER, Scott DW, Miller WH, Erb HN. Efficacy of tetracycline and niacinamide for the treatment of cutaneous lupus erythematosus in 17 dogs (1997-2011). Jpn J Vet Dermatol. 2014;20:9–15.

46. Balazs V. Caso clínico: Lupus eritematoso mucocutáneo en un perro (case report: mucocutaneous lupus in a dog). Rev Hosp Vet. 2017;9:6–11.

47. Rothfield N, Sontheimer RD, Bernstein M. Lupus erythematosus: systemic and cutaneous manifestations. Clin Dermatol. 2006;24:348–62.

48. Oberkirchner U, Linder KE, Olivry T. Successful treatment of a novel generalized variant of canine discoid lupus erythematosus with oral hydroxychloroquine. Vet Dermatol. 2012;23:65,70, e15–6.

49. Banovic F, Olivry T, Linder KE. Ciclosporin therapy for canine generalized discoid lupus erythematosus refractory to doxycycline and niacinamide. Vet Dermatol. 2014;25:483–e79.

50. Rossi MA, Messinger LM, Linder KE, Olivry T. Generalized canine discoid lupus erythematosus responsive to tetracycline and niacinamide therapy. J Am Anim Hosp Assoc. 2015;51:171–5.

51. Messinger L, Strauss T, Jonas L. A randomized, double-blinded, placebo controlled crossover study evaluating 0.03% tacrolimus ointment monotherapy in the treatment of discoid lupus erythematosus in dogs. SOJ. Vet Sci. 2017;3:1–6.

52. Scott DW. Lichenoid reactions in the skin of dogs: clinicopathologic correlations. J Am Anim Hosp Assoc. 1982;20:305–17.

53. Costner MI, Sontheimer RD, Provost TT. Lupus erythematosus. In: Sontheimer RD, Provost TT, editors. *Cutaneous manifestations of rheumatic diseases. Volume 2nd*. Philadelphia: Lippincott Williams and Wilkins; 2004. p. 15–64.

54. Scott DW, Miller WH. Squamous-cell carcinoma arising in chronic discoid lupus-erythematosus nasal lesions in 2 German shepherd dogs. Vet Dermatol. 1995;6:99–104.

55. Fernandes MS, Girisha BS, Viswanathan N, Sripathi H, Noronha TM. Discoid lupus erythematosus with squamous cell carcinoma: a case report and review of the literature in Indian patients. Lupus. 2015;24:1562–6.

56. Chong BF, Song J, Olsen NJ. Determining risk factors for developing systemic lupus erythematosus in patients with discoid lupus erythematosus. Br J Dermatol. 2012;166:29–35.

57. Olivry T, Linder KE. Bilaterally symmetrical alopecia with reticulated hyperpigmentation: a manifestation of cutaneous lupus erythematosus in a dog with systemic lupus erythematosus. Vet Pathol. 2013;50:682–5.

58. Hutt JH, Dunn KA, Scase TJ, Shipstone MA. A preliminary survey of the histopathological features of skin from the planum nasale and adjacent skin of dogs unaffected by dermatological or respiratory disease. Vet Dermatol. 2015;26:359,62,e78–9.

59. Hutt JH, Dunn KA, Scase TJ, Shipstone MA. Pigmentary incontinence in the skin of the planum nasale from normal dogs. Vet Dermatol. 2016;27:324–5.

60. De Lucia M, Mezzalira G, Bardagi M, Fondevila DM, Fabbri E, Fondati A. A retrospective study comparing histopathological and immunopathological features of nasal planum dermatitis in 20 dogs with discoid lupus erythematosus or leishmaniosis. Vet Dermatol. 2017;28:200–e46.

61. Wiemelt SP, Goldschmidt MH, Greek JS, Jeffers JG, Wiemelt AP, Mauldin EA. A retrospective study comparing the histopathological features and response to treatment in two canine nasal dermatoses, discoid lupus erythematosus and mucocutaneous pyoderma. Vet Dermatol. 2004;15:341–8.

62. Kossard S. Lymphocytic mediated alopecia: histological classification by pattern analysis. Clin Dermatol. 2001;19:201–10.

63. Jessop S, Whitelaw DA, Grainge MJ, Jayasekera P. Drugs for discoid lupus erythematosus. Cochrane Database Syst Rev. 2017;5:CD002954.

64. White SD, Rosychuk RAW, Reinke SI, Paradis M. Use of tetracycline and niacinamide for treatment of autoimmune skin disease in 31 dogs. J Am Vet Med Assoc. 1992;200:1497–500.

65. Mueller RS, Rosychuk RAW, Jonas LD. A retrospective study regarding the treatment of lupoid onychodystrophy in 30 dogs and literature review. J Am Anim Hosp Assoc. 2003;39:139–50.

66. Griffies JD, Mendelsohn CL, Rosenkrantz WS, Muse R, Boord MJ, Griffin CE. Topical 0.1% tacrolimus for the treatment of discoid lupus erythematosus and pemphigus erythematosus in dogs. J Am Anim Hosp Assoc. 2004;40:29–41.

67. Fournel C, Chabanne L, Caux C, Faure J, Rigal D, Magnol JP, Monier JC. Canine systemic lupus erythematosus. I: a study of 75 cases. Lupus. 1992;1:133–9.

68. Yell J, Allen J, Wojnarowska F, Kirtschig G, Burge S. Bullous systemic lupus erythematosus: revised criteria for diagnosis. Br J Dermatol. 1995;132:921–8.

18

Cyclooxygenase-2 immunoexpression in intestinal epithelium and lamina propria of cats with inflammatory bowel disease and low grade alimentary lymphoma

Jorge Castro-López[1,2]* (iD), Antonio Ramis[3], Marta Planellas[1,2], Mariana Teles[4] and Josep Pastor[1,2]

Abstract

Background: Cyclooxygenase 2 (COX-2) is an inducible isoform by cellular activation, proinflammatory cytokines and growth factors. The aims of the current study were to evaluate COX-2 immunoexpression in epithelial and lamina propria (LP) of cats with inflammatory bowel disease (IBD) and low grade alimentary lymphoma (LGAL), as well as to correlate them with clinical signs and histopathological scoring. Cats diagnosed with IBD and LGAL (2007–2013) were included in the current study. Feline chronic enteropathy activity index (FCEAI) was calculated for all cases. Control group was composed by 3 healthy indoor cats and 5 sick cats died or were euthanized (non-gastrointestinal illness). Diagnosis and classification of IBD and LGAL was established according to the WSAVA gastrointestinal standardization group template and the National Cancer Institute formulation, respectively. Furthermore, a modified WSAVA template was applied for LGAL evaluation. Immunolabelling for COX-2 (polyclonal rabbit anti-murine antibody) was performed on biopsy samples. Epithelial and LP (inflammatory or neoplastic cells) COX-2 immunolabelling was calculated according to the grade and intensity. The most representative segment scored by the WSAVA and the modified WSAVA were used for statistical analysis.

Results: Significant difference was found regarding COX-2 intensity overexpression in the epithelial cells of IBD and LGAL groups when compared to control cats, but not between the groups of sick cats, whereas no differences were found regarding the grade of immunoreactivity between groups. No difference was found for COX-2 immunoexpression at the LP between all groups. However, 3 cats from LGAL group showed COX-2 expression in neoplastic cells at the LP. There were no correlations between epithelial or LP COX-2 expression and FCEAI and histological alterations.

Conclusions: Increased COX-2 intensity at the epithelial cells observed in cats with IBD and LGAL may be secondary to the inflammatory response or a protective function in the intestinal reparation. COX-2 expression at the LP was presented in 33% of LGAL. This result provides a reason for further investigation concerning the role of COX-2 expression in feline alimentary lymphoma.

Keywords: Feline, Chronic enteropathy, Inflammatory bowel disease, Alimentary lymphoma, Cyclooxigenase 2, COX-2

* Correspondence: jorgecastro77@gmail.com
[1]Departament de Medicina i Cirurgia Animals, Universitat Autònoma de Barcelona, 08193 Barcelona, Spain
[2]Fundació Hospital Clínic Veterinari de la Universitat Autònoma de Barcelona, 08193 Barcelona, Spain
Full list of author information is available at the end of the article

Background

Inflammatory bowel disease (IBD) and low grade alimentary lymphoma (LGAL) are common causes of chronic enteropathies (CEs) in cats [1–6]. IBD is a chronic immune-mediated disease whose cause remains unknown but is likely multifactorial [1–3, 6]. Currently, alimentary lymphoma (AL) is the most common anatomic form of lymphoma and its cause is also unknown [5, 7–12]. IBD and LGAL can affect any segments of the gastrointestinal (GI) tract and clinical differentiation between them may be a challenge. Therefore histopathological diagnosis is always needed though overlapping may also occur, complicating the definitive diagnosis [3, 5, 13–16]. In addition, evolution from chronic intestinal inflammation to AL has been proposed in cats but definitive proof is lacking [9, 17].

Cyclooxygenase 2 (COX-2) is an inducible inflammatory regulator isoform by cellular activation, proinflammatory cytokines, growth factors, tumour promoters and prostaglandin mediator [18–21]. Prostaglandin E$_2$, a COX-2 metabolite, has many biological roles including mediating pain, modulation of cytokine production, induction of regulators of angiogenesis, production of proinflammatory mediators and promotes tumourigenesis [22, 23]. Furthermore, overexpression of COX-2 may be a consequence of inflammation leading to increased levels of Bcl-2 and resistance to apoptosis of the cells, thus enhancing the risk of cancer [24, 25]. To the author's knowledge, there is only one available study in cats that included 6 cases of intestinal lymphoma and described negative COX-2 immunoexpression [26], and there is no study describing COX-2 immunoexpression in feline IBD and LGAL.

The aim of the present study was to evaluate COX-2 immunoexpression at the epithelium and lamina propria (LP) of cats with IBD and LGAL. The second objective was to correlate the COX-2 immunolabelling with clinical signs and histopathological scoring.

Methods
Study population
Control group was composed of 3 healthy control indoor female cats (HCC, median age = 2 years; range = 1–5 years) owned by the personal staff were submitted to endoscopy prior to ovariohysterectomy and duodenal biopsies were obtained, and 5 sick cats (SC, median age = 7 years; range = 1–18 years) who died or were euthanized for unrelated GI diseases and full thickness biopsies (FTB) from duodenum, jejunum and ileum were obtained within 1 h. Cats had not received glucocorticoids (GC), chemotherapy, non-steroidal anti-inflammatory drugs (NSAIDs) or antibiotics with immunomodulatory action such as doxycycline and azithromycin previously. All these cats were recruited from the Fundació Hospital Clínic Veterinari of the Universitat Autònoma de Barcelona.

Approval consent was signed and accepted by the owners and procedures were approved by the Ethical Committee from the Faculty of Veterinary Medicine and Bioscience Engineering of Universitat Autònoma de Barcelona (CEAAH 2354).

IBD and LGAL cases of the study were collected between 2007 and 2013 from the Fundació Hospital Clínic Veterinari of the Universitat Autònoma de Barcelona. The inclusion criteria was the presence of chronic GI signs (> 3 weeks duration), complete medical history and no previous GC, chemotherapy, NSAIDs or antibiotics with immunomodulatory action treatments 6 months before the presentation. Information obtained from all cats included signalment (age, breed, sex, body weight), history, physical examination, clinicopathological testing (complete blood count, biochemistry profile and total T4 and abdominal ultrasonography). All patients were negative to feline leukaemia virus antigen and immunodeficiency virus antibodies. Cats with mild to moderate clinical signs were treated at the beginning with antiparasitic for 5 days, followed by elimination diet (novel protein or hydrolysed elimination diets) for at least 14 days to rule out parasitism and food response enteropathy, respectively. Posteriorly, endoscopy or FTB were obtained. Otherwise, severely compromised patients were submitted to intestinal biopsy after blood works and ultrasonography. These patients did not receive antiparasitics or placed on diet trials at presentation, but did during treatment in cats with IBD. Biopsies were obtained by laparotomy (duodenum, jejunum and/or ileum) or endoscopy (duodenum). Stomach and colonic biopsies were not considered in this study. Cats with extra-GI diseases were excluded from the study.

Chronic enteropathy activity index
The feline chronic enteropathy activity index (FCEAI) was applied to all studied cats [2]. This index gave a scoring to GI signs (vomiting, diarrhoea, anorexia, weight loss, lethargy; 0 to 3 points for each sign according to severity), hyperproteinaemia (yes = 1 point, no = 0 point), hypophosphataemia (yes = 1 point, no = 0 point), increased serum alanine aminotransferase (ALT) and/or alkaline phosphatase (ALP) activities (yes = 1 point, no = 0 point). Endoscopic lesions parameter was not included because FTB were performed in most of the cats and endoscopy was not repeated. A questionnaire was filled by the owners at the first visit or phone calls. A composite score was subsequently calculated yielding values for mild (2 to 5), moderate (6 to 11) and severe (12 or greater) CE [27].

Histopathological classification
Biopsy samples were fixed in neutral-buffered formalin and embedded in paraffin wax. Tissue was sectioned

(3 μm) and stained with haematoxylin and eosin. Single board-certified pathologist (AR) reviewed all sections and was blinded to the clinical information. Previously published diagnostic algorithm was used to differentiate IBD from LGAL [16].

Biopsies from the control and IBD groups were evaluated according to the world small animal veterinary association (WSAVA) GI Standardization Group template [28]. This template only assesses the duodenal morphological features (villous stunting, epithelial injury, crypt distension, lacteal dilation and mucosal fibrosis) and inflammation changes (intraepithelial lymphocytes, LP lymphocytes and plasma cells, eosinophils, neutrophils, other cells) from the duodenum. They were scored as absent = 0, mild = 1, moderate = 2, or severe = 3. Finally, histologic severity scores were recorded and determined to be normal (score 0), mild (1–6), moderate (7–13), severe (14–20), and very severe (> 20) [29]. Jejunal and ileal biopsies were scored according to the WSAVA template as Casamian-Sorrosal and colleagues described in these segments [30].

Modified WSAVA (MWSAVA) score was used for LGAL cases that included morphological features (villous stunting, epithelial injury and crypt distension) and applied to duodenum, jejunum and ileum [31]. These features were scored as absent = 0, mild = 1, moderate = 2, or severe = 3. Total scores were classified as normal (score = 0), mild (1–3), moderate (4–6), severe (7–9), and very severe (> 10) according to a calculated proportion of the classification mentioned above.

LGAL cases were classified according to the National Cancer Institute working formulation. The number of mitoses between 0 and 5 at high-power field and small nuclear size (< 1.5X the size of a red blood cell) correspond to LGAL [32]. Furthermore, CD3 and CD20 immunophenotyping was performed in LGAL and severe IBD cases as previously described [16].

For statistical evaluation, the small intestinal segment with the higher or modified histological score of each individual was considered.

COX-2 immunohistochemistry

Sections (3 μm) were routinely deparaffinised, rehydrated and antigen retrieval at pH 6 was performed by PT-Link Automatic System (Dako Glostup, Denmark). Immunostaining was performed on a Dako Autostainer Plus, using procedures, buffers and solutions provided by the manufacturer. Primary antibody binding was detected with a standard two-layer indirect method (EnVision; DakoCytomation). Chromogen staining was developed with diaminobenzidine. Slides were counterstained with haematoxylin. The primary antibody (polyclonal rabbit anti-murine COX-2; Cayman Chemical, Ann Arbor, Michigan, USA) at a 1 in 500 dilution was used. A rabbit

polyclonal antibody against *Leishmania infantum*, kindly provided by Instituto de Salud Carlos III (Madrid, Spain), was used for negative control purposes (1:3000). Sections of feline foetal kidney (Fig. 1) and cutaneous squamous cell carcinoma were used as positive controls [33–35]. COX-2 immunohistochemical staining was performed on a normal feline lymph node as a negative control.

Epithelial, inflammatory and/or neoplastic cells COX-2 immunolabelling was evaluated by a semi-quantitative assessment which included staining grade (percentage of positive cells) and intensity. Five 10X fields from each slide were evaluated. The grade (percentage) was evaluated by the following scoring system: 0 = negative; 1 = < 10% of cells staining positive; 2 = 10–30%; 3 = 31–60%; 4= > 60%. Intensity was evaluated by the following scoring system: 0 = negative; 1 = weak staining; 2 = moderately intense staining; and 3 = marked intense staining. Intensity of positive control cells was considered marked staining [26]. The final expression score was calculated multiplying the intensity with percentage and classified as weak (1–2), moderate (3–5), marked (6–8) and very marked (> 9).

Statistical analysis

Statistical analysis was performed using SPSS statistics software (SPSS 17.0 version, Chicago, IL, USA) adopting a level of significance of $p < 0.05$. Shapiro-Wilk test were used for tested normality of the data. Non-parametric tests were applied for data that did not present a normal distribution, and median and range were used for summary. The Kruskal-Wallis test was used to compare continuous variables (FCEAI, WSAVA and MWSAVA scores, epithelial and LP COX-2 expression) between

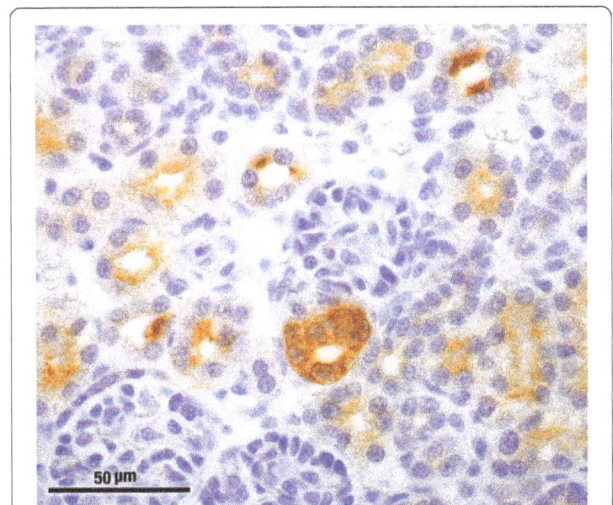

Fig. 1 Macula densa from a foetal kidney showing marked intensity of COX-2 immunoexpression and apical border of renal tubular cells expressing moderate intensity

groups. The Mann-Whitney test was used as post-test analysis for the evaluation of the variation between the different groups.

Results

A total of 28 cats met the inclusion criteria but 8 cats were eliminated because biopsy samples were unavailable. Therefore, 11 cats with IBD and 9 cats with LGAL were studied. The median age was 5 years (range = 2–12) for IBD group and 12 years (range = 8–15) for the LGAL group. LGAL group presented a slightly higher body weight (median = 4.2 kg; range = 3.00–6.26) than IBD group (median = 3.88 kg; range = 2.00–6.00). All cats were neutered, except 1 intact female and 1 intact male from the IBD group. There were 5 (45%) female and 6 (55%) male cats in the IBD group and 1 (11%) female and 8 (89%) male cats in the LGAL group. Breeds represented in the IBD group were Domestic Shorthair (DSH, 4), Domestic Longhair (3), Siamese (2), Persian (1) and Norwegian Forest (1) cats. All cats belonging to the LGAL group were DSH cats.

Endoscopy biopsies were obtained from 3 cats and FTB from 8 cats of the IBD group. Samples were obtained mostly from the duodenum (9 cats). Regarding the inflammatory cells infiltration at the LP, 8 cases had lymphoplasmacytic (73%) and 3 eosinophilic (27%) inflammation. FTB were collected in all cats with LGAL except for 1 patient. All LGAL animals were T cell lymphoma and it was most commonly diagnosed in the jejunum (6 cats out of 9), followed by duodenum (2) and ileum (1).

Median of FCEAI score obtained by LGAL group was 11 (range = 5–14) and IBD group was 9 (range = 4–12) corresponding to moderate CE, but no statistical significant difference was found ($p = 1.000$) (Table 1).

According to the WSAVA template, IBD group showed a significant statistically higher score of morphological and inflammatory changes compared to the control group ($p = 0.011$, Table 1 and Fig. 2). Considering the MWSAVA score, that only includes the morphological features of the WSAVA template, LGAL group presented a significantly higher value than the IBD ($p = 0.011$) and control group ($p < 0.001$, Table 1 and Fig. 2). No significant difference was found between IBD and control group according to the MWSAVA score ($p = 0.156$, Table 1 and

Fig. 2). No lineal correlation was found between FCEAI and total WSAVA, and MWSAVA scores ($p > 0.05$).

COX-2 epithelial immunoexpression was observed in all studied cats, except 3 SC that belong to the control group. Regarding the intensity of expression, 82% of cats with IBD (9 out of 11) and 67% with LGAL (6 out of 9 cats) presented a marked intensity; remaining cats presented a moderate intensity. No significant difference was detected between these groups ($p = 1.000$, Table 1). Sixty-three per cent of cats from the control group showed a moderate epithelial COX-2 intensity, but the other ones did not present staining as mentioned above. Furthermore, control group presented lower intensity in comparison with the IBD ($p = 0.001$) and LGAL group ($p = 0.008$, Table 1 and Fig. 2). Regarding the percentage of cells, all cats from the IBD, 67% (6 out of 9) from the LGAL and 63% (5 out of 8) from the control group showed immunolabelling in more than 60% of the enterocytes, and no statistically significant difference was observed concerning to staining grade ($p = 0.081$, Table 1). COX-2 immunoexpressions are presented in Fig. 3a, b, c and d.

COX-2 expression at the LP was absent in all cats from the control and IBD group (Table 1). In the LGAL group, 2 cats presented moderate intensity and 1 cat a marked intensity immunolabelling of neoplastic, however the immunoreactivity was presented in less than 10% of cells (Table 1 and Fig. 4a, b and c). Regardless, no statistical significant differences were observed according to intensity, staining grade and final score of COX-2 expression at the LP between the three groups ($p > 0.05$, Table 1).

Statistically significant lineal correlations were not observed between epithelial or LP COX-2 expression and FCEAI and histological alterations ($p > 0.05$; Spearman's $\rho < 0.354$).

Discussion

The population of animals used in the present study confirmed previous findings showing that IBD affects younger cats compared to AL, although overlap was present. Male cats were overrepresented in LGAL group as well as DSH cats in both studied groups in agreement to previous reports [1–6, 16, 31].

Lymphoplasmacytic inflammation has been the most common inflammatory pattern defined in cats with IBD

Table 1 FCEAI, modified and total WSAVA scores and COX-2 immunoexpression of Control, IBD and LGAL group

Group	FCEAI	Modified WSAVA score	Total WSAVA score	Intensity Epithelium	% Epithelium	Total Epithelium	Intensity LP	% LP	Total LP
Control (median)	–	0[a]	1[a]	2[a]	4[a]	8[a]	0[a]	0[a]	0[a]
IBD (median)	9[a]	1[a]	5[b]	3[b]	4[a]	12[a]	0[a]	0[a]	0[a]
LGAL (median)	11[a]	2[b]	–	3[b]	4[a]	12[a]	0[a]	0[a]	0[a]

FCEAI feline chronic enteropathy activity index, WSAVA world small animal veterinary association; % percentage, LP lamina propria, IBD inflammatory bowel disease, LGAL low grade alimentary lymphoma, – non score. Different letters show a significant difference (p < 0.05)

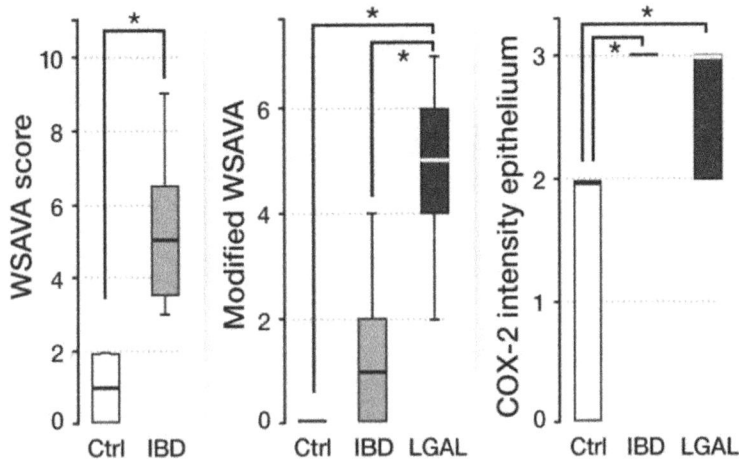

Fig. 2 (left) WSAVA scores comparison between Control (Ctrl) and IBD group (*: significant difference ($p < 0.05$) between Control and IBD group), (center) modified WSAVA scores comparison between Control, IBD and LGAL group (*: significant difference ($p < 0.05$) between Control and LGAL group; between IBD and LGAL group) and (right) COX-2 intensity in the epithelium (*: significant difference ($p < 0.05$) between Control and IBD group; between Control and LGAL group). Box plots represent median, 25th percentil, 75th percentil, maximum and minimum. WS AVA : world small animal veterinary association; IBD: inflammatory bowel disease; LGAL: low grade alimentary lymphoma; COX-2: cyclooxygenase 2

and was localized most frequently in duodenum [6, 15, 36]. Duodenum is the most common GI segment evaluated, but it is unlikely that IBD is restricted to this segment. This location is probably overrepresented due to limitations of endoscopy to obtain samples from lower small intestine segments. Furthermore, FTBs are likely more obtained from the duodenum as well than the jejunum and ileum like the present study. According to previous reports, T cell LGAL was more frequently localized in the jejunum [5, 6, 11, 16, 37].

In contrast to our findings, a study in cats found correlation between the WSAVA template and the FCEAI [2], however no correlation was observed in studies performed in dogs [1, 29, 38]. These discrepancies might be due to the FCEAI was calculated retrospectively in most of the cats. Furthermore, pancreatitis and hypocobalaminaemia that could worsen clinical signs, was not completely ruled out. Also, in the present study we used FTB from different intestinal segments that have been evaluated by a single pathologist, which might have influenced WSAVA scores.

Maunder and colleagues [31] observed severe duodenal morphological changes applying the MWSAVA scoring in LGAL and herein moderate changes were found. Nevertheless, a significant difference was observed between LGAL and IBD group in the present study regarding MWSAVA scoring. Further studies are needed to determinate whether this histological scoring might help to differentiate between CE.

To our knowledge, this is the first report regarding COX-2 expression in the intestinal epithelium and LP of cats with IBD and LGAL. COX-2 is classically considered an inducible enzyme, but it is also considered a constitutive enzyme expressed in the GI tract [39]. Moreover, COX-2 products might be involved in maintaining the integrity of intestinal mucosa [39]. Differences between species have been described about epithelial COX-2 expression along the GI tract in normal individuals. COX-2 is expressed in the ileocoecal junction and colon in rodents, in all the GI tract in dogs and in the stomach and colon in humans [40–47]. In the present study, cats of the control group presented epithelial COX-2 expression in duodenum, jejunum and ileum (data not shown). Therefore, this supports the need of more studies to clarify COX-2 expression and role in normal individuals.

Regarding immunoreactivity in healthy feline GI tract, only one study described COX-2 immunoexpression in basal granulated cells of the epithelium using a polyclonal antiprostaglandin H synthetase-2 (COX-2) human C terminus antibody [48]. Some differences may be found depending on the antibody used, in our study, immunolabelling was found in the cytoplasm of the enterocytes in 5 cats of the control group (3 HCC and 2 SC). The discordance on inmunoexpression may be explained by the different anti-reagent used, or different affinity of the antibody, however the antibody used herein was previously used in cats [33–35, 45, 46, 49–51]. The presence of COX-2 positive and negative enterocytes in SC of the control group might be explained by the degree of epithelial autolysis in the samples. However, SC were necropsied within 1 h. Even though epithelial autolysis was not observed in the histopathology, molecular autolysis cannot be totally ruled out that could influence on the COX-2 expression. Another possible explanation is the individual variability, it has been demonstrated that only 50 to 80% of healthy humans presents COX-2 expression in colon and stomach

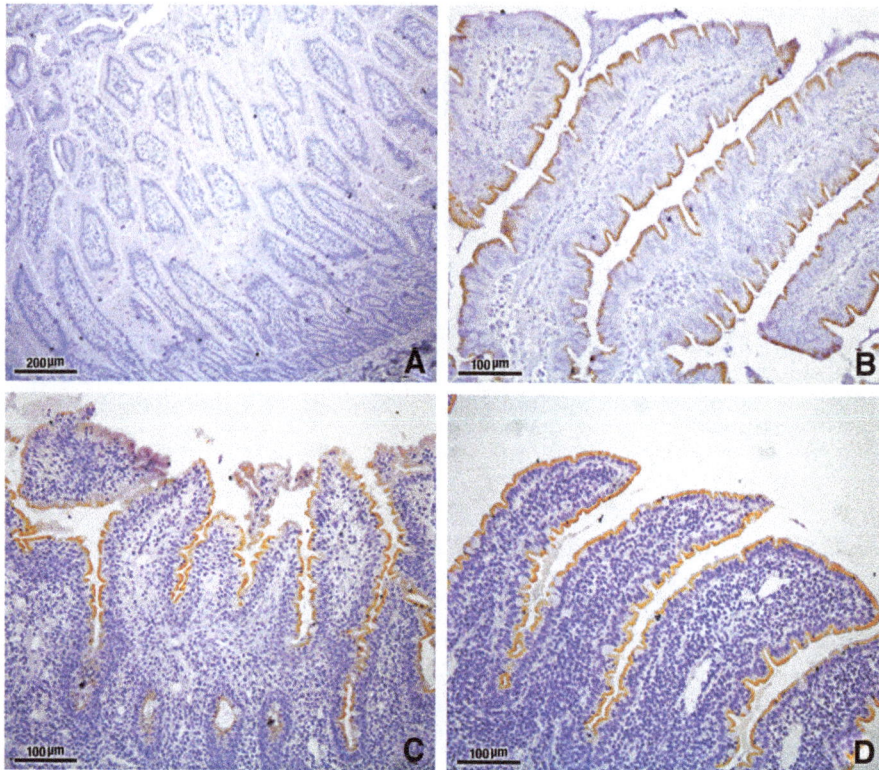

Fig. 3 a Absence of COX-2 immunolabelling in the apical membrane of the epithelium from duodenum of a sick cat from the control group (score 0); scale bar, 200 μm. **b** Moderate epithelial COX-2 immunoexpression of the apical membrane of enterocytes from the duodenum of healthy control cats (score 2); scale bar, 100 μm. **c** Marked epithelial COX-2 labelling of the apical membrane of enterocytes from the jejunum of severe lymphoplasmacytic enteritis (score 3); scale bar, 100 μm. **d** Marked epithelial COX-2 labelling of the apical membrane of enterocytes from the jejunum of severe lymphoplasmacytic enteritis (score 3); scale bar, 100 μm

[45–47, 52]. Further studies with larger number of cats are needed to obtain conclusions about normal COX-2 expression in the GI tract.

Epithelial intensity immunoexpression in IBD and LGAL groups was significantly higher in comparison with control group though no statistical difference was found between the group of cats with IBD and LGAL. Higher epithelial COX-2 immunolabelling has been reported in humans with gastritis induced by *Helicobacter pylori*, ulcerative colitis or Crohn's disease compared to normal epithelium. These observations agree with the present study [45–47, 49, 52]. The increased COX-2 expression may be due to GI epithelial ulceration, however in our study only 2 cats with LGAL presented epithelial ulceration (data not shown) [45, 49]. Furthermore, it has been described that COX-2 expression increases after feeding in feline duodenum, but this is unlikely since the cats used in the present study were fasted for anaesthetic procedure or were anorectics [48]. Increased mucosal levels of prostaglandin E_2 in humans and interleukin-1β

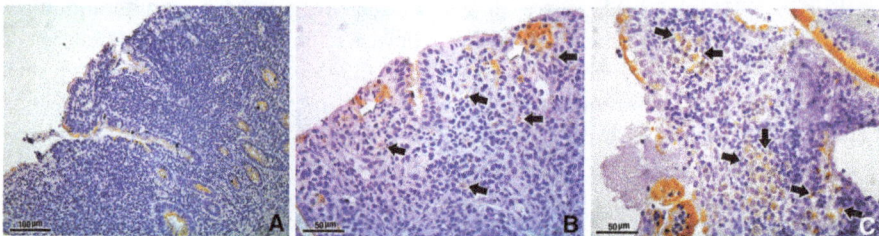

Fig. 4 a No expression of COX-2 at the neoplastic lymphocytes at the lamina propria of a low grade alimentary lymphoma (intensity 0); scale bar, 100 μm. **b** Moderate COX-2 expression of a few neoplastic cells at the lamina propria (black arrows) and enterocytes with marked reactivity (white arrows) from a cat with low grade alimentary lymphoma (intensity 2); scale bar, 50 μm. **c** Marked expression of COX-2 at some neoplastic lymphocytes at the lamina propria (black arrows) in a cat with low grade alimentary lymphoma (intensity 3); scale bar, 100 μm

in dogs with IBD and food responsive diarrhoea have been linked to an increased COX-2 immunoexpression or upregulation [44, 49]. Based on these studies, it has been suggested that cytokines and prostaglandins induced by an inflammatory response increase COX-2 in the intestinal mucosa as a protective mechanism [44, 49]. Regarding LP, no expression was found in any cat from control or IBD groups. At the same time, the normal feline lymph node did not presented COX-2 expression (data not shown), as previously described in dogs [53]. In humans with IBD, macrophages and polymorphs are stained by COX-2 at the LP [46, 47, 49, 52, 54]. However, those inflammatory cells are not present in feline IBD, and probably for this reason immunolabelling was not found in our cases. Association between COX-2 upregulation and development of lymphoma, as occurs in some tumours, remains unknown but COX-2 overexpression is associated with cell proliferation and angiogenesis [50, 51, 55, 56]. In this study, only 3 cats with LGAL presented COX-2 expression in lymphoid tumour cells. Conversely, Beam and colleagues [26] did not find COX-2 immunoexpression in 6 cats with AL. This disagreement may be due to a different immunohistochemical technique. A recent report stated that 15% of canine lymphoma presented COX-2 overexpression which agrees with the present findings [57]. However, other studies in canine lymphoma did not find COX-2 immunoreactivity [53, 56]. Furthermore, studies in humans revealed that most of non-Hodgkin's lymphoma (> 50% of cases) had COX-2 expression by tumour cells [58–60]. Thus, COX-2 upregulation in lymphomas has been associated with the aggressiveness, relapsed, worst response to therapy and less overall survival [58–61]. This latter could not be determined in our study because not all cats had available follow-up. Prospective studies are needed in cats with different lymphoma phenotypes and anatomical locations to further understand the role of COX-2 in feline AL. No correlations were observed between FCEAI, histological alterations, IBD and LGAL with COX-2 expression. Similar results have been obtained in canine IBD, and human lymphoma and IBD [44, 46, 58–60].

This study presented some limitations, most of the cases were recruited retrospectively and FCEAI was calculated by record data or owner interview by phone calls, therefore subjectivity may be an uncontrolled variable. Although intraobserver variation among histopathologic evaluations of intestinal tissues were not present due to one pathologist evaluated all biopsies, an intraobserver variation could have existed [62]. Cases of triaditis were not included, however feline specific pancreatic lipase was not available in all cases and pancreatitis was ruled out by ultrasound. Moreover, all histopathological diagnosis was made prior to the availability of polymerase chain reaction for antigen receptor rearrangements;

thereby a misdiagnosis could have occurred. However, FTB was available in almost all cats and immunohistochemistry was performed by increasing the sensitivity and specificity [16].

Conclusions

Increased COX-2 intensity at the epithelial cells observed in cats with IBD and LGAL may be secondary to the inflammatory response or a protective function in the intestinal reparation. COX-2 expression at the LP was presented in only 33% of LGAL cats, thus further investigation of COX-2 expression in feline AL are needed to clarify its importance in prognostic and response to therapy.

Abbreviations

AL: Alimentary lymphoma; ALP: Alkaline phosphatise; ALT: Alanine aminotransferase; CEs: Chronic enteropathies; COX-2: Cyclooxygenase 2; FCEAI: Feline chronic enteropathy activity index; FTB: Full thickness biopsies; GC: Glucocorticoids; GI: Gastrointestinal; HCC: Healthy control indoor female cats; IBD: Inflammatory bowel disease; LGAL: Low grade alimentary lymphoma; LP: Lamina propria; MWSAVA: Modified WSAVA; SC: Sick cats; WSAVA: World small animal veterinary association

Acknowledgements

L. Fresno, L. Santos and A. Burballa for the endoscopies performed and all clinicians and residents of the internal medicine service and interns of the FHCV-UAB. J.C. Balasch is thankfully acknowledged for the graphic design of the figures.

Funding

No financial support was provided for this study. M. Teles has a post-doctoral fellowships from FCT (SFRH/BPD/109219/2015) supported by the European Social Fund and national funds from the "Ministério da Educação e Ciência (POPH – QREN – Tipologia 4.1)" of Portugal. J. Castro-López had a grant from the Chilean government (Becas CONICYT) for his PhD studies.

Authors' contributions

Design of the study: J. Pastor, M. Planellas. Assesment of the histopathological biopsies and immunohistochemistry: A. Ramis and J. Castro-López. Data analysis: J. Castro-López, J. Pastor, M. Teles. Preparation of the manuscript: J. Castro-López, M. Teles, J. Pastor, M. Planellas. All authors read and approved the final manuscript.

Competing interests

The authors declare that they have no competing interests.

Author details

[1]Departament de Medicina i Cirurgia Animals, Universitat Autònoma de Barcelona, 08193 Barcelona, Spain. [2]Fundació Hospital Clínic Veterinari de la Universitat Autònoma de Barcelona, 08193 Barcelona, Spain. [3]Servei de Diagnòstic de Patologia Veterinària, Departament de Sanitat i d'Anatomia Animals, Universitat Autònoma de Barcelona, 08193 Barcelona, Spain. [4]Department de Biologia Cel·lular, Fisiologia i d'Immunologia, Universitat Autònoma de Barcelona, 08193 Barcelona, Spain.

References

1. Guilford WG, Jones BR, Markwell PJ, Arthur DG, Collett MG, Harte JG. Food sensitivity in cats with chronic idiopathic gastrointestinal problems. J Vet Intern Med. 2001;15:7–13.

2. Jergens AE, Crandell JM, Evans R, Ackermann M, Miles KG, Wang C. A clinical index for disease activity in cats with chronic enteropathy. J Vet Intern Med. 2010;24:1027–33.

3. Jergens AE. Feline idiopathic inflammatory bowel disease: what we know and what remains to be unravelled. J Feline Med Surg. 2012;14:445–58.

4. Richter KP. Feline gastrointestinal lymphoma. Vet Clin North Am Small Anim Pract. 2003;33:1083–98.

5. Barrs VR, Beatty JA. Feline alimentary lymphoma: 1. Classification, risk factors, clinical signs and non-invasive diagnostics. J Feline Med Surg. 2012;14:182–90.

6. Norsworthy GD, Scot Estep J, Kiupel M, Olson JC, Gassler LN. Diagnosis of chronic small bowel disease in cats: 100 cases (2008-2012). J Am Vet Med Assoc. 2013;243:1455–61.

7. Vail DM, Moore AS, Ogilvie GK, Volk LM. Feline lymphoma (145 cases): proliferation indices, cluster of differentiation 3 immunoreactivity, and their association with prognosis in 90 cats. J Vet Intern Med. 1998;12:349–54.

8. Bertone ER, Snyder LA, Moore AS. Environmental tobacco smoke and risk of malignant lymphoma in pet cats. Am J Epidemiol. 2002;156:268–73.

9. Louwerens M, London CA, Pederson NC, Lyons LA. Feline lymphoma in the post-feline leukemia virus era. J Vet Intern Med. 2005;19:329–35.

10. Milner RJ, Peyton J, Cooke K, Fox LE, Gallagher A, Gordon P, Hester J. Response rates and survival times for cats with lymphoma treated with the University of Wisconsin-Madison chemotherapy protocol: 38 cases (1996-2003). J Am Vet Med Assoc. 2005;227:1118–22.

11. Lingard AE, Briscoe K, Beatty JA, Moore AS, Crowley AM, Krockenberger M, Churcher RK, Canfield PJ, Barrs VR. Low-grade alimentary lymphoma: clinicopathological findings and response to treatment in 17 cases. J Feline Med Surg. 2009;11:692–700.

12. Stützer B, Lutz H, Majzoub M, Hermanns W, Hirschberger J, Sauter-Louis C, Hartmann K. Incidence of persistent viraemia and latent feline leukemia virus infection in cats with lymphoma. J Feline Med Surg. 2011;13:81–7.

13. Moore PF, Woo JC, Vernau W, Kosten S, Graham PS. Characterization of feline T cell receptor gamma (TCRG) variable region genes for the molecular diagnosis of feline intestinal T cell lymphoma. Vet Immunol Immunopathol. 2005;106:167–78.

14. Barrs VR, Beatty JA. Feline alimentary lymphoma: 2. Further diagnostics, therapy and prognosis. J Feline Med Surg. 2012;14:191–201.

15. Briscoe KA, Krockenberger M, Beatty JA, Crowley A, Dennis MM, Canfield PJ, Dhand N, Lingard AE, Barrs VR. Histopathological and immunohistochemical evaluation of 53 cases of feline lymphoplasmacytic enteritis and low-grade alimentary lymphoma. J Comp Pathol. 2011;145:187–98.

16. Kiupel M, Smedley RC, Pfent C, Xie Y, Xue Y, Wise AG, DeVaul JM, Maes RK. Diagnostic algorithm to differentiate lymphoma from inflammation in feline intestinal biopsy specimens. Vet Pathol. 2011;48:212–22.

17. Mahony OM, Moore AS, Cotter SM, Engler SJ, Brown D, Penninck DG. Alimentary lymphoma in cats: 28 cases (1988-1993). J Am Vet Med Assoc. 1995;207:1593–8.

18. Vane JR, Bakhle YS, Botting RM. Cyclooxygenases 1 and 2. Annu Rev Pharmacol Toxicol. 1998;38:97–120.

19. Williams CS, Mann M, DuBois RN. The role of cyclooxygenases in inflammation, cancer and development. Oncogene. 1999;18:7908–16.

20. Yu Y, Fan J, Hui Y, Rouzer CA, Marnett LJ, Klein-Szanto AJ, FitzGerald GA, Funk CD. Targeted cyclooxygenase gene (ptgs) exchange reveals discriminant isoform functionality. J Biol Chem. 2007;282:1498–506.

21. Ghosh N, Chaki R, Mandal V, Mandal SC. COX-2 as a target for cancer chemotherapy. Pharmacol Rep. 2010;62:233–44.

22. Funk CD. Prostaglandins and leukotrienes: advances in eicosanoid biology. Science. 2001;294:1871–5.

23. Charlier C, Michaux C. Dual inhibition of cyclooxygenase-2 (COX-2) and 5-lipoxygenase (5-LOX) as a new strategy to provide safer non steroidal anti-inflammatory drugs. Eur J Med Chem. 2003;38:645–59.

24. Tsujii M, Kawano S, Tsuji S, Sawaoka H, Hori M, DuBois RN. Cyclooxygenase regulates angiogenesis induced by colon cancer cells. Cell. 1998;93:705–16.

25. Sakamoto T, Uozaki H, Kondo K, Imauchi Y, Yamasoba T, Sugasawa M, Kaga K. Cyclooxygenase-2 regulates the degree of apoptosis by modulating bcl-2 protein in pleomorphic adenoma and mucoepidermoid carcinoma of the parotid gland. Acta Otolaryngol. 2005;125:191–5.

26. Beam SL, Rassnick KM, Moore AS, McDonough SP. An immunohistochemical study of cyclooxygenase-2 expression in various feline neoplasms. Vet Pathol. 2003;40:496–500.

27. Bailey S, Benigni L, Eastwood J, Garden OA, McMahon L, Smith K, Steiner JM, Suchodolski JS, Allenspach K. Comparisons between cats with normal and increased fPLI concentrations in cats diagnosed with inflammatory bowel disease. J Small Anim Pract. 2010;51:484–9.

28. Day MJ, Bilzert T, Mansell J, Wilcock B, Hall EJ, Jergens A, Minami T, Willard M, Washabau R. Histopathological standards for the diagnosis of gastrointestinal inflammation in endoscopic biopsy samples from the dog and cat: a report from the world small animal veterinary association gastrointestinal standardization group. J Comp Pathol. 2008;138:S1–S40.

29. Procoli F, Môtskûla PF, Keyte SV, Priestnall S, Allenspach K. Comparison of histopathologic findings in duodenal and ileal endoscopic biopsies in dogs with chronic small intestinal enteropathies. J Vet Intern Med. 2013;27:268–74.

30. Casamian-Sorrosal D, Willard MD, Murray JK, Hall EJ, Taylor SS, Day MJ. Comparison of histopathological findings in biopsies from the duodenum and ileum of dogs with enteropathy. J Vet Intern Med. 2010;24:80–3.

31. Maunder CL, Day MJ, Hibbert A, Steiner JM, Suchodolski JS, Hall EJ. Serum cobalamin concentrations in cats with gastrointestinal signs: correlation with histopathological findings and duration of clinical signs. J Feline Med Surg. 2012;14:686–93.

32. Valli VE, San Myint M, Barthel A, Bienzle D, Caswell J, Colbatzky F, Durham A, Ehrhart EJ, Johnson Y, Jones C, Kiupel M, Labelle P, Lester S, Miller M, Moore P, Moroff S, Roccabianca P, Ramos-Vara J, Ross A, Scase T, Tvedten H, Vernau W. Classification of canine malignant lymphomas according to the World Health Organization criteria. Vet Pathol. 2011;48:198–211.

33. Hayes A, Scase T, Miller J, Murphy S, Sparkes A, Adams V. COX-1 and COX-2 expression in feline oral squamous cell carcinoma. J Comp Pathol. 2006;135:93–9.

34. Newman SJ, Mrkonjich L. Cyclooxygenase-2 expression in feline pancreatic adenocarcinomas. J Vet Diagn Investig. 2006;18:590–3.

35. Bardagí M, Fondevila D, Ferrer L. Immunohistochemical detection of COX-2 in feline and canine actinic keratoses and cutaneous squamous cell carcinoma. J Comp Pathol. 2012;146:11–7.

36. Daniaux LA, Laurenson MP, Marks SL, Moore PF, Taylor SL, Chen RX, Zwingenberger AL. Ultrasonographic thickening of the muscularis propria in feline small intestinal small cell T-cell lymphoma and inflammatory bowel disease. J Feline Med Surg. 2014;16:89–98.

37. Moore PF, Rodriguez-Bertos A, Kass PH. Feline gastrointestinal lymphoma: mucosal architecture, immunophenotype, and molecular clonality. Vet Pathol. 2012;49:658–68.

38. Allenspach K, Wieland B, Gröne A, Gaschen F. Chronic enteropathies in dogs: evaluation of risk factors for negative outcome. J Vet Intern Med. 2007;21:700–8.

39. Kefalakes H, Stylianides TJ, Amanakis G, Kolios G. Exacerbation of inflammatory bowel diseases associates with the use of nonsteroidal anti-inflammatory drugs: myth or reality? Eur J Clin Pharmacol. 2009;65:963–70.

40. Porcher C, Horowitz B, Ward SM, Sanders KM. Constitutive and functional expression of cyclooxygenase 2 in the murine proximal colon. Neurogastroenterol Motil. 2004;16:785–99.

41. Haworth R, Oakley K, McCormack N, Pilling A. Differential expression of COX-1 and COX-2 in the gastrointestinal tract of the rat. Toxicol Pathol. 2005;33:239–45.

42. Wilson JE, Chandrasekharan NV, Westover KD, Eager KB, Simmons DL. Determination of expression of cyclooxygenase-1 and -2 isozymes in canine tissues and their differential sensitivity to non-steroidal anti-inflammatory drugs. Am J Vet Res. 2004;65:810–8.

43. Amorim I, Taulescu MA, Ferreira A, Rêma A, Reis CA, Faustino AM, Cătoi C, Gärtner F. An immunohistochemical study of canine spontaneous gastric polyps. Diagn Pathol. 2014;9:166.

44. Dumusc SD, Ontsouka EC, Schnyder M, Hartnack S, Albrecht C, Bruckmaier RM, Burgener IA. Cyclooxygenase-2 and 5-lypoxygenase in dogs with chronic enteropathies. J Vet Intern Med. 2014;28:1684–91.

45. Jackson LM, Wu KC, Mahida YR, Jenkins D, Hawkey CJ. Cyclooxygenase (COX) 1 and 2 in normal, inflamed, and ulcerated human gastric mucosa. Gut. 2000;47:762–70.

46. Paiotti AP, Artigiani Neto R, Forones NM, Oshima CT, Miszputen SJ, Franco M. Immunoexpression of cyclooxygenase-1 and -2 in ulcerative colitis. Braz J Med Biol Res. 2007;40:911–8.

47. Romero M, Artigiani R, Costa H, Oshima CT, Miszputen S, Franco M. Evaluation of the immunoexpression of COX-1, COX-2 and p53 in Crohn's disease. Arq Gastroenterol. 2008;45:295–300.

48. Satoh H, Amagase K, Ebara S, Akiba Y, Takeuchi K. Cyclooxygenase (COX)-1 and COX-2 both play an important role in the protection of the duodenal mucosa in cats. J Pharmacol Exp Ther. 2013;344:189–95.

49. Singer II, Kawka DW, Schloemann S, Tessner T, Riehl T, Stenson WF. Cyclooxygenase 2 is induced in colonic epithelial cells in inflammatory bowel disease. Gastroenterology. 1998;115:297–306.

50. Joo YE, Oh WT, Rew JS, Park CS, Choi SK, Kim SJ. Cyclooxygenase-2 expression is associated with well-differentiated and intestinal-type pathways in gastric carcinogenesis. Digestion. 2002;66:222–9.

51. Joo YE, Rew JS, Seo YH, Choi SK, Kim YJ, Park CS, Kim SJ. Cyclooxygenase-2 overexpression correlates with vascular endothelial growth factor expression and tumor angiogenesis in gastric cancer. J Clin Gastroenterol. 2003;37:28–33.

52. Dai L, King DW, Perera DS, Lubowski DZ, Burcher E, Liu L. Inverse expression of prostaglandin E2-related enzymes highlights differences between diverticulitis and inflammatory bowel disease. Dig Dis Sci. 2015;60:1236–46.

53. Rodrigues LCS, Cogliati B, Guerra JL, Dagli MLZ, Lucas RR. An immunohistochemical study of cyclooxygenase-2 expression in canine multicentric lymphoma. An Vet (Murcia). 2011;27:43–9.

54. Roberts PJ, Morgan K, Miller R, Hunter JO, Middleton SJ. Neuronal COX-2 expression in human myenteric plexus in active inflammatory bowel disease. Gut. 2001;48:468–72.

55. Ohsawa M, Fukushima H, Ikura Y, Inoue T, Shirai N, Sugama Y, Suekane T, Kitabayashi C, Nakamae H, Hino M, Ueda M, et al. Expression of cyclooxygenase-2 in Hodgkin's lymphoma: its role in cell proliferation and angiogenesis. Leuk Lymphoma. 2006;47:1863–71.

56. Mohammed SI, Khan KNM, Sellers RS, Hayek MG, DeNicola DB, Wu L, Bonney PL, Knapp DW. Expression of cyclooxygenase-1 and 2 in naturally-ocurring canine cancer. Prostaglandins Leukot Essent Fatty Acids. 2004;70:479–83.

57. Asproni P, Vignoli M, Cancedda S, Millanta F, Terragni R, Poli A. Immunohistochemical expression of cyclooxygenase-2 in normal, hyperplastic and neoplastic canine lymphoid tissues. J Comp Pathol. 2014;151:35–41.

58. Hazar B, Ergin M, Seyrek E, Erdoğan S, Tuncer I, Hakverdi S. Cyclooxygenase-2 (COX-2) expression in lymphoma. Leuk Lymphoma. 2006;45:1395–9.

59. Paydas S, Ergin M, Erdogan S, Seydaoglu G. Cyclooxygenase-2 in non-Hodgkin's lymphomas. Leuk Lymphoma. 2007;48:389–95.

60. Ma SP, Lin M, Liu HN, Yu JX. Lymphangiogenesis in non-Hodgkin's lymphoma and its correlation with cyclooxygenase-2 and vascular endothelial growth factor-C. Oncol Lett. 2012;4:695–700.

61. Sugita Y, Komatani H, Ohshima K, Shigemori M, Nakashima A. Expression of cyclooxygenase-2 and vascular endothelial growth factor in primary central nervous system lymphomas. Oncol Rep. 2007;18:617–22.

62. Willard MD, Jergens AE, Duncan RB, Leib MS, McCracken MD, DeNovo RC, Helman RG, Slater MR, Harbison JL. Interobserver variation among histopathologic evaluations of intestinal tissues from dogs and cats. J Am Vet Med Assoc. 2002;220:1177–82.

19

Characterization of respiratory dendritic cells from equine lung tissues

Yao Lee, Matti Kiupel and Gisela Soboll Hussey[*] ⓘ

Abstract

Background: Dendritic cells (DCs) are professional antigen-presenting cells that have multiple subpopulations with different phenotypes and immune functions. Previous research demonstrated that DCs have strong potential for anti-viral defense in the host. However, viruses including alphaherpesvirinae have developed strategies to interfere with the function or maturation of DCs, causing immune dysfunction and avoidance of pathogen elimination. The goal of the present study was to isolate and characterize equine lung-derived DCs (L-DCs) for use in studies of respiratory viruses and compare their features with equine blood-derived DCs (B-DCs), which are currently used for these types of studies.

Results: We found that L-DCs were morphologically similar to B-DCs. Overall, B-DCs demonstrated higher expression of CD86 and CD172α than L-DCs, but both cell types expressed high levels of MHC class II and CD44, as well as moderate amounts of CD163, CD204, and Bla36. In contrast, the endocytic activity of L-DCs was elevated compared to that of B-DCs. Finally, mononuclear cells isolated from lung (L-MCs), which are used as precursors for L-DCs, expressed more antigen-presenting cell-associated markers such as MHC class II and CD172α compared to their counterparts from blood.

Conclusions: Our results indicate that L-DCs may be in an earlier differentiation stage compared to B-DCs. Concurrent with this observation, L-MCs possessed significantly more antigen-uptake capacity compared to their counterparts from blood. It is likely that L-DCs play an important role in antigen uptake and processing of respiratory pathogens and are major contributors to respiratory tract immunity and may be ideal tools for future in vitro or ex vivo studies.

Keywords: Equine, Blood dendritic cells, Lung dendritic cells, Antigen-presenting cells

Background

Dendritic cells (DCs) are the most important antigen-presenting cells (APCs) in the body. They act as a surveillance system to detect foreign antigens and shape immunogenic or tolerogenic responses [1]. There are many subsets of DCs with different phenotypes derived from either conventional or lymphoid lineages. Lymphoid lineage DCs primarily differentiate into plasmacytoid DCs and occupy approximately 0.5% of peripheral blood mononuclear cells (PBMCs) in humans [2], but the cell population percentage is unclear in horses. Conventional lineage DCs generally differentiate into myeloid DCs which originally come from tissues, such as epithelial or interstitial DCs. Blood monocyte-derived DCs (B-DCs), as one group of myeloid DCs, can be generated by incubation of monocytes that are isolated from PBMCs with exogenous granulocyte macrophage colony-stimulating factor (GM-CSF) and interleukin-4 (IL-4) for 6–7 days [3]. This approach produces a highly-differentiated DC population, which is specialized in antigen presentation and T cell priming [3–5].

Studies in humans and mice have shown that conventional DCs isolated and cultured from different tissues including bone marrow, lung, gut, and other organs, possessed slightly different phenotypes compared to B-DCs [6–10]. As one example, the respiratory tract represents one of the largest surface areas in the body and acts as an interface with the external environment that is frequently exposed to foreign particles or pathogens. For immune defense, the respiratory tract contains DCs

* Correspondence: husseygi@msu.edu
Department of Pathobiology & Diagnostic Investigation, College of Veterinary Medicine, Michigan State University, 784 Wilson Rd, A13, East Lansing, MI 48824, USA

that function as a robust antigen presentation system. Human lung DCs are localized within the airway epithelium, alveolar septae, or connective tissues of the pulmonary parenchyma [7]. Lung DCs are typically isolated from either bronchoalveolar lavage fluid (BALF) or by lung tissue digestion, resulting in a number of phenotypes and sub-populations [11, 12]. Interestingly, airway derived DCs were found to possess better antigen presenting capacity than DCs isolated from the blood [7]. It has also been shown that lung DCs, which reside in the intraepithelial region, can extend their processes through the luminal surface into the airway to detect any foreign antigens [13]. More recent studies suggested that DCs derived from tissues without "danger" signal stimulation should be regarded as immature DCs, based on their major role in antigen uptake and endocytosis of antigens [11, 14]. However, at this point, the phenotype and function of DC from different sources is not well understood for many veterinary species including horses, and most studies use B-DCs for investigating veterinary diseases.

As the bridge between the innate and adaptive immunity, DCs can direct the outcome of infectious diseases such as bacteria, fungi, parasites or viruses [15–17]. However, many viruses, including herpesviruses, have strategies to interfere with DC function through the down regulation of the host immune response. Human herpes simplex virus (HSV) inhibits DC maturation by modulating the expression of co-stimulatory molecules on DC, which consequently leads to the absence of cytokine production and lack of migration back to lymphoid organs [18]. Virion host shut-off protein from the tegument of HSV-1 has been found to impair DC activation via a Toll-like receptor-independent pathway [19]. Equine herpesvirus-1 (EHV-1) is a major viral pathogen of horses and the cause of rhinopneumonitis, abortion, and central nervous system disorders. Because the respiratory epithelium is the first site of contact between host and pathogen, as well as the initial site for viral replication, it is important to understand respiratory tract immunity including the sentinel network of DCs if we are to understand immunity to EHV-1. Recent research has shown that EHV-1 interferes with the migration of monocytes and DCs isolated from the airway mucosa and uses these cells for transport from the apical side of the respiratory epithelium to the lamina propria and for establishment of viremia [20]. However, the exact mechanism of this process has yet to be identified and protocols for isolating respiratory dendritic cells at numbers sufficient for further in vitro or ex vivo use are needed, particularly in veterinary species.

Because it is likely that characteristics of blood-derived DCs will be different from those of lung-derived DCs, the objective of the current study was to culture lung-derived DCs by adapting the protocol used for isolating blood DCs and to characterize the isolated cells in addition to comparing them with blood-derived DCs. For this purpose, mononuclear cells from equine lung tissue were isolated and cultivated with equine recombinant GM-CSF and IL-4 to generate lung DCs. Isolated cells were then characterized using common markers for APCs [3, 4] and endocytosis was evaluated.

Methods

Animals and sample collections

Lungs from 3 adult horses, and blood from 4 different adult horses were collected for this study. None of the horses showed signs of respiratory diseases, and horses used for lung collection were euthanized for unrelated reasons. Horses were of mixed breed, both genders and ranged in age from 2 to 23 years. Euthanasia was performed by an overdose of 0.22 ml/kg of a 39 mg/ml sodium pentobarbital solution as previously described [21]. All experimental protocols were reviewed and approved under number AUF 10/15–160-00 and AUF 05/13–111-00 by the Michigan State University Institutional Animal Care and Use Committee. During the necropsy procedure, a sample of lung tissue from the diaphragmatic lobe measuring approximately 20 × 20 × 20 cm was collected from each horse. Tissues were washed with cold phosphate buffered saline (PBS) [Gibco, Carlsbad, CA, USA] and deposited in cold DMEM [Gibco, USA] for transportation. Five-hundred ml of 0.1% heparin (1000 U/ml) [Sagent Pharmaceuticals, Schaumburg, IL, USA]-anticoagulated blood was collected from each horse for PBMC isolation.

Lung tissue processing

Freshly collected lung tissue was processed as previously described with some modifications [12, 14]. The tissue was washed with sterile cold PBS several times to remove blood. Tissue was then minced to small pieces (approximately 0.2 × 0.2 × 0.2 cm) and soaked in digestion media (1 mg/ml collagenase type 2 [Sigma-Aldrich, St. Louis, MO, USA], 0.02 mg/ml DNase I [Life technologies, Carlsbad, CA, USA], 5% fetal bovine serum (FBS) [Gibco, USA] and 1% penicillin/ streptomycin [Gibco, USA] dissolved in RPMI-1640 with L-glutamine and 2-mercaptoethanol [Gibco, USA]) for 2–4 h at 37 °C. The digestion media was replaced one time during the incubation to enhance the digestion effect. Following this incubation period, cold 10% FBS was added to the tissue suspension to inactivate the digestion media enzymes. The tissue suspension was then passed through a 100 μm sieve followed by 40 μm cell strainers [Greiner Bio-One, Monroe, NC, USA] to remove tissue debris, and centrifugation was performed on the flow-through at 300 g for 10 min at room temperature. After discarding the supernatant, the cell pellet was re-suspended in PBS and was subject to mononuclear cell isolation (see section 2.4).

Isolation of peripheral blood mononuclear cells, monocytes, and differentiation of monocyte-derived dendritic cells from blood samples

The protocol for isolating different subsets of cells from equine whole blood has been described previously [3]. Briefly, PBMCs were isolated from heparinized whole blood by density centrifugation at 600 g for 45 min at room temperature with Histopaque (∂ = 1.077) [Sigma, USA]. Then, PBMCs were re-suspended and cultured in culture media (cRPMI) (RPMI 1640 with 4 mM L-glutamine, 10% FBS, and 1% penicillin / streptomycin [Gibco, USA]) at a concentration of 1×10^7 cells/ml for 4 h in 200 mm tissue culture-treated dishes at 37 °C. Following the incubation period, adherent blood monocytes (B-MOS) were separated from non-adherent mononuclear cells by washing off non-adherent cells with cRPMI. To collect the adherent B-MOS for flow cytometry, the B-MOS were subjected to treatment of cold Versene EDTA solution [ThermoFisher, Rockford, IL, USA] to detach, followed by gently scraping to collect the cells. For B-DC culture, dendritic cell culture media (RPMI-DC) (RPMI 1640 with 4 mM L-glutamine, 10% heat-inactivated heterologous horse serum, 50 uM β-mercaptoethanol [Sigma, USA], 1% penicillin / strepto-mycin, and 2.5 µg/ml amphotericin B [Gibco, USA], supplemented with recombinant equine GM-CSF (10 ng/ml or 1000 U/ml) as well as recombinant equine IL-4 (10 ng/ml or 1000 U/ml) [KingFisher Biotech, St. Paul, MN, USA], was added and adherent B-MOS were incubated for 4 days, at which point cells differentiated into B-DCs. Loosely adherent B-DCs were separated from firmly attached cells, and purified by further density centrifugation at 600 g for 15 min with Nycoprep (∂ = 1.068) [Progen Biotechnik, Heidelburg, Germany] [4]. Low-density DCs were then collected and cultured in RPMI-DC supplemented with GM-CSF and IL-4 for 3 more days.

Isolations of mononuclear cells, monocytes, and dendritic cells from lung tissues

Similar to the procedure applied for isolation of B-MOS and B-DCs (section 2.3), density centrifugation was performed on the cell suspension obtained from lung tissues at 600 g for 45 min with Histopaque (∂ = 1.077). Cells isolated in this manner were defined as lung mononuclear cells (L-MCs), which were then further cultured in cRPMI for 4 h to separate adherent lung monocytes (L-MOS) from non-adherent cells. For flow cytometry of adherent L-MOS, cells were subjected to treatment of cold Versene EDTA solution [Thermo-Fisher, USA] followed by gently scrapping for collection.

For generation of L-DCs, adherent L-MOS were con-tinuously cultured with RPMI-DC supplemented with GM-CSF and IL-4 for a total of 5 days, with a one-time replenishment of fresh media during cultivation. Cells were collected as lung-derived dendritic cells (L-DCs) after 5 days of cultivation.

Antibodies for flow cytometric analysis and immunocytochemical (ICC) labeling

Different cell types were characterized using antibodies to cell antigens that are generally regarded as monocytic and dendritic cell markers (Table 1). Equine-specific monoclonal antibodies (mAb) recognizing equine MHC class II (clone CVS10) and CD44 mAb (clone CVS18) have previously been described [22]. An anti-CD172α mAb, produced by Washington State University (clone DG-DH59B) [Cat. No. DG-BOV2049] has shown cross-reactivity with multiple animal species [23]. Furthermore, anti-human mAbs with cross-reactivity to equine CD86 (clone IT2.2) [Cat No. 555663; BD Pharmingen, San Jose, CA, USA]) [3], CD163 (clone AM-3 K) [Cat. No. KT-013; Trans Genic, Kobe, Japan], CD204 (clone SRA-E5) [Cat. No. KT-022; Trans Genic, Japan], and anti-B Lymphocyte antigen 36 mAb (Bla 36, clone A7–42) [Cat. No. MU231-UC; Biogenex, Fremont, CA, USA] were used. Mouse IgG1 and IgG2b isotype antibodies [ThermoFisher, USA] were applied as isotype controls. A fluorescein FITC Affi-niPure goat anti-mouse IgG H + L [Jackson ImmunoRe-search, West Grove, PA, USA] was used as the secondary antibody for flow cytometric analysis.

Flow cytometric analysis for detection of cell surface antigens

Flow cytometric analysis was performed to quantify expression of MHC class II, CD44, CD86, and CD172α. Cells were collected and re-suspended in FACS buffer

Table 1 The summary of antigens applied to characterize various types of cells isolated from blood and lung tissues in the present study

Antigen	Function
MHC class II	Antigen presenting protein on antigen presenting cells
CD44	Cell adhesion molecule on lymphocytes, monocytes, and DCs
CD86	T cell co-stimulating molecule on DCs
CD163	Macrophage scavenger receptor on cells of monocytic lineage
CD172α	Signal-regulatory protein on myeloid cells
CD204	Macrophage scavenger receptor on cells of monocytic lineage
Bla36	Glycoprotein on B cell lineage, macrophages, and DCs
IgG1&2b	Isotype controls

(PBS with 0.4% bovine serum albumin and 0.1% sodium azide) [Sigma, USA] prior to incubation with the respective primary antibodies or isotype control for 1 h at 4 °C, at appropriate concentrations: mAbs for MHC class II and CD44: no dilution; CD86: 1:10 dilution; CD172α: 1:100 dilution. Isotype controls were applied at the same concentration as mAbs. After 3 washes, cells were re-suspended in 1:300 diluted goat anti-mouse IgG secondary antibody and incubated for 1 h at 4 °C, before analysis via BD Accuri™ C6 cytometer [BD Biosciences, San Jose, CA, USA]. Gating was applied in forward scatter versus side scatter (FSC/SSC) dot plots to exclude cell debris. Autofluorescence or background was excluded by examining the fluorescence of unstained cells and isotype controls.

Endocytosis tracer assay

An endocytosis tracer assay was used to determine the antigen uptake and endocytic capacity of the different isolated cell types [24]. A total number of 4×10^5 cells was suspended in 200 μl of RPMI-1640 blank or fluorescently tagged antigens (50 μg ovalbumin conjugated with Alexa Fluor 647™ [Molecular Probes, Eugene, OR, USA]) and incubated for 1.5 h at 37 °C or 4 °C, in which the latter were considered as the negative control. Cold FACS buffer was added to terminate the endocytosis reaction, followed by 3 washes in FACS buffer. Flow cytometric analysis was conducted using a BD Accuri™ C6 cytometer [BD Biosciences, San Jose, CA, USA]. For analysis of the results, both percentage of cells stained positive compared to controls and the mean fluorescence intensity (MFI) of cells incubated at 37 °C standardized against the MFI of cells incubated at 4 °C were evaluated. Results were presented as MFI of experimental samples compared to MFI of controls as previously described [24].

Immunocytochemical (ICC) labeling

For ICC labeling, mAb for CD163, CD204, and Bla36 were used. Specific cell-types were re-suspended in PBS, and subjected to an 800 rpm, 10 min centrifugation with a Cyto-Tek° Cytocentrifuge [Electron Microscopy Sciences, Hatfield, PA, USA] to generate cytospin slides, with 5×10^4 cells per slide. Slides were fixed by immersion in acetone at -20 °C for 5 min. Slides were then submitted to the Michigan State University Diagnostic Center for Population and Animal Health for ICC labeling. An EnVision FLEX+ detecting system [Dako, Carpinteria, CA, USA] including peroxidase block, non-biotin polymerized horseradish peroxidase (HRP), 3,3'-Diaminobenzidine (DAB) with DAB plus chromogen solution, and FLEX+ mouse linker, were applied with an autostainer [Dako, USA] as previously described [25]. Hematoxylin [Dako, USA] was used as the counter stain. Finally, cytological inspection

was performed on a light microscope [Leica, Buffalo Grove, IL, USA] and evaluated by a board certified pathologist. The general microscopic observation was performed under 100× magnification to inclusively evaluate the positive staining of the whole cell population. A grading system was used to determine the positive percentage of the detected surface antigens, as follows: one plus for less than 30% positive cells, double plus for 30% to 60% positive cells, triple plus for more than 60% cells that were positive, minus for no positive cells (negative result).

Statistical analysis

Data was graphed using Excel 2016 [Microsoft, Redmond, WA, USA]. For the endocytosis assay, one-way ANOVA followed by post-hoc Tukey's multiple comparisons test [Graphpad Prism 6.01 for Windows, La Jolla, CA, USA] was used to compare the values of mean fluorescence intensity (MFI) in a log scale among different cell types. Statistical significance was considered at $p < 0.05$.

Results

Morphology of mononuclear cells and dendritic cells

Microscopically, freshly isolated PBMCs were round-shaped with a moderate amount of cytoplasm and an euchromatic nucleus (data not shown). Approximately 5–10% of PBMCs, which were considered B-MOS, adhered to the bottom of the tissue culture plate after 2–4 h incubation at 37 °C while the remaining cells were non-adherent were removed after 4 h of incubation. The B-MOS had similar morphology when compared to PBMCs in suspension, but were slightly larger in cell size (data not shown). Upon evaluation by flow cytometry in FSC/SCC plots, PBMCs consisted of mainly lymphocytes characterized by small size (FSC^{low}) and low granularity (SSC^{low}), and a small portion of monocytes characterized by larger size ($FSC^{moderate}$) and higher granularity ($SSC^{moderate}$) (Fig. 1a). After 4 h attachment, an increased number of monocytes, which were $FSC^{moderate}$ and $SSC^{moderate}$ was observed (Fig. 1b),

Initially there were no visible projections on the cell surface of B-MOS. However, projections, or pseudopods, became visible after several days in the presence of GM-CSF and IL-4, suggesting that the cells were transforming into DCs. Dendritic cells were polymorphic during the culture period. They possessed numerous short projections on the cell surface (Fig. 2a, hollow arrow), sometimes with single or multiple extremely extended dendrites (Fig. 2a, solid arrows) aligned by several nodes (Fig. 2a, arrow head). The cells became loosely attached or floated by day 4, and could be easily separated from firmly attached remaining cells. By the end of 7 days in culture, B-DCs were identified as non-adherent, polymorphic and veiled in shape, with several pseudopods projecting around the cell surface (Fig. 2b, solid arrow).

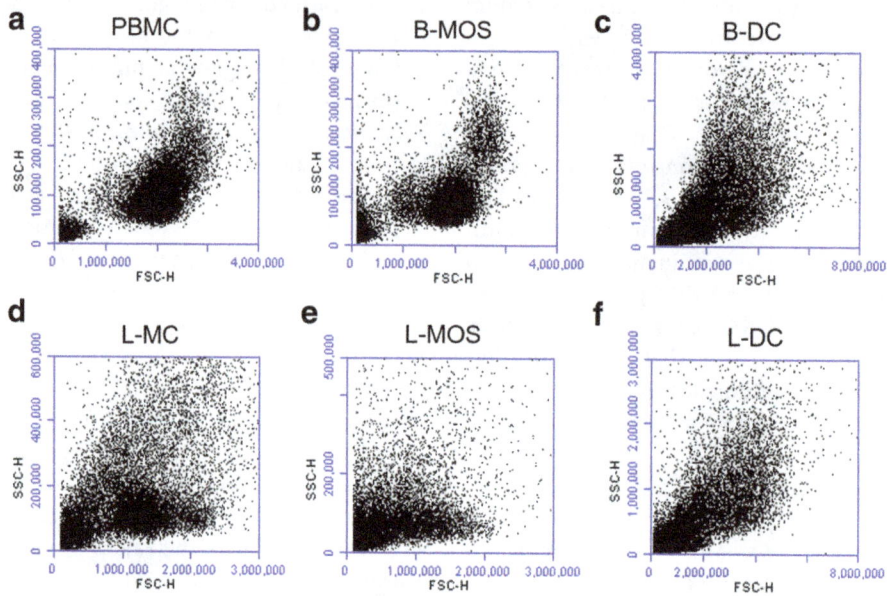

Fig. 1 The dot plots of forward scatter-height (FSC-H) versus side scatter-height (SSC-H) from the representative sample, respectively, for all the cell types isolated in this study (**a**. PBMCs, **b**. B-MOS, **c**. B-DC, **d**. L-MC, **e**. L-MOS, **f**. L-DC

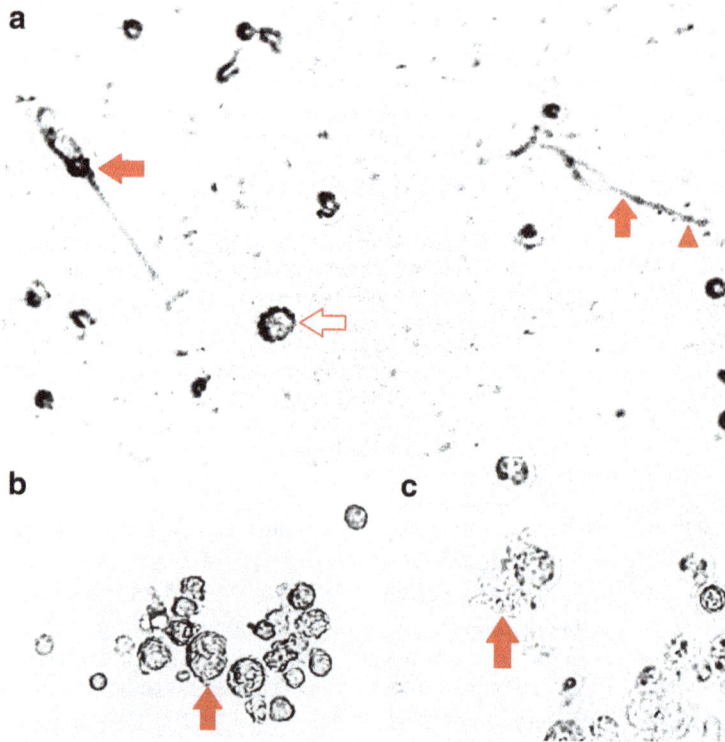

Fig. 2 Microscopic images of dendritic cells following cultivation with recombinant granulocyte macrophage colony-stimulating factor (GM-CSF) and recombinant interleukin-4 (IL-4). All of the images were taken at 200× magnification. **a**) Blood dendritic cells (B-DCs) collected after 3 days of incubation with recombinant proteins of GM-CSF and IL-4. Solid arrows show cells with extended dendrites, one of which possessed several nodes aligning (indicated by arrowhead). Some cells had short projections on the surface (indicated by hollow arrow). **b**) B-DCs collected after 7 days of incubation with recombinant GM-CSF and IL-4. The cells were veiled with pseudopods (indicated by solid arrow). **c**) Lung dendritic cells (L-DCs) after 5 days of incubation with GM-CSF and IL-4. Cells demonstrated visible pseudopods (indicated by solid arrow)

Upon evaluation by flow cytometry in FSC/SCC plots, live B-DCs were mostly large in cell size (FSC^high) and moderate to high in granularity (SSC^high) compared to lymphocytes and monocytes (Fig. 1c).

The morphology of cells isolated from the lungs was comparable with those from blood samples. L-MCs isolated by Histopaque [Sigma, USA] centrifugation were small, round, non-adherent cells, with scarce to moderate cytoplasm and medium size nuclei. The flow cytometry results showed a main cell population characterized by small size (FSC^low) and low granularity (SSC^low), and a small group of cells characterized by slightly larger size (FSC^moderate) and low granularity (SSC^low) (Fig. 1d). After a 2–4 h incubation at 37 °C, adherent L-MOS had identical morphology when compared to B-MOS. Similar to L-MCs, flow cytometry for L-MOS revealed a main population characterized by small size (FSC^low) and low granularity (SSC^low), and few cells exhibiting larger size (FSC^moderate) and low granularity (SSC^low) (Fig. 1e).

L-DCs did not exhibit pseudopods until cultivation with GM-CSF and IL-4 for several days. Like B-DCs, L-DCs were loosely attached or floating, polymorphic, with either remarkably extended or short projections around cell surface (Fig. 2c, solid arrow). Upon evaluation by flow cytometry using FSC/SCC plots, the live cell population of L-DCs was characterized by large cell size (FSC^high) and moderate to high granularity (SSC^high) (Fig. 1f).

Immunophenotypes of mononuclear cells, monocytes, and dendritic cells isolated from blood and lungs

The immunophenotypes of the different isolated cell types were examined by flow cytometry and immunocytochemical (ICC) labeling. The average background staining for flow cytometry assays ranged from 3 to 10% depending on cell type. Results with values below 10% were considered negative.

A summary of the results of the flow cytometric analysis is shown in Fig. 3, with percentage of cells expressing each cell marker for each cell group shown as a bar chart (Fig. 3a). Mean fluorescence intensity (MFI) generally correlated with percentage values. Figure 3b shows representative dot plots of FSC (cell size) versus immunofluorescence (FL1) of each cell marker for each cell group isolated from blood and lung cells, respectively. The dot plots highlight a trend for cells becoming more uniform in phenotype following the cell adherence step and cultivation with GM-CSF and IL-4 (Fig. 2b B-DCs and L-DCs).

Furthermore, we show that PBMCs had low expression of MHC class II (21.8%), high expression of CD44 (86.0%), and no expression of CD86 and CD172α (Fig. 3a). In contrast, expression of MHC class II and CD172a was elevated in B-MOS while CD44 and CD86 stayed

the same. Immunocytochemically, PBMCs expressed similar cell surface molecules when compared to B-MOS, which were positive for Bla36^+ but only mildly positive for macrophage scavenger receptors e.g. CD163 and CD204 (Fig. 4-a, –e, –i). B-DCs strongly expressed MHC class II (98%), CD44 (99%), and CD172α (93%), as well as moderately expressed CD86 (52.3%) (Fig. 3a). B-DCs were also Bla36^+++, and some of the giant cells with multiple nuclei were positive for CD163 and CD204 (Fig. 4-b, –f, –j).

For cells isolated from the lung, a moderate to high percentage of L-MCs expressed MHC class II (84.8%), CD44 (61.3%), and CD172α (31.5%), but were negative for CD86 using flow cytometric analysis (Fig. 3). Immunocytochemically, L-MCs also showed moderate expression of CD163^+, CD204^+, and Bla36^+ (data not shown). Results of L-MOS were similar to L-MCs; L-MOS expressed MHC class II (56.8%), CD44 (72.9%), and CD172α (44.1%), but were negative for CD86 (Fig. 2), as well as CD163^+, CD204^+, and Bla36^+ (Fig. 4-c, –g, –k). Expression of most markers was increased on L-DCs, which showed a high percentage of cells expressing MHC class II (88.3%), CD44 (92.7%), CD172α (73.1%), and moderate percentage of cells expressing CD86 (25.3%) using flow cytometric analysis (Fig. 3). L-DCs were also positive for CD163^++, CD204^+, and Bla36^++ (Fig. 4-d, –h, –l).

Antigen uptake by dendritic cells isolated from lung and blood

For endocytosis assays, PBMCs and B-MOS were isolated from 4 horses, and B-DCs were isolated from 3 horses. L-MCs and L-DCs were isolated from 3 additional horses. Percentage of cells that stained positive and MFIs were compared among different cell types and trends between percentage of positive cells and MFI were similar (data not shown). L-DCs demonstrated significantly higher antigen uptake when compared to any other cell type ($p < 0.05$). The antigen uptake of B-DCs was significantly higher than PBMCs or B-MOS ($p < 0.05$) but there was no significant difference compared to L-MCs ($p = 0.5895$) (Fig. 5). An endocytosis assay was not performed on L-MOS because of limited cell numbers.

Discussion

The majority of studies that investigate viral interactions with host DCs have used cells derived from blood leukocytes because of the relative ease of obtaining appropriate cell numbers and generating cells with DC phenotype [3, 4]. However, DCs derived from respiratory tissues may have distinct immunological phenotypes as well as better capacity for antigen processing when compared to blood-derived cells [26, 27]. Thus, it may be advantageous to use lung-derived DCs particularly

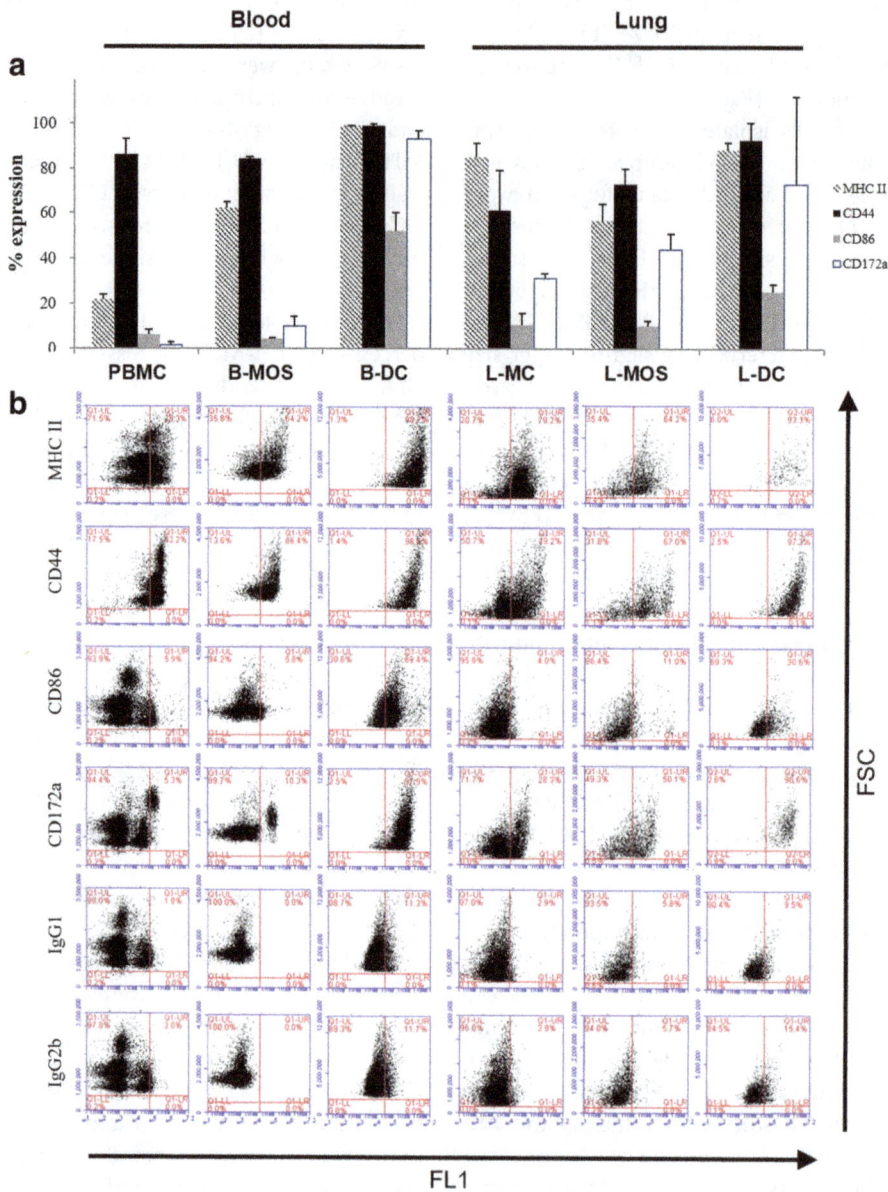

Fig. 3 Results of flow cytometric analysis. **a**. Bar chart showing mean values of immunofluorescence of MHC class II (box filled with diagonal pattern), CD44 (solid black box), CD86 (solid gray box), and CD172a (white box) expression in peripheral blood mononuclear cell (PBMCs), blood monocyte (B-MOS), and blood dendritic cell (B-DC), as well as lung mononuclear cell (L-MC), lung monocyte (L-MOS), and lung dendritic cell (L-DC). The error bars indicate standard deviation. **b**. Representative results showing dot plots of blood cells (PBMC, B-MOS, and B-DC) from one horse and lung cells (L-MC, L-MOS, and L-DC) from another horse. The X-axis for each dot plot is a logarithmic scale of immunofluorescence parameter (FL1) for MHC class II, CD44, CD86, CD172a, and isotype controls including IgG1 and IgG2b; the y-axis for each dot plot is forward scatter (FSC), indicating the size of the cells

when studying the interaction between pathogens and antigen-presenting cells that infect via mucosal routes, or when considering pathogens that can affect DC function [18–20]. We developed a protocol for isolating L-DCs from lung mononuclear cells by adapting a commonly used equine B-DC protocol [3]. While the L-DC derived using this protocol maybe distinct from tissue resident lung DCs isolated directly from tissue lysates [7, 11, 14, 28], the number of tissue resident lung DCs isolated from

lysates is often scarce and cells die quickly without supplement of GM-CSF [29]. Our protocol is the first to generate cytokine-activated lung DCs from horses at sufficient numbers that are phenotypically similar to B-DCs and have improved endocytic capacity.

More specifically, we isolated and cultivated L-DCs by using a protocol similar to isolation of B-DC with small modifications. Comparing DCs derived from blood and lung, we demonstrated that the morphology of DCs was

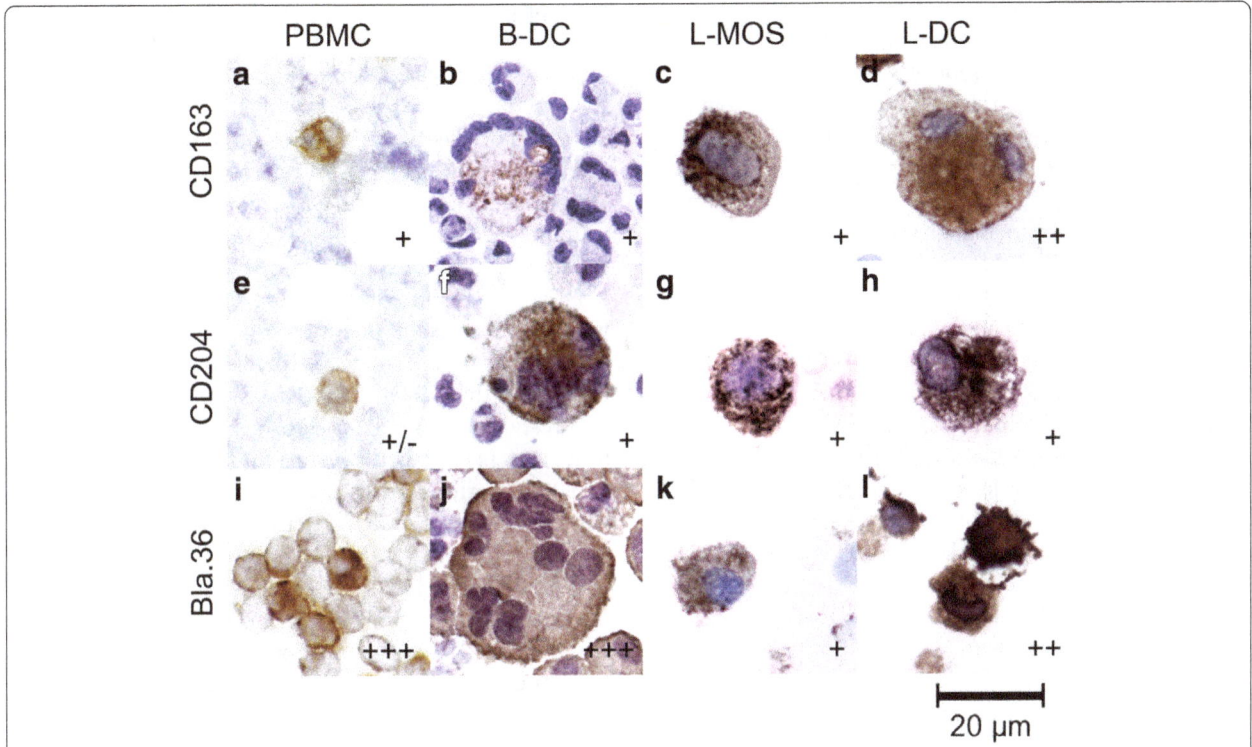

Fig. 4 Microscopic images of immunocytochemical staining for CD163 (**a-d**), CD204 (**e-h**), and Bla36 (**i-l**) expression on blood monocytes (B-MOS) and blood dendritic cells (B-DCs), as well as lung monocytes (L-MOS) and lung dendritic cells (L-DCs). All of the images were taken at 400× magnification

similar; however, the immunological profiles of L-DCs were different compared to B-DCs. L-DCs expressed high levels of MHC class II and CD44 that were similar compared to the expression profiles of B-DCs, though the expression level of CD86 was higher on B-DCs (52.3%) than on L-DCs (25.3%). MHC class II is responsible for antigen presentation and a marker found in many cell types; high levels of this marker are indicative of antigen presenting cells, in particular DCs. CD44 is a cell surface glycoprotein involved in lymphocyte/monocyte activation, cell-to-cell interaction and migration. When there is antigen present, the expression of CD44 is triggered to bind extracellular matrix, inducing an inflammatory cell response [30]. The expression of CD44 on DCs can also be enhanced by antigen stimulation, which results in DC migration and mediates T cell activation [31]. CD86 facilitates DC stimulation and contact with the T cell receptor [32]. Peripheral DCs are typically immature DCs, generally in charge of antigen uptake through receptor-mediated endocytosis and function in the transport from sites of infection to lymph nodes. Once they arrive in the lymph nodes, DCs present processed antigen to T cells via MHC class II molecules and provide co-stimulation signals via CD86 and T cell receptor CD28 [33]. L-DCs isolated in our study expressed less CD86 than B-DCs did, suggesting that L-DCs may be less mature when compared to B-DCs. We also observed that initially the isolated mononuclear cells (B-MOS or L-MOs) were of a mixed cell type; however, the phenotype of cells became more uniform after cultivation with GM-CSF and IL-4, suggesting a role of these cytokines in the maturation of B-DCs and L-DCs (Fig. 3b).

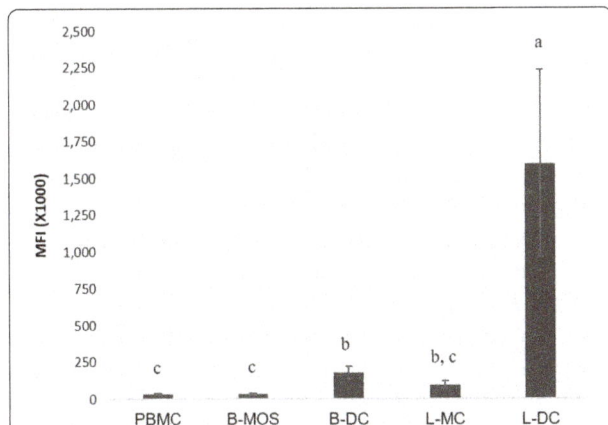

Fig. 5 Flow cytometric analysis showing antigen uptake capacity of blood mononuclear cell (PBMC), blood monocyte (B-MOS), blood dendritic cell (B-DC), as well as lung mononuclear cell (L-MC) and lung dendritic cell (L-DC). Mean values are shown for each cell type with error bars indicating standard errors of the mean (SEM). Different alphabetic letters represent significant differences ($p < 0.05$) using Tukey's multiple comparison tests. MFI: mean fluorescence intensit

CD172α belongs to a family of signal regulatory proteins and is primarily expressed on myeloid cells including monocytes, DCs, and macrophages, though the expression is different among different DC subtypes or in different tissues [34–36]. A recent equine study further illustrated that APCs isolated from airway epithelium had both CD172α$^+$ and CD172α$^-$ cells [26]. L-DCs in our study expressed moderate to high level of CD172α, but with remarkable variability when compared to B-DCs. CD172α is involved in DC migration and activation of Th2 cells [37] and can be used as an indicator of differentiation and maturation of DCs. In general, our results suggest that L-DCs showed similar expressions of markers that were expressed on B-DCs, but at lower levels. This could be due to there being multiple cell sub-types within each cell population or due to a lesser degree of maturation of L-DCs when compared to B-DCs. More experiments using dual or triple staining of classical DC markers such as CD11c, CD86, CD172a and CD14 could be performed to further subtype these populations but this went beyond the scope of the current study [5].

L-MCs and L-MOS shared similar marker profiles, with moderate to high level of MHC class II and CD44 expressions, moderate levels of CD172α, and low expression of CD86, indicating that mononuclear cells and monocytes isolated from lung tissues express the molecules associated with antigen presentation and DC maturation and that there is already a number of L-MOS present in the isolated L-MCs. In contrast and as expected, PBMCs demonstrated a distinct profile with high expression of CD44, but low to no expression of DC markers such as MHC class II, CD86, and CD172α. It was also noticed that mononuclear cells isolated from lung tissues possessed more features consistent with antigen presentation than their counterparts isolated from blood prior to stimulation with cytokines. Studies in either human or animal species have demonstrated isolation of different DC subpopulations directly from lung tissue digests without further cultivation [12, 14, 24, 27], verifying that naïve APCs are widely distributed in tissues, but less so in blood.

Cytokine supplementation during DC cultivation and differentiation is critical to produce differentiated cell populations for ex vivo cell culture. Continuous replenishment of GM-CSF and IL-4 in culture was found essential to keep high expression of MHC I and II on DCs, as well as to increase the level of antigen uptake via receptor-mediated endocytosis [38]. In our study, equine DCs isolated from digested lung tissues cultured with GM-CSF and IL-4 showed higher capacity of endocytosis than those without GM-CSF and IL-4 supplementation. Previous studies have demonstrated that the endocytic abilities of CD172α$^+$ APCs and CD172α$^-$ APCs were not different from each other when no cytokines were added to cell culture [26]. It is likely that immature DCs prior to stimulation by danger signals such as CpG or LPS [39] have good endocytic ability to internalize antigens. After migrating to lymph nodes, they require inductive signals, including GM-CSF, TNFα, and CD40L, for further maturation to full antigen presenting capacity and activation of T cells [28]. Our results suggest that GM-CSF and IL-4 play a role in inducing coordination of DC maturation. Moreover, the endocytosis level of L-DCs was higher than that of B-DCs. The results of the endocytosis assay, in parallel with the results of phenotyping, suggest that B-DCs are possible more mature/differentiated than L-DCs, though both L-DCs and B-DCs are still considered relatively immature DCs due to lack of danger signal induction [11]. It is however important to consider incubation periods with GM-CSF and IL-4 for L-DCs were only 5 days rather than 7 days for the B-DCs, due to poor cell viability of L-DCs after more than 5-days of culture. This may explain the lesser degree of maturation/differentiation of L-DC. Previous studies demonstrated that a continuous supplement of GM-CSF and IL-4 for 6–7 days is required to generate stable phenotype of DCs [40]. Therefore, different phenotypes of B-DCs and L-DCs may be attributed to discrepancy of duration of cytokine stimulation, aside from differences in cell origin.

CD163 and CD204 are members of a super family of scavenger receptors; CD163 belongs to class B, whereas CD204 belongs to class A (also known as SRA). Both CD163 and CD204 are considered to be specific markers for tissue-resident macrophages [41, 42], particularly anti-inflammatory macrophages M2 [43, 44]. More recent studies have shown expression of CD163 and CD204 on ex vivo generated DCs [44–46]. In our study, cells exhibiting APC phenotypes, including B-DCs, L-MOS, and L-DCs, stained positive for CD163 and CD204. Within these cell types a small portion of cells, which showed multinucleated giant cell morphology expressed strong signals for CD163 and CD204. Considering that M2 macrophages can be generated from PBMCs by stimulation with macrophage colony stimulating factor (M-CSF), IL-4, and IL-10 [47], which are similar to the cytokines used for culture of DCs, it might be possible that our isolated cell populations contained a portion of M2-associated macrophages. BLA36, on the other hand, is a surface glycoprotein that has been reported primarily on activated B lymphocytes, Reed–Sternberg cells and their mononuclear variants isolated from human Hodgkin's lymphoma [48], as well as DCs in dog skin [49]. Our present study shows that a portion of equine mononuclear cells and DCs from equine tissues were BLA36 positive, which has been shown to also label macrophages and dendritic cells in horses [50]. Further cell sorting plus characterization will be required to identify sub-populations of L-DCs.

Conclusions

The phenotypes and functions of lung-derived DCs isolated in our study will be particularly helpful for future research of respiratory diseases. Our study used an already established protocol for isolating B-DCs by culture with GM-CSF and IL-4 and generated a population of cells from the horse lung that shares phenotypic features with B-DCs but has higher endocytic capacity. Unlike blood cells, mononuclear cells freshly isolated from lung digests exhibited markers of APCs. Furthermore, GM-CSF and IL-4 supplementation during DC cultivation induced DC differentiation and significantly increased the endocytic capacity of L-DCs. Although our L-DCs likely do not represent pure tissue resident DCs and were exposed to cytokine supplementation, we nevertheless identified an alternative way to generate airway DCs that share features with primary tissue resident DCs and may be an ideal tool for studying respiratory disease in horses.

Abbreviations
ANOVA: Analysis of variance; APC: Antigen-presenting cells; B-DC: Blood dendritic cells; BLA 36: B lymphocyte antigen 36; B-MOS: Adherent blood monocytes; DC: Dendritic cells; EDTA: Ethylenediaminetetraacetic acid; FACS: Fluorescence-activated cell sorting; FSC: Forward scatter; GM-CSF: Granulocyte macrophage-colony stimulating factor; ICC: Immunocytochemistry; IgG: Immunoglobulin G; IL-4: Interleukin-4; L-DC: Lung dendritic cells; L-MC: Lung mononuclear cells; L-MOS: Adherent lung monocytes; mAb: Monoclonal antibodies; M-CSF: Macrophage-colony stimulating factor; MFI: Mean fluorescence intensity; MHC I & II: Major histocompatibility complex class I & II; PBMC: Peripheral blood mononuclear cells; PBS: Phosphate-buffered saline; SSC: Side scatter; TNFα: Tumor necrosis factor alpha

Acknowledgements
We acknowledge Dr. Thomas Wood at the Veterinary Diagnostic Laboratory at Michigan State University for assisting with immunocytochemical staining.

Funding
This project was supported by Agriculture and Food Research Initiative competitive grant no. 2012–67,015-20,498. Funding was used to support the design of the study, analysis and interpretation of the data as well as preparation of the manuscript.

Authors' contributions
YL contributed to the experimental design, data collection, data analysis, drafting and writing of this manuscript. MK contributed to conception, supervision, and revision of the manuscript. GSH contributed to the acquisition of funds, conception, experimental design, supervision and mentoring of YL and revision of the manuscript. All authors have read and approved the final manuscript.

Consent for publication
Not applicable.

Competing interests
The authors declare that they have no competing interests.

References
1. Mellman I, Steinman RM. Dendritic cells: specialized and regulated antigen processing machines. Cell. 2001;106:255–8.
2. Robinson SP, Patterson S, English N, Davies D, Knight SC, Reid CD. Human peripheral blood contains two distinct lineages of dendritic cells. Eur J Immunol. 1999;29:2769–78.
3. Hammond SA, Horohov D, Montelaro RC. Functional characterization of equine dendritic cells propagated ex vivo using recombinant human GM-CSF and recombinant equine IL-4. Vet Immunol Immunopathol. 1999;71:197–214.
4. Siedek E, Little S, Mayall S, Edington N, Hamblin A. Isolation and characterisation of equine dendritic cells. Vet Immunol Immunopathol. 1997;60:15–31.
5. Sallusto F, Lanzavecchia A. Efficient presentation of soluble antigen by cultured human dendritic cells is maintained by granulocyte/macrophage colony-stimulating factor plus interleukin 4 and downregulated by tumor necrosis factor alpha. J Exp Med. 1994;179:1109–18.
6. Egner W, McKenzie JL, Smith SM, Beard ME, Hart DN. Identification of potent mixed leukocyte reaction-stimulatory cells in human bone marrow. Putative differentiation stage of human blood dendritic cells. J Immunol. 1993;150:3043–53.
7. Sertl K, Takemura T, Tschachler E, Ferrans VJ, Kaliner MA, Shevach EM. Dendritic cells with antigen-presenting capability reside in airway epithelium, lung parenchyma, and visceral pleura. J Exp Med. 1986;163:436–51.
8. Pavli P, Maxwell L, Van de Pol E, Doe F. Distribution of human colonic dendritic cells and macrophages. Clin Exp Immunol. 1996;104:124–32.
9. Prickett TC, McKenzie JL, Hart DN. Characterization of interstitial dendritic cells in human liver. Transplantation. 1988;46:754–61.
10. Hart DN, Fabre JW. Demonstration and characterization of Ia-positive dendritic cells in the interstitial connective tissues of rat heart and other tissues, but not brain. J Exp Med. 1981;154:347–61.
11. van Haarst JM, Hoogsteden HC, de Wit HJ, Verhoeven GT, Havenith CE, Drexhage HA. Dendritic cells and their precursors isolated from human bronchoalveolar lavage: immunocytologic and functional properties. Am J Respir Cell Mol Biol. 1994;11:344–50.
12. Gong JL, McCarthy KM, Telford J, Tamatani T, Miyasaka M, Schneeberger EE. Intraepithelial airway dendritic cells: a distinct subset of pulmonary dendritic cells obtained by microdissection. J Exp Med. 1992;175:797–807.
13. Jahnsen FL, Strickland DH, Thomas JA, Tobagus IT, Napoli S, Zosky GR, Turner DJ, Sly PD, Stumbles PA, Holt PG. Accelerated antigen sampling and transport by airway mucosal dendritic cells following inhalation of a bacterial stimulus. J Immunol. 2006;177:5861–7.
14. Gonzalez-Juarrero M, Orme IM. Characterization of murine lung dendritic cells infected with mycobacterium tuberculosis. Infect Immun. 2001;69:1127–33.
15. Steinbach F, Borchers K, Ricciardi-Castagnoli P, Ludwig H, Stingl G, Elbe-Burger A. Dendritic cells presenting equine herpesvirus-1 antigens induce protective anti-viral immunity. J Gen Virol. 1998;79:3005–14.
16. Morel PA, Butterfield LH. Dendritic cell control of immune responses. Front Immunol. 2015;6:42.
17. Ramirez-Ortiz ZG, Means TK. The role of dendritic cells in the innate recognition of pathogenic fungi (a. Fumigatus, C. Neoformans and C. Albicans). Virulence. 2012;3:635–46.
18. Salio M, Cella M, Suter M, Lanzavecchia A. Inhibition of dendritic cell maturation by herpes simplex virus. Eur J Immunol. 1999;29:3245–53.
19. Cotter CR, Nguyen ML, Yount JS, Lopez CB, Blaho JA, Moran TM. The virion host shut-off (vhs) protein blocks a TLR-independent pathway of herpes simplex virus type 1 recognition in human and mouse dendritic cells. PLoS One. 2010;5:e8684.
20. Baghi HB, Nauwynck HJ. Impact of equine herpesvirus type 1 (EHV-1) infection on the migration of monocytic cells through equine nasal mucosa. Comp Immunol Microbiol Infect Dis. 2014;37:321–9.
21. Quintana AM, Landolt GA, Annis KM, Hussey GS. Immunological characterization of the equine airway epithelium and of a primary equine airway epithelial cell culture model. Vet Immunol Immunopathol. 2011;140:226–36.
22. Lunn DP, Holmes MA, Antczak DF, Agerwal N, Baker J, Bendali-Ahcene S, Blanchard-Channell M, Byrne KM, Cannizzo K, Davis W, et al. Report of the second equine leucocyte antigen workshop, squaw valley, California, July 1995. Vet Immunol Immunopathol. 1998;62:101–43.
23. Cobbold SP, Metcalfe SM. Monoclonal antibodies that define canine homologues of human CD antigens: summary of the first international canine leukocyte antigen workshop (CLAW). Tissue Antigens. 1994;43:137–54.

24. Loving CL, Brockmeier SL, Sacco RE. Differential type I interferon activation and susceptibility of dendritic cell populations to porcine arterivirus. Immunology. 2007;120:217–29.

25. Barnes KJ, Garner MM, Wise AG, Persiani M, Maes RK, Kiupel M. Herpes simplex encephalitis in a captive black howler monkey (Alouatta Caraya). J Vet Diagn Investig. 2016;28:76–8.

26. Baghi HB, Laval K, Favoreel H, Nauwynck HJ. Isolation and characterization of equine nasal mucosal CD172a + cells. Vet Immunol Immunopathol. 2014;157:155–63.

27. Demedts IK, Brusselle GG, Vermaelen KY, Pauwels RA. Identification and characterization of human pulmonary dendritic cells. Am J Respir Cell Mol Biol. 2005;32:177–84.

28. Holt PG, Oliver J, Bilyk N, McMenamin C, McMenamin PG, Kraal G, Thepen T. Downregulation of the antigen presenting cell function(s) of pulmonary dendritic cells in vivo by resident alveolar macrophages. J Exp Med. 1993; 177:397–407.

29. Mauel S, Steinbach F, Ludwig H. Monocyte-derived dendritic cells from horses differ from dendritic cells of humans and mice. Immunology. 2006; 117:463–73.

30. Johnson P, Ruffell B. CD44 and its role in inflammation and inflammatory diseases. Inflamm Allergy Drug Targets 2009;8:208–220.

31. Weiss JM, Sleeman J, Renkl AC, Dittmar H, Termeer CC, Taxis S, Howells N, Hofmann M, Kohler G, Schopf E, et al. An essential role for CD44 variant isoforms in epidermal Langerhans cell and blood dendritic cell function. J Cell Biol. 1997;137:1137–47.

32. Rissoan MC, Soumelis V, Kadowaki N, Grouard G, Briere F, de Waal Malefyt R, Liu YJ. Reciprocal control of T helper cell and dendritic cell differentiation. Science. 1999;283:1183–6.

33. Shahinian A, Pfeffer K, Lee KP, Kundig TM, Kishihara K, Wakeham A, Kawai K, Ohashi PS, Thompson CB, Mak TW, Differential T. cell costimulatory requirements in CD28-deficient mice. Science. 1993;261:609–12.

34. Seiffert M, Brossart P, Cant C, Cella M, Colonna M, Brugger W, Kanz L, Ullrich A, Buhring HJ. Signal-regulatory protein alpha (SIRPalpha) but not SIRPbeta is involved in T-cell activation, binds to CD47 with high affinity, and is expressed on immature CD34(+)CD38(−) hematopoietic cells. Blood. 2001; 97:2741–9.

35. Bimczok D, Sowa EN, Faber-Zuschratter H, Pabst R, Rothkotter HJ. Site-specific expression of CD11b and SIRPalpha (CD172a) on dendritic cells: implications for their migration patterns in the gut immune system. Eur J Immunol. 2005;35:1418–27.

36. Epardaud M, Bonneau M, Payot F, Cordier C, Megret J, Howard C, Schwartz-Cornil I. Enrichment for a CD26hi SIRP- subset in lymph dendritic cells from the upper aero-digestive tract. J Leukoc Biol. 2004;76:553–61.

37. Raymond M, Rubio M, Fortin G, Shalaby KH, Hammad H, Lambrecht BN, Sarfati M. Selective control of SIRP-alpha-positive airway dendritic cell trafficking through CD47 is critical for the development of T(H)2-mediated allergic inflammation. J Allergy Clin Immunol. 2009;124:1333–42. e1331

38. Basak SK, Harui A, Stolina M, Sharma S, Mitani K, Dubinett SM, Roth MD. Increased dendritic cell number and function following continuous in vivo infusion of granulocyte macrophage-colony-stimulating factor and interleukin-4. Blood. 2002;99:2869–79.

39. Sparwasser T, Koch ES, Vabulas RM, Heeg K, Lipford GB, Ellwart JW, Wagner H, Bacterial DNA. Immunostimulatory CpG oligonucleotides trigger maturation and activation of murine dendritic cells. Eur J Immunol. 1998;28:2045–54.

40. Romani N, Reider D, Heuer M, Ebner S, Kampgen E, Eibl B, Niederwieser D, Schuler G. Generation of mature dendritic cells from human blood. An improved method with special regard to clinical applicability. J Immunol Methods. 1996;196:137–51.

41. Zeng L, Takeya M, Takahashi K. AM-3K, a novel monoclonal antibody specific for tissue macrophages and its application to pathological investigation. J Pathol. 1996;178:207–14.

42. Becker M, Cotena A, Gordon S, Platt N. Expression of the class a macrophage scavenger receptor on specific subpopulations of murine dendritic cells limits their endotoxin response. Eur J Immunol. 2006;36:950–60.

43. Hogger P, Dreier J, Droste A, Buck F, Sorg C. Identification of the integral membrane protein RM3/1 on human monocytes as a glucocorticoid-inducible member of the scavenger receptor cysteine-rich family (CD163). J Immunol. 1998;161:1883–90.

44. Ohnishi K, Komohara Y, Fujiwara Y, Takemura K, Lei X, Nakagawa T, Sakashita N, Takeya M. Suppression of TLR4-mediated inflammatory response by macrophage class a scavenger receptor (CD204). Biochem Biophys Res Commun. 2011;411:516–22.

45. Maniecki MB, Moller HJ, Moestrup SK, Moller BK. CD163 positive subsets of blood dendritic cells: the scavenging macrophage receptors CD163 and CD91 are coexpressed on human dendritic cells and monocytes. Immunobiology. 2006;211:407–17.

46. Yi H, Yu X, Gao P, Wang Y, Baek SH, Chen X, Kim HL, Subjeck JR, Wang XY. Pattern recognition scavenger receptor SRA/CD204 down-regulates toll-like receptor 4 signaling-dependent CD8 T-cell activation. Blood. 2009;113:5819–28.

47. Verreck FA, de Boer T, Langenberg DM, van der Zanden L, Ottenhoff TH. Phenotypic and functional profiling of human proinflammatory type-1 and anti-inflammatory type-2 macrophages in response to microbial antigens and IFN-gamma- and CD40L-mediated costimulation. J Leukoc Biol. 2006;79:285–93.

48. Imam A, Stathopoulos E, Taylor CRBLA. 36: a glycoprotein specifically expressed on the surface of Hodgkin's and B cells. Anticancer Res. 1990;10:1095–104.

49. Gache Y, Pin D, Gagnoux-Palacios L, Carozzo C, Meneguzzi G. Correction of dog dystrophic epidermolysis bullosa by transplantation of genetically modified epidermal autografts. J Invest Dermatol. 2011;131:2069–78.

50. Valli V, Kiupel M, Bienzle D. Hematopoietic system. In: Maxie M, editor. Jubb, Kennedy, and Palmer's pathology of domestic animals. 6th ed. St. Louis, MO: Elsevier; 2016. p. 237.

20

Novel insights into the host immune response of chicken Harderian gland tissue during Newcastle disease virus infection and heat treatment

Perot Saelao[1,2,3†], Ying Wang[2,3†], Rodrigo A. Gallardo[4], Susan J. Lamont[5], Jack M. Dekkers[5], Terra Kelly[2,6] and Huaijun Zhou[2,3*] [iD]

Abstract

Background: Newcastle disease virus, in its most pathogenic form, threatens the livelihood of rural poultry farmers where there is a limited infrastructure and service for vaccinations to prevent outbreaks of the virus. Previously reported studies on the host response to Newcastle disease in chickens have not examined the disease under abiotic stressors, such as heat, which commonly experienced by chickens in regions such as Africa. The objective of this study was to elucidate the underlying biological mechanisms that contribute to disease resistance in chickens to the Newcastle disease virus while under the effects of heat stress.

Results: Differential gene expression analysis identified genes differentially expressed between treated and non-treated birds across three time points (2, 6, and 10 days post-infection) in Fayoumi and Leghorn birds. Across the three time points, Fayoumi had very few genes differentially expressed between treated and non-treated groups at 2 and 6 days post-infection. However, 202 genes were differentially expressed at 10 days post-infection. Alternatively, Leghorn had very few genes differentially expressed at 2 and 10 days post-infection but had 167 differentially expressed genes at 6 days post-infection. Very few differentially expressed genes were shared between the two genetic lines, and pathway analysis found unique signaling pathways specific to each genetic line. Fayoumi had significantly lower viral load, higher viral clearance, higher anti-NDV antibody levels, and fewer viral transcripts detected compared to Leghorns. Fayoumis activated immune related pathways including SAPK/JNK and p38 MAPK signaling pathways at earlier time points, while Leghorn would activate these same pathways at a later time. Further analysis revealed activation of the GP6 signaling pathway that may be responsible for the susceptible Leghorn response.

Conclusions: The findings in this study confirmed our hypothesis that the Fayoumi line was more resistant to Newcastle disease virus infection compared to the Leghorn line. Within line and interaction analysis demonstrated substantial differences in response patterns between the two genetic lines that was not observed from the within line contrasts. This study has provided novel insights into the transcriptome response of the Harderian gland tissue during Newcastle disease virus infection while under heat stress utilizing a unique resistant and susceptible model.

Keywords: Newcastle disease virus, Heat stress, Harderian gland, RNA-Seq, Disease resistance

* Correspondence: hzhou@ucdavis.edu
†Perot Saelao and Ying Wang contributed equally to this work.
2Genomics to Improve Poultry Innovation Lab, University of California, Davis, CA 95616, USA
3Department of Animal Science, University of California, Davis, CA 95616, USA
Full list of author information is available at the end of the article

Background

Newcastle disease virus (NDV) is a negative-sense, single stranded RNA virus in the family *Paramyxoviridae* that infects a wide range of avian species. There exist several different strains of the virus, each defined by their pathogenicity and grouped as: asymptomatic, lentogenic (nonvirulent), mesogenic (intermediate virulence), and velogenic (highly virulent) [1]. Outbreaks of virulent strains of NDV in poultry farms can result in 80–90% mortality [2]. Globally, the virus represents a major threat to food security in rural areas, and represents a huge economic drain during outbreaks [3]. Although vaccines exist for NDV, the lack of infrastructure and "cold chain" in under-developed countries limits the protection that vaccination can offer to address Newcastle disease. Genetic improvement of disease resistance provides an alternative approach to further reduce the likelihood of Newcastle disease outbreaks in less developed countries.

In addition to the threat of biotic factors, abiotic factors such as heat stress threaten have become one of the most economically devastating factors for poultry farmers. The overall impact of heat stress on poultry flocks is estimated to result in a loss of $165 millions dollars annually to the poultry industry in the U.S. [4]. Heat stress is characterized as the result of a net energy imbalance between an organism's body and its environment [5]. This energy in the form of heat is unable to dissipate into the environment and thus accumulates in the host resulting in high internal temperatures that cause a dysregulation of neuroendocrine, behavioral, and metabolic systems [5]. In chickens, this physiological impairment can result in an overall decrease in production quality traits such as egg yield, egg quality, body weight, and reduced immune function [6, 7]. Bartlett and Smith reported that heat stress reduced the total level of circulating IgM and IgG antibodies during primary and secondary immune response [7]. In HD11 cell lines however, Slawinska et al. found that heat stress of LPS treated cell lines resulted in an up regulation of some immune related genes potentially due to the increase abundance of heat shock proteins and chaperones [8]. A few studies have suggested that host genetic makeup plays a significant role in response to heat stress in chickens [9, 10]. The increasing impact of climate change on global temperatures necessitates a greater emphasis on understanding the role of abiotic factors have on host physiology and immune response.

To develop novel methods to limit economic losses due to biotic and abiotic stress factors in poultry, it is essential to gain a deeper understanding of the immune response elicited under the simultaneous effects of these two factors. Transcriptome profiling offers the potential to gain insight into the host's entire gene expression profile and the complex biological processes underlying the host immune response. Several studies on the transcriptome of the chicken immune system during NDV infection have focused on the trachea, lung, and spleen [11–13]. Nuss et al. highlighted the importance of tissue-specific expression profiling in understanding infection specific functions regulating the host-pathogen transcriptome [14]. In chickens, the Harderian gland is a key immune organ and major site of infection for NDV due to its proximity to the eye. The Harderian gland is located within the inner orbit of the eye and functions as a major component of the head associated lymphoid tissues (HALT) containing secretory bodies of antibodies and other immune cells [15]. In addition to its function as an immune organ, the Harderian gland also plays a role in thermoregulation and the production of thermal regulator secretions [15]. Despite its critical role as an essential immune organ, very few studies have attempted to profile the Harderian gland specific host response to pathogen infection at the transcriptome level.

The genetic makeup of the host has a significant impact on disease resistance and heat tolerance. Previous research in chickens has investigated the genetics of resistance to pathogens by utilizing two highly inbred chicken lines, Fayoumi and Leghorn. The Fayoumi line has been used to understand relative resistance to a wide range of pathogens including, avian influenza virus (AIV), Marek's disease virus, coccidiosis, and *Salmonella* [16–19]. Wang et al. demonstrated that the Fayoumi line was relatively more resistant to AIV when compared to Leghorns, with Fayoumis having a reduced AIV viral titer and an increase in signaling pathways associated with immune function [16]. Furthermore, Fayoumi is believed to be relatively more heat tolerant when compared to Leghorn based on blood chemistry analysis comparing the two genetic lines [20].

We hypothesized that Fayoumi birds were more NDV resistant while under the effects of heat stress relative to Leghorn. The specific objective of this study was to profile the host immune response to NDV infection under heat stress, and to identify genes and signaling pathways associated with disease resistance of the Harderian gland transcriptome at three time post-infection points during NDV infection and heat stress in both Fayoumi and Leghorn.

Results

The Fayoumi line was more resistant to NDV than leghorns while under heat stress

NDV viral load was measured by qRT-PCR from extracted chicken lachrymal fluid determined that Fayoumi chickens had significantly lower NDV titers than Leghorns at both 2 and 6 dpi ($p = 1.23E-05$, $p = 1.46E-10$, respectively, Fig. 1). In addition, there was a significant

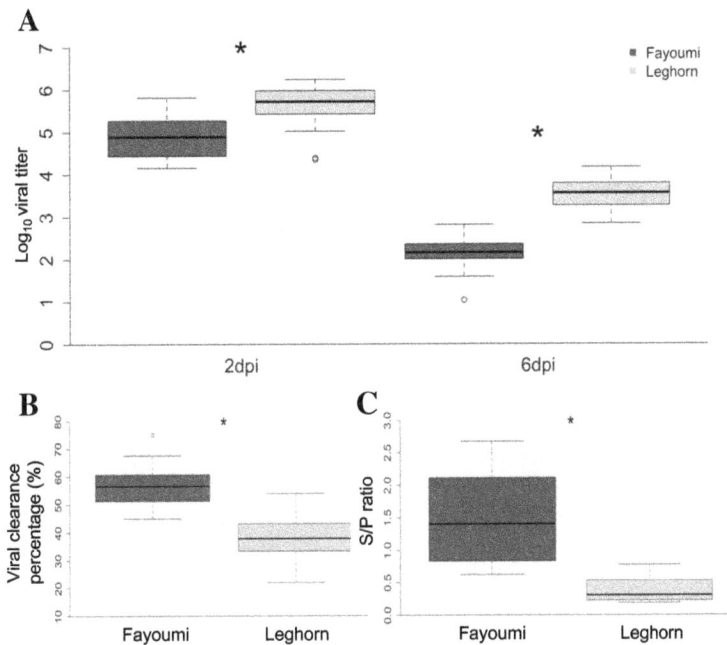

Fig. 1 Box plots for viral titer, viral clearance, and anti-NDV antibody level of Fayoumi and Leghorn birds by days post-infection. Significance ($p <$ 0.05) of the differences is indicated by *. **a** Log_{10} viral titer measured by qPCR in Fayoumi and Leghorn birds at 2 dpi ($p = 1.23E-05$) and 6 dpi ($p = 1.46E-10$). **b** Viral clearance rate of Fayoumi and Leghorn birds measured as the percent change in viral load from 2 to 6 dpi ($p = 3.57E-07$). **c** Anti-NDV antibody S/P ratio at 10 dpi ($p = 1.5E-03$)

difference in virus clearance rate from 2 to 6 dpi between the two lines ($p = 3.57E-07$). On average, the Fayoumi chickens line were able to clear 56% of the virus from 2 to 6 dpi, while the Leghorn line only cleared 37% of the virus from 2 to 6 dpi. Furthermore, anti-NDV antibody titers measured by ELISA in 10 dpi serum samples revealed that Fayoumis produced significantly more anti-NDV antibodies than Leghorn birds ($p = 1.5E-03$).

Viral genome alignment identifies less NDV gene expression at the site of infection in Fayoumi than leghorn

Viral transcripts extracted from the Harderian gland transcriptome sequences of NDV-infected individuals from both lines were aligned to the NDV La Sota strain genome. In Fayoumi chickens, NDV transcripts were only detected at 2 dpi and but not at 6 and 10 dpi, while Leghorn chickens had significantly higher quantities of the NDV transcripts detected at 2 dpi, with detectable quantities of the virus transcripts at 6 dpi and none at 10 (Fig. 2).

Differential gene expression analysis within lines identified time specific responses to NDV infection under heat treatment

To understand the difference in the host gene expression response to the combined effect of NDV and heat stress within Fayoumis and Leghorns, contrasts were made comparing treated and non-treated birds across

three time points (2, 6, and 10 dpi). In the Fayoumi line, only 12 and 10 genes were differentially expressed between treated and non-treated birds at 2 and 6 dpi, respectively (Fig. 3). However, at 10 dpi the overall number of differentially expressed genes (DEGs) substantially increased to 202 at 10 dpi, with 111 genes up regulated and 91 genes down regulated. Within the Leghorn line, 23 genes were differentially expressed at 2 dpi, with 21 genes up regulated (Fig. 3). However, at 6 dpi the total number of DEGs increased to 167, with 130 genes up regulated and 37 genes down regulated. Finally, at 10 dpi the number of DEGs decreased to only 9.

Comparison of DEGs identified in response to NDV and heat within line demonstrated very little overlap between Fayoumi and Leghorn. Across time points, 1, 4, and 3 DEGs were shared between the two lines at 2, 6, and 10 dpi, respectively (Fig. 4).

Pathway analysis of the DEGs identified between treated and non-treated birds from within line contrasts was used to identify signaling pathways that were enriched at each time point. For Fayoumi at 2 dpi, 22 pathways were significantly enriched (Fig. 5a, c, e), of which 14 were associated with immune-related functions, which include pathways such as RIG1-like receptors in antiviral innate immunity, IRF activation, SAPK/JNK signaling, and p38 MAPK signaling. At 6 dpi, only 9 pathways were enriched between treated and non-treated Fayoumi birds, including immune pathways such as T lymphocyte activity and

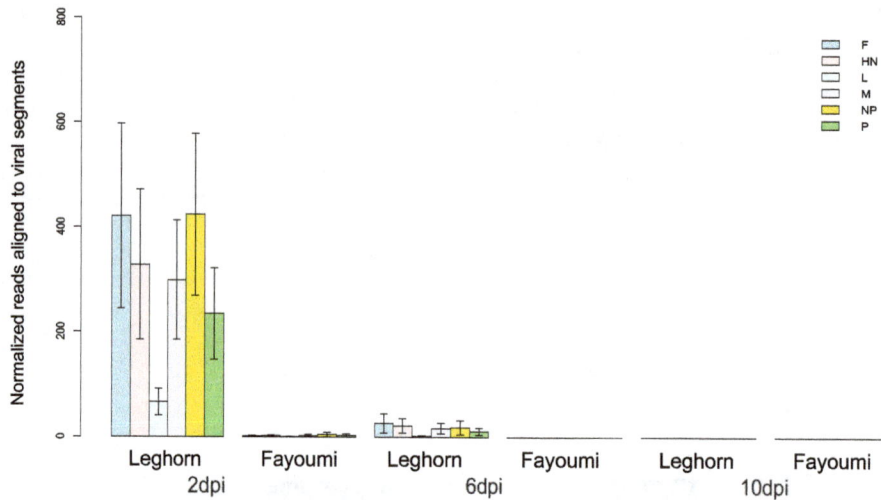

Fig. 2 Normalized number of reads that aligned to the La Sota viral genome and to specific gene segments: Fusion glycoprotein (F), Hemagglutinin-neuraminidase (HN), RNA-directed RNA polymerase L (L), Matrix protein (M), Nucleoprotein (NP), and Phophoprotein (P). Reads were extracted from treated individuals by genetic line and time point and aligned to the NDV La Sota genome. Bars indicate normalized number of reads with standard error. A higher number of reads aligned to the viral genome in Leghorn at 2 dpi and 6 dpi, with no reads detectable in either line at 10 dpi

cytokine signaling were significantly different between treated and non-treated Fayoumi birds. At 10 dpi, there was a substantial increase in the total number of enriched pathways (23), with the majority of genes involved in these processes down regulated. Interestingly, pathways such as Nur77 signaling in T lymphocytes and gas signaling were significantly enriched across 6 and 10 dpi.

Similar to Fayoumi, pathway analysis was performed for DEGs identified between treated and non-treated Leghorns across all three time points (Fig. 5b, d, f). At 2 dpi, 30 enriched pathways were significantly enriched among DEGs. At 6 dpi, 28 pathways were significantly enriched, with GP6 signaling pathway having a positive activation z-score of 2.0. Two genes in this pathway, LAMA4 and COL4A1 were significantly up regulated in

the treated compared to non-treated birds (Fig. 6). At 10 dpi, only three significant pathways were enriched among DEGs, which included superoxide radicals degradation, TCA cycle II, and PEDF signaling functions. The entire list of DEGs between treated and non-treated birds within each line and time point are included in Additional file 1.

Interaction analysis of treatment by genetics revealed unique and line-specific response patterns to NDV during heat treatment

While genes associated with NDV infection under heat stress within each line are important to understand the host immune response to pathogen infection, genes that differ between lines that are associated with resistance to NDV infection are more critical in elucidating the

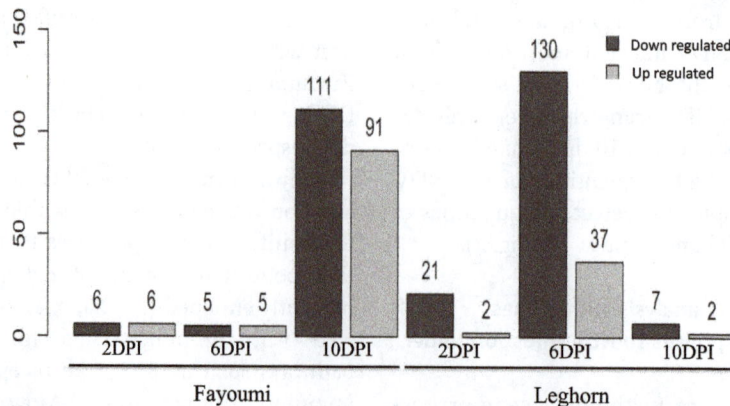

Fig. 3 Number of differentially expressed genes identified between treated and non-treated birds by genetic line and time point. A false discovery rate < 0.05 was used to classify genes as differentially expressed. Genes are signified by color as up regulated (dark grey) or down regulated (light grey)

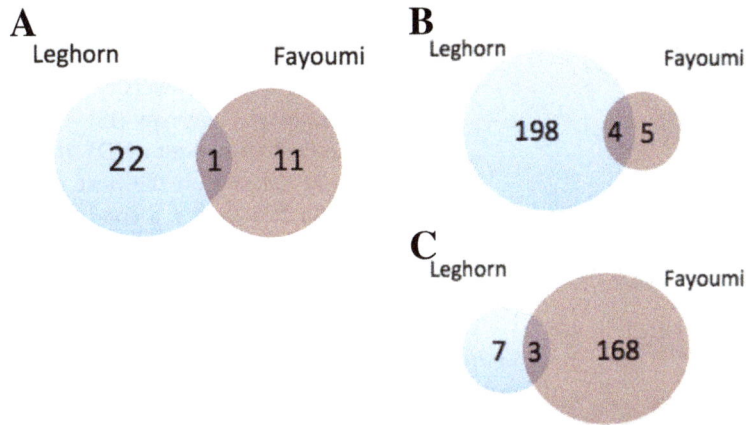

Fig. 4 Venn diagrams displaying the number of overlapping differentially expressed genes that overlap between genetic line by time point when comparing treated vs. non-treated birds. **a** Overlapped DEGs between Fayoumi (22) and Leghorn (11) genes at 2 dpi. **b** Overlapped DEGs between the two genetic lines at 6 dpi and **c** Overlapped DEGs between the two genetic lines at 10 dpi

underlying mechanisms that contribute to differences between the Fayoumi and Leghorn lines. To identify such genes and signaling pathways, interaction analysis of treatment by line was conducted, resulting in 757, 194, and 403 DEGs for this interaction at 2, 6, and 10 dpi, respectively. Further, pathway analysis identified many pathways that were significantly enriched among these DEGs that were not found for the within line contrasts (Fig. 7). In total, 26 pathways were enriched at 2 dpi, with 15 enriched in Leghorn including NF-Kappa B signaling and activation, p38 MAPK, and IL-1 mediated inhibition of RXR function and 11 for Fayoumi including PPARa/RXRa activation and G beta gamma signaling, which had the highest absolute Z-score value of all significant pathways. At 6 dpi, all significant pathways identified were enriched in Leghorn that include: GP6 signaling, GNRH signaling,

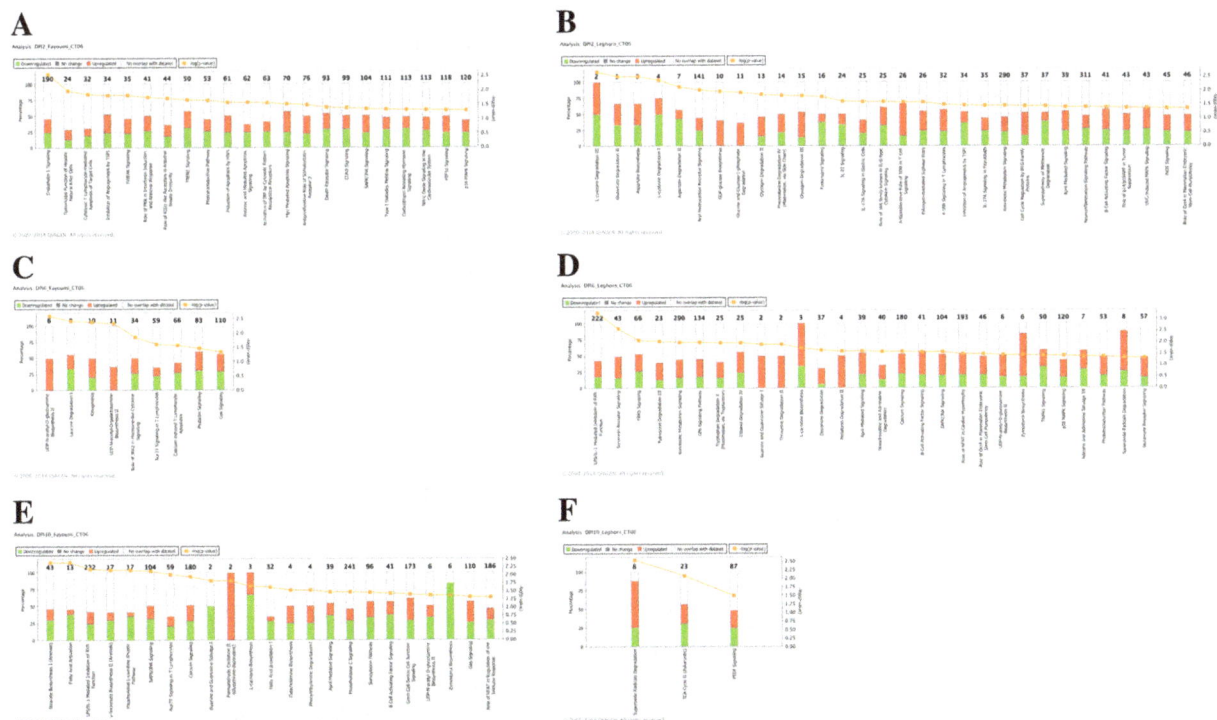

Fig. 5 Significantly enriched pathways identified through Ingenuity Pathway Analysis among differentially expressed genes by dpi and genetic line. **a** Fayoumi at 2 dpi, **b** Leghorn at 2 dpi, **c** Fayoumi at 6 dpi, **d** Leghorn at 6 dpi, **e** Fayoumi at 10 dpi, and **f** Leghorn at 10 dpi. Figures identify the number of genes in each pathway shown in black, if the gene is up (red) or down (green) regulated in the pathway, and its significant −log(p value) shown in orange

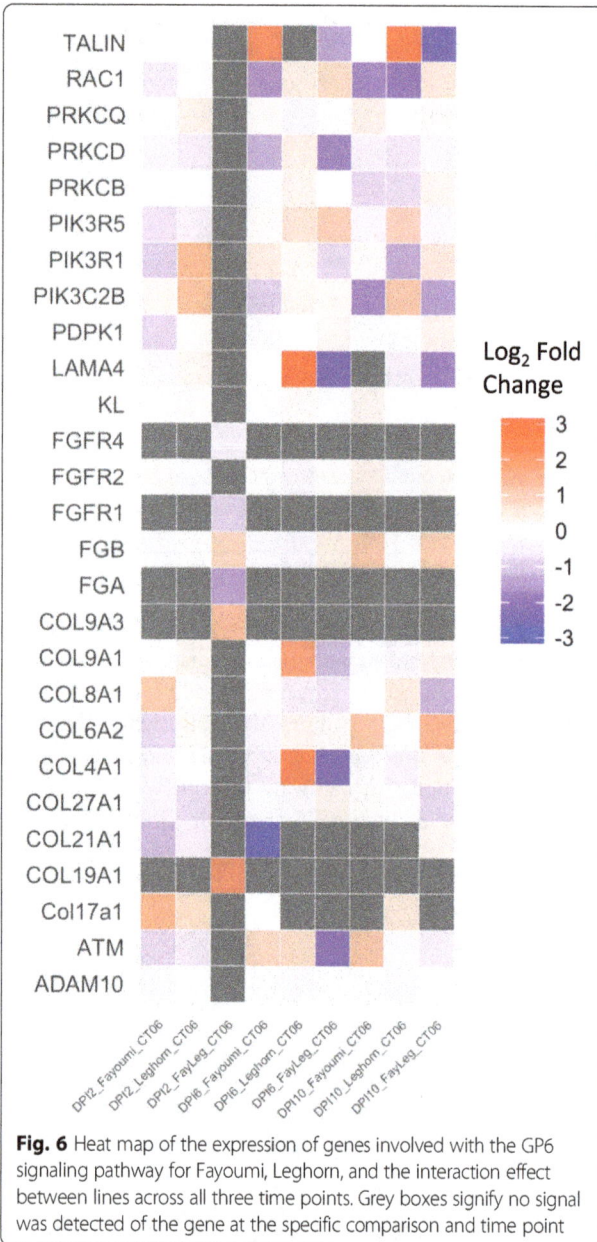

Fig. 6 Heat map of the expression of genes involved with the GP6 signaling pathway for Fayoumi, Leghorn, and the interaction effect between lines across all three time points. Grey boxes signify no signal was detected of the gene at the specific comparison and time point

calcium signaling, acute phase response signaling, phospholipase C signaling, and sirtuin signaling. Finally at 10 dpi, 13 pathways were enriched with 8 enriched in Leghorns and 5 in Fayoumis. HGF signaling was the most significant pathway identified at 10 dpi, and it was the only pathway significant across all three time points in Leghorns. HGF signaling and its respective genes play a role in regulating apoptotic processes and activates STAT3 and PI-3 kinase activity to affect inflammation and other cell phenotypes [21].

Discussion

The study presented is part of the Feed the Future Innovation Lab for Genomics to Improve Poultry program to further the body of knowledge regarding the genetic

basis of disease resistance to NDV in chickens. Two parallel animal-pathogen challenge experiments using the same inbred lines (Fayoumi and Leghorn chickens) were conducted at the University of California, Davis (UCD) and Iowa State University (ISU). The study at ISU focused on the host response to NDV inoculation, while the study at UCD focused on the host response to NDV inoculation under heat stress, a condition commonly experienced by village poultry flocks Africa. In the present study, Fayoumi birds had significantly lower levels of NDV in the chicken lachrymal fluid at both 2 dpi and 6 dpi, along with a much higher viral clearance rate than Leghorn birds. Anti-NDV antibody titers were also significantly higher in Fayoumis than in Leghorns. These results were consistent with NDV expression in the Harderian gland at both time points (Fig. 2). Significant differences in viral load between the two lines were only observed at 6 dpi in previous studies comparing NDV infected Fayoumi and Leghorn birds without heat stress [11]. This result further suggests that environmental stress could significantly differentiate the host response to NDV infection between two genetic lines. We speculate that Fayoumis were able to have significantly lower viral titer levels than Leghorns at the initial stage of the infection. This difference suggests either that Fayoumi may be mounting a more robust early immune response while under the effects of heat stress, or that the heat treatment has significantly impacted Leghorns' ability to respond the infection as effectively as Fayoumis. Other studies in avian influenza have indicated that heat stress could reduce the viral load of the host [22]. Activation of heat stress proteins could play a protective role during virus infection [23, 24]. The strategy of utilizing heat stress to alleviate infection has been the basis of fomentation, infrared therapies, and saunas therapies to some positive effect [24]. The mechanism by which heat stress is leading to improved viral clearance in Fayoumi warrants further investigation to understand how an effective immune response is modulated during heat stress.

RNA-seq analysis has demonstrated a time-specific host response to NDV while under heat stress at the genome-wide level. Three time points (2, 6, and 10 dpi) at which the Harderian gland was profiled, captured the host innate, adaptive, and the transition between the responses throughout the course of NDV infection during heat stress. Distinct line and stage specific responses were observed (Fig. 3) based on the number of DEGs at the three different stages of infection. A single gene, protein kinase C delta (PRKCD), was the only gene that was differentially expressed across all three time points in Fayoumi. PRKCD encodes for a protein kinase that is a regulator of cell apoptosis and is often highly expressed in lymphoid tissue in humans [25]. A limited early response in both Fayoumi and Leghorn lines occurred at 2 dpi, although the Leghorn line had relatively more DEGs

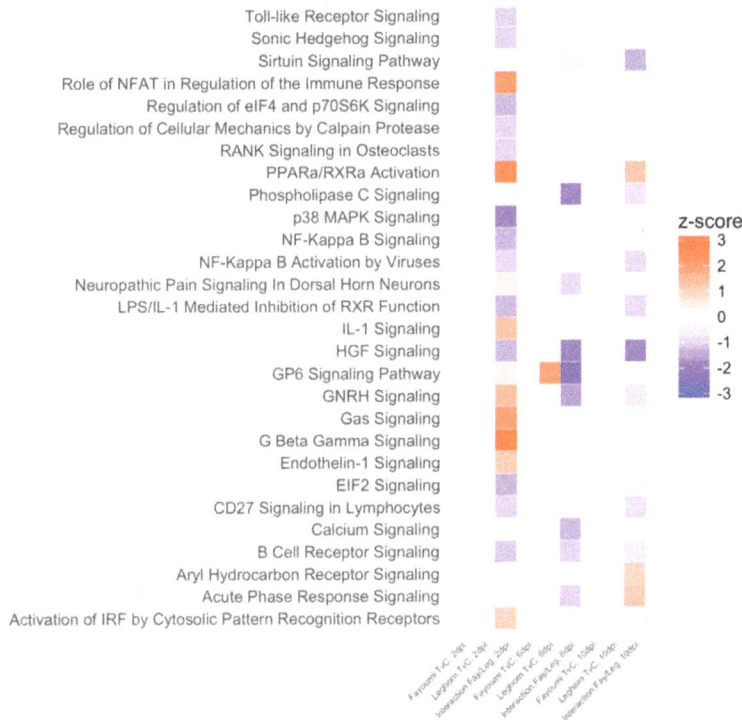

Fig. 7 Heat map of predicted activation or inhibition of significant pathways from Ingenuity Pathway Analysis that were significantly (−log(p value) > 1.3) enriched and that had a Z-score > |1| for the effect of treatment within each genetic line and for the interaction effect between line and treatment for each time point. Complete names of the pathways show the predicted activation of the pathway (Z-score > 1) or inhibition of the pathways (Z-score < − 1). Predicted Z-score for the interaction effect identify pathways primarily enriched in Fayoumi (Z-score > 1) or Leghorn (Z-score < − 1)

than Fayoumi. Leghorns eventually had a substantially stronger response at 6 dpi, while Fayoumi had a robust response at the later stages of infection under heat stress. In addition, very few differentially expressed genes overlapped between the lines at each time point suggesting a distinct, line-specific host response to NDV. A similar gene expression profile in terms of the number of DEGs observed in Harderian gland tissue was found in a parallel study in chickens under NDV infection only conducted at ISU by Deist et al. (Personal communication). However, the specific genes and signaling pathways identified in their study did not appear to have overlap with genes identified in this study. This suggests that understand the effects of both the combination of NDV and heat stress is critical to deepening our understanding of disease resistance to NDV in varying environments.

Several immune related DEGs (FADD, MAPK15, and GUCY1A2) in Fayoumi at 2 dpi, had been previously identified to be important in the host response to viral infection and the inflammatory response in cell lines [26–28]. FADD is of particular interest as it encodes for a protein that interfaces with cell surface receptors to mediate cell apoptotic signals that can help mitigate viral infections by disrupting mammalian cell replication [26]. Furthermore, knockout studies in mice suggest that this gene is crucial in

promoting early T cell development and T cell activation [29]. Notably, FADD and MAPK15 were both up regulated (log2(fold change): 1.783 and 3.378) at 2 dpi in Fayoumi and down regulated (log2(fold change): − 1.854 and − 1.046) in Leghorns at 6 dpi. This suggests that following an infection by NDV, Fayoumis might have initiated T cell activation at 2 dpi, while this may have been inhibited in Leghorns at 6 dpi.

Interestingly, immune related pathways such as SAPK/JNK signaling and p38 MAPK signaling identified in Fayoumis at 2 dpi were also identified in Leghorns at 6 dpi, suggesting that these shared pathways were activated more rapidly in Fayoumi than in Leghorn. The most significant pathway identified within the Fayoumi line was related to Endothelin-1 signaling, which has previously has been identified as being important in the modulation of the inflammation response by immune cells [30]. Significantly fewer DEGs identified in Fayoumi compared to Leghorns at 6 dpi indicate that Fayoumis had not be experienced the infection as intensely as the Leghorn birds had and therefore required a lesser response to NDV infection. This was consistent with viral titer results measured through both the chicken lachrymal fluid and virus extracted reads from the Harderian gland at 6 dpi (Figs. 1 and 2).

At 10 dpi, there was a substantial increase in the overall number of DEGs in Fayoumi birds. Down regulation of genes such as GNB1, MAP3K1, CD247, and TNFRSF13B ($\log_2$(fold change): -5.988, -6.022, -3.846, -3.632) in immune-related pathways including SAPK/JNK signaling, Nur77 signaling in T lymphocytes, and B cell activation, suggest that Fayoumis may have begun to down modulate various processes associated with immunity in an attempt to restore homeostatic functions. However, treatment by line interaction analysis at 10 dpi showed that Leghorns had significantly higher activation of immune pathways such as NF-Kappa B activation by viruses, CD27 signaling, and B cell receptor signaling, which suggest that Leghorn birds may not have completely cleared the virus by 10 dpi. This prolonged immune response could be detrimental to the overall health of the host.

The observed global gene expression patterns observed by this study are wholly based on RNA-seq gene expression data. Functional assessment of candidate genes identified here (potentially by qPCR) may be needed in order to further understand the functional role of many of these genes that may be playing roles in regulating the chickens' response to NDV while under heat stress. Ideally, we would desire to re-validate our findings through a separate cohort of samples, however due to the difficulty in accessing these samples, these experiments were not conducted at this study. In addition, the Ingenuity Pathway Analysis software uses primarily human and mouse biology curated database of pathways. The data was calculated using this background, however IPA supports the upload of genomic identifiers from a variety of species which includes chicken.

Only one pathway (GP6 signaling pathway), found in Leghorn birds at 6 dpi, was significantly enriched based on Z score when comparing the within line effects across all three time points (Fig. 7). The GP6 signaling pathway is involved with the activity of a protein in the immunoglobulin superfamily and is expressed in platelets and megakaryocytes [31]. GP6 proteins are also involved in collagen formation and function [31]. Previous research suggests that down regulation of collagen was associated with apoptosis, immune cell migration, and T cell activation [32–34]. Two genes, LAMA4 and COL4A1, were significantly up-regulated in this pathway and both these genes function in cell adhesion and play a role in regulating the migration cells such as neutrophils in mammals [35, 36]. One study revealed that gene expression of collagen genes in the trachea were lower in resistant birds infected with infectious bronchitis virus [29]. In addition, a parallel study at ISU investigating the host response to NDV infection without heat treatment found significantly lower expression of these genes in Fayoumi birds at 2 dpi compared to Leghorn birds [11]. Collectively, activation of the GP6 signaling pathway, through increase collagen gene expression, at 6 dpi could be partially responsible for the Leghorn lines susceptible phenotype.

The interaction analysis of treatment by genetic line would provide further insights into the resistant and susceptible phenotypes of the Fayoumi and Leghorn lines. While only one signaling pathway was identified in the within line contrasts, a number of significant signaling pathways were enriched from the interaction analysis of treatment by genetic line. The majority of enriched pathways were found at 2 dpi and 10 dpi, with 6 dpi have the least enrichment. This suggests that distinct signaling pathways were enriched between the two lines but were undetectable when only investigating for within line effects.

Conclusion

Transcriptome analysis of two unique genetic lines has helped identify line and time specific gene expression patterns related to NDV infection under the effects of heat stress. The Harderian gland demonstrated very unique response profiles between the two genetic lines, both in the number of DEGs identified, and the pathways that were enriched within each line. The overall lower viral titer levels, detectable viral transcripts, and increased viral clearance rate observed in Fayoumi suggest that the birds were effectively responding to NDV infection while under heat stress than the Leghorn birds. Fayoumis appeared to have activated immune related pathways that were in line with a more robust immune response at an earlier time point, while Leghorns were clearly responding up to 6 dpi. Additional candidate genes such as FADD, MAPK11, and MAPK15 that were identified as critically important genes in regulating the chickens' response to NDV infection during abiotic stress. Future investigations on these novel candidate genes and signaling pathways will allow us to elucidate the different regulatory mechanisms of disease resistance to NDV under heat stress. More importantly, these efforts will lay solid foundation on achieving the overall goal of Genomics to Improve Poultry Innovation Lab: improve poultry production by genetically enhancing disease resistance to NDV infection in Africa.

Methods
Experimental populations and design
The experimental design of this study has been previously described by Wang et al. [20]. Fayoumi (M15.2) and Leghorn (GHs 6) chicken lines from Iowa State University poultry farm (Ames, IA) were used in this study. On day of hatch, 56 Fayoumi and 55 Leghorn chicks were transported from Iowa State University to Davis, CA. Upon arrival, the chicks were housed in temperature and humidity-controlled chambers at the biosafety level 2 animal facility at the University of California, Davis. Twenty-five individuals from each genetic line were randomly selected and housed in a separate chamber to be used as the control group. From day 1 to day 13 both

groups were reared at 29.4 °C and 60% humidity. At 14 days of age, the experimental group was exposed to 38 °C for 4 h, then decreased to 35 °C and maintained at this temperature until the conclusion of the trial. The control group was maintained at 25 °C. On day 21 the heat treated birds were inoculated with 200 μL 10^7 EID$_{50}$ of the La Sota strain of NDV through both ocular and nasal passages. The control group was mock inoculated with 200 μL of 1X phosphate-buffered saline (PBS). At 2, 6, and 10 days post-infection (dpi), 4 birds per treatment group per genetic line were randomly selected and euthanized with CO$_2$ and Harderian gland tissue was harvested then, quickly placed into RNA*later* (ThermoFisher Cat#AM7024) and kept at − 80 °C. The experiment's procedures were performed according to the guidelines approved by the Institutional Animal Care and Use Committee at the University of California, Davis (IACUC #17853).

Viral titer measurement

Viral RNA was extracted from chicken lachrymal fluid at 2 and 6 dpi from both control and infected groups and extracted using the MagMAX-96 viral RNA isolation kit (Life Technologies Cat#AMB18365). Quantification of the virus was conducted using qRT-PCR using the TaqMan Newcastle Disease Virus Real-Time PCR kit (Life Technologies Cat#44006874) and measured on the ABI 7500 fast Real-Time PCR system (Thermofisher Cat#4351107, Carlsbad, CA). A standard curve was generated from a log copy number dilution of the virus from 10^5 to 10^2 EID$_{50}$ and used to calculate the viral titer in tears. Viral clearance was calculated as the difference in viral log copy number from 2 to 6 dpi divided by the viral log copy number at 2 dpi.

Anti-NDV antibody measurement

Serum samples were extracted from whole blood collected at pre-challenge (day 20) and 10 dpi (day 31). Antibodies in the serum were then measured using the IDEXX NDV ELISA kit for chickens (IDEXX Laboratories Cat#99–09263). The Sample to Positive ratio (S/P) was calculated by the average absorbance of each sample divided by the recorded measurement of the provided kit control.

RNA-isolation and library construction

Total RNA was extracted from the Harderian gland of four individuals per treatment and genetic line for each of

the three time points. The Harderian gland was homogenized in ice cold TRIzol (ThermoFisher Cat#15596026) and processed using a standard phenol:chloroform method and precipitated in 100% ethanol. The RNA pellet was then dissolved into water and treated with DNase I (ThermoFisher Cat#EN0521). Strand specific RNA library preparation was prepared exactly as stated in the NEBNext Ultra Directional RNA Library Prep Kit for Illumina (NEB Cat#E7420S). Library validation and quantification was done using the Agilent Bioanalyzer High Sensitivity Kit (Agilent Cat#5067–4626) and Qubit dsDNA HS Assay kit (ThermoFisher Cat#Q32854). The 100 base pair, paired-end sequencing was performed on the Illumina HiSeq2500 system with a minimum sequencing depth of 30 million reads. Sequence data have been submitted through the Sequence Read Archive (https://www.ncbi.nlm.nih.gov/sra/) under accession number: SRP135507.

NDV viral genome alignment

Unaligned transcript reads from the chicken genome of the treated individuals were aligned to the NDV La Sota reference genome using the Burrows-Wheeler Aligner (BWA) [37].Default settings were used and gene counts from the NDV genome were calculated using HTSeq [38].

Data analysis

Analysis of viral titer and anti-NDV S/P ratio differences between the two lines was analyzed using a least squares regression analysis with the main effects including line, day, and line by day. A Student's T-test was used to determine significance, with a $p < 0.05$ considered statistically significant between comparisons. Statistical analysis and visualization of the viral titers was performed using the statistical data analysis software R with standard packages [39].

Four major factors were included for analysis: condition (treated, non-treated), line (Leghorn, Fayoumi), sex (male, female), and time point (2, 6, and 10 dpi). Data at each time point consisted of 16 individuals, 4 per treatment and genetic line. Raw reads from RNA-seq were trimmed using FastQC [40] to remove duplicates, reads with base quality scores < 30, and adapter contamination. These reads were then aligned using Tophat2 [41] to the galGal5 reference genome and Ensembl annotation using default settings and a summary of the alignment statistics can be found in Table 1. Gene counts were calculated using HTSeq and differential gene

Table 1 Summary statistics of RNA-Seq alignment

		Average number of reads mapped (bp)	Average % of reads mapped
Fayoumi	Treated	21,285,421	75.59
	Non-Treated	24,270,472	76.70
Leghorn	Treated	21,092,774	72.31
	Non-Treated	18,515,551	70.92

analysis was done using edgeR [42]. The statistical model design included the effects of line, condition, sex, and time point, along with the interactions between condition and line. In addition, in order to identify genes that were differentially expressed between genetic lines in response to treatment and, therefore, potentially associated with disease resistance to NDV, the interaction between condition and genetic line was included. Genes were identified as differentially expressed (DEGs) if they had a false discovery rate (FDR) < 0.05, and an average transcript count > 10. Pathway analysis using the DEGs of between line contrasts and the interaction effect was performed using Qiagen's Ingenuity Pathway Analysis software [43]. Z-score cutoff of |z| > 1 identified significantly up or down regulated pathways [43].

Abbreviations
DEG: Differentially expressed gene; dpi: Days post-infection; FDR: False Discovery Rate; LFC: Log$_2$(fold change); NDV: Newcastle disease virus

Acknowledgements
The authors would like to thank the members of the Zhou and Gallardo lab for their assistance in collecting and preparing samples from the live bird trial. This study was funded by the US Agency for International Development Feed the Future Innovation Lab for Genomics to Improve Poultry AID-OAA-A-13-00080. Partial support was provided by the United States Department of Agriculture, National Institute of Food and Agriculture, Multistate Research Project NRSP8 and NE1334 (HZ) and the Calfornia Agricultural Experimental Station (HZ).

Funding
This study was funded by the US Agency for International Development Feed the Future Innovation Lab for Genomics to Improve Poultry AID-OAA-A-13-00080.

Authors' contributions
PS: Collected samples, isolated RNA, constructed libraries, processed and analyzed data, wrote manuscript; YW: Collected samples, isolated viral RNA, performed qRT-PCR, reviewed and edited manuscript; RAG: Experimental design, viral isolate preparation, collected samples, reviewed and edited manuscript. JMD, SJL, TRK: Experimental design, reviewed and edited paper; HZ: Experimental design, reviewed and edited manuscript, oversaw data analysis and sample collection. All authors read and approved the final manuscript.

Consent for publication
Not applicable.

Competing interests
The authors declare that they have no competing interests.

Author details
Integrative Genetics and Genomics Graduate Group, University of California, Davis, CA 95616, USA. [2]Genomics to Improve Poultry Innovation Lab, University of California, Davis, CA 95616, USA. [3]Department of Animal Science, University of California, Davis, CA 95616, USA. [4]School of Veterinary Medicine, University of California, Davis, CA 95616, USA. [5]Department of Animal Science, Iowa State University, Ames, IA 50011, USA. [6]One Health Institute, University of California, Davis, CA 95616, USA.

References
1. Aldous E, Manvell R, Cox W, Ceeraz V, Harwood D, Shell W, et al. Outbreak of Newcastle disease in pheasants (Phasianus colchicus) in south-East England in July 2005. Vet Rec. 2007;160:482–4.
2. Alexander DJ. Gordon Memorial Lecture. Newcastle disease. Br Poult Sci. 2001;42:5–22.
3. Spickler AR. Newcastle Disease. Cent Food Secur Public Health. 2016. Available from: http://www.cfsph.iastate.edu/Factsheets/pdfs/newcastle_disease.pdf
4. St-Pierre NR, Cobanov B, Schnitkey G. Economic losses from heat stress by US livestock industries. J Dairy Sci. 2003;86:E52–77.
5. Lara LJ, Rostagno MH. Impact of heat stress on poultry production. Anim Open Access J MDPI. 2013;3:356–69.
6. Lu Q, Wen J, Zhang H. Effect of chronic heat exposure on fat deposition and meat quality in two genetic types of chicken. Poult Sci. 2007;86:1059–64.
7. Bartlett JR, Smith MO, Yan Q, Li L. Effects of different levels of selenium on growth performance and immunocompetence of broilers under heat stress. Poult Sci. 2003;82:1580–8.
8. Slawinska A, Hsieh JC, Schmidt CJ, Lamont SJ. Heat stress and lipopolysaccharide stimulation of chicken macrophage-like cell line activates expression of distinct sets of genes. PLoS One. 2016;11:1–17.
9. Lamont SJ, Cobl DJ, Bjorkquis A, Rothschil MF, Persi M, Ashwel C, et al. Genomics of heat stress in chickens. In: Proc 10th World Congr Genet Appl Livest Prod; 2014. Available from: https://asas.confex.com/asas/WCGALP14/webprogram/Paper10350.html.
10. Bjorkquis A, Ashwel C, Persi M, Rothschil MF, Schmid C, Lamon SJ. QTL for body composition traits during heat stress revealed in an advanced intercross line of chickens. In: Proc 10th World Congr Genet Appl Livest Prod; 2014. p. 3–5.
11. Deist MS, Gallardo RA, Bunn DA, Kelly TR, Dekkers JCM, Zhou H, et al. Novel mechanisms revealed in the trachea transcriptome of resistant and susceptible chicken lines following infection with Newcastle disease virus. Clin Vaccine Immunol. 2017:CVI.00027–17.
12. Deist MS, Gallardo RA, Bunn DA, Dekkers JCM, Zhou H, Lamont SJ. Resistant and susceptible chicken lines show distinctive responses to Newcastle disease virus infection in the lung transcriptome. BMC Genomics. 2017;18:1–15.
13. Zhang J, Kaiser MG, Deist MS, Gallardo RA, Bunn DA, Kelly TR, et al. Transcriptome Analysis in Spleen Reveals Differential Regulation of Response to Newcastle Disease Virus in Two Chicken Lines. Sci Rep. 2018:8. [cited 2018 Mar 6] Available from: http://www.nature.com/articles/s41598-018-19754-8
14. Nuss AM, Beckstette M, Pimenova M, Schmühl C, Opitz W, Pisano F, et al. Tissue dual RNA-seq allows fast discovery of infection-specific functions and riboregulators shaping host–pathogen transcriptomes. Proc Natl Acad Sci. 2017;114:E791–800.
15. Payne AP. The harderian gland: a tercentennial review. J Anat. 1994;185(Pt 1):1–49.
16. Wang Y, Lupiani B, Reddy SM, Lamont SJ, Zhou H. RNA-seq analysis revealed novel genes and signaling pathway associated with disease resistance to avian influenza virus infection in chickens. Poult Sci. 2014;93:485–93.
17. Lakshmanan N, Kaiser MG, Lamon SJ. Marek's disease resistance in MHC-congenic lines from leghorn and Fayoumi breeds. In: Curr res Mareks Dis Proc 5th Int Symp. Kennet Square. Pennsylvania: American Association of Avian Pathologists; 1996.
18. Cheeseman JH, Kaiser MG, Ciraci C, Kaiser P, Lamont SJ. Breed effect on early cytokine mRNA expression in spleen and cecum of chickens with and without Salmonella enteritidis infection. Dev Comp Immunol. 2007;31:52–60.
19. Pinard-Van Der Laan MH, Monvoisin JL, Pery P, Hamet N, Thomas M. Comparison of outbred lines of chickens for resistance to experimental infection with coccidiosis (Eimeria tenella). Poult Sci. 1998;77:185–91.
20. Wang Y, Saelao P, Chanthavixay K, Gallardo R, Bunn D, Lamont SJ, et al. Physiological responses to heat stress in two genetically distinct chicken inbred lines. Poult Sci. 2017:1–11.
21. Organ SL, Tsao MS. An overview of the c-MET signaling pathway. Ther Adv Med Oncol. 2011;3:S7–19.
22. Xue J, Fan X, Yu J, Zhang S, Xiao J, Hu Y, et al. Short-term heat shock affects host-virus interaction in mice infected with highly pathogenic avian influenza virus H5N1. Front Microbiol. 2016;7:1–8.

23. Basu S, Srivastava PK. Heat shock proteins: the fountainhead of innate and adaptive immune responses. Cell Stress Chaperones. 2000;5:443.

24. Anderson KM, Srivastava PK. Heat, heat shock, heat shock proteins and death: a central link in innate and adaptive immune responses. Immunol Lett. 2000;74:35–9.

25. Salzer E, Santos-Valente E, Keller B, Warnatz K, Boztug K. Protein kinase C δ: a gatekeeper of immune homeostasis. J Clin Immunol. 2016;36:631–40.

26. Balachandran S, Thomas E, Barber GN. A FADD-dependent innate immune mechanism in mammalian cells. Nature. 2004;432:401–5.

27. Colecchia D, Strambi A, Sanzone S, Iavarone C, Rossi M, Dall'Armi C, et al. MAPK15/ERK8 stimulates autophagy by interacting with LC3 and GABARAP proteins. Autophagy. 2012;8:1724–40.

28. Del Rey MJ, Izquierdo E, Usategui A, Gonzalo E, Blanco FJ, Acquadro F, et al. The transcriptional response of normal and rheumatoid arthritis synovial fibroblasts to hypoxia. Arthritis Rheum. 2010;62:3584–94.

29. Smith J, Sadeyen J-R, Cavanagh D, Kaiser P, Burt DW. The early immune response to infection of chickens with Infectious Bronchitis Virus (IBV) in susceptible and resistant birds. BMC Vet Res. 2015:11. [cited 2018 Mar 7] Available from: http://www.biomedcentral.com/1746-6148/11/256

30. Elisa T, Antonio P, Giuseppe P, Alessandro B. Endothelin receptors expressed by immune cells are involved in modulation of inflammation and in fibrosis: relevance to the pathogenesis of systemic sclerosis. J Immunol. 2015:2015. Available from: http://www.hindawi.com/journals/jir/aa/147616/abs/

31. Horii K. Structural basis for platelet collagen responses by the immune-type receptor glycoprotein VI. Blood. 2006;108:936–42.

32. Frisch SM, Francis H. Disruption of epithelial cell-matrix interactions induces apoptosis. J Cell Biol. 1994;124:619–26.

33. Gunzer M, Schäfer A, Borgmann S, Grabbe S, Zänker KS, Bröcker E-B, et al. Antigen presentation in extracellular matrix: interactions of T cells with dendritic cells are dynamic, short lived, and sequential. Immunity. 2000;13:323–32.

34. Lämmermann T, Germain RN. The multiple faces of leukocyte interstitial migration. Semin Immunopathol. 2014;36:227–51.

35. Wondimu Z, Geberhiwot T, Ingerpuu S, Juronen E, Xie X, Lindbom L, et al. An endothelial laminin isoform, laminin 8 (α4β1γ1), is secreted by blood neutrophils, promotes neutrophil migration and extravasation, and protects neutrophils from apoptosis. Blood. 2004;104:1859–66.

36. Miyake M, Hori S, Morizawa Y, Tatsumi Y. Collagen type IV alpha 1 (COL4A1) and collagen type XIII alpha 1 (COL13A1) produced in cancer cells promote tumor budding at the invasion front in human urothelial carcinoma of the bladder. Oncotarget. 2017;8:36099–114.

37. Li H, Durbin R. Fast and accurate short read alignment with burrows-wheeler transform. Bioinformatics. 2009;25:1754–60.

38. Anders S, Pyl PT, Huber W. HTSeq - a Python framework to work with high-throughput sequencing data. Bioinformatics. 2015;31(2):166–169. https://doi.org/10.1093/bioinformatics/btu638

39. R Core Team. R: A language and environment for statistical computing. Austria: R Found Stat Comput Vienna; 2018. Available from: https://www.R-project.org/.

40. Andrew, Simon. FastQC: a quality control tool for high throughput sequence data. Available from: http://www.bioinformatics.babraham.ac.uk/projects/fastqc

41. Kim D, Pertea G, Trapnell C, Pimentel H, Kelley R, Salzberg SL. TopHat2: accurate alignment of transcriptomes in the presence of insertions, deletions and gene fusions. Genome Biol. 2013;14:R36.

42. Robinson MD, McCarthy DJ, Smyth GK. edgeR: a Bioconductor package for differential expression analysis of digital gene expression data. Bioinformatics. 2010;26:139–40.

43. Krämer A, Green J, Pollard J, Tugendreich S. Causal analysis approaches in ingenuity pathway analysis. Bioinformatics. 2014;30:523–30.

21

Prognostic efficacy of the human B-cell lymphoma prognostic genes in predicting disease-free survival (DFS) in the canine counterpart

Mohamad Zamani-Ahmadmahmudi[1*], Sina Aghasharif[2] and Keyhan Ilbeigi[2]

Abstract

Background: Canine B-cell lymphoma is deemed an ideal model of human non-Hodgkin's lymphoma where the lymphomas of both species share similar clinical features and biological behaviors. However there are some differences between tumor features in both species. In the current study, we sought to evaluate the prognostic efficacy of human B-cell lymphoma prognostic gene signatures in canine B-cell lymphoma.

Methods: The corresponding probe sets of 36 human B-cell lymphoma prognostic genes were retrieved from 2 canine B-cell lymphoma microarray datasets (GSE43664 and GSE39365) (76 samples), and prognostic probe sets were thereafter detected using the univariate and multivariate Cox proportional-hazard model and the Kaplan–Meier analysis. The two datasets were employed both as training sets and as external validation sets for each other. Results were confirmed using quantitative real-time PCR (qRT-PCR) analysis.

Results: In the univariate analysis, *CCND1*, *CCND2*, *PAX5*, *CR2*, *LMO2*, *HLA-DQA1*, *P53*, *CD38*, *MYC-N*, *MYBL1*, and *BIRCS5* were associated with longer disease-free survival (DFS), while *CD44*, *PLAU*, and *FN1* were allied to shorter DFS. However, the multivariate Cox proportional-hazard analysis confirmed *CCND1* and *BIRCS5* as prognostic genes for canine B-cell lymphoma. qRT-PCR used for verification of results indicated that expression level of *CCND1* was significantly higher in B-cell lymphoma patients with the long DFS than ones with the short DFS, while expression level of *BIRCS5* wasn't significantly different between two groups.

Conclusion: Our results confirmed *CCND1* as important gene that can be used as a potential predictor in this tumor type.

Keywords: Canine B-cell lymphoma, Prognosis, Cox proportional-hazard analysis, Survival

Background

Lymphoma is one of the most common malignancies in dogs and occurs in different forms, including multicentric, mediastinal (thymic), alimentary, cutaneous, and solitary types [1, 2]. Investigators have proposed canine B-cell lymphoma as a suitable model of human non-Hodgkin lymphoma (NHL) because the tumors of both species have common clinical manifestations and biological properties. However there are some differences between tumor features in both species [3, 4].

Some clinical and histological features have been proposed as prognostic factors in canine lymphoma [2, 5, 6]. For example, there are conflicting data on the use of the Kiel and Working Formulation classifications insofar as studies have revealed that both classifications are unreliable prognosticators [2, 5]. Nonetheless, in a study by Teske et al. (1994), the Working Formulation classification and Kiel classification were suggested as prognostic factors for the overall survival and time-to-relapse in treated dogs with malignant lymphoma, respectively [7]. Moreover, investigations have reported that such clinical parameters

* Correspondence: zamani_2012@alumni.ut.ac.ir
[1]Department of Clinical Science, Faculty of Veterinary Medicine, Shahid Bahonar University of Kerman, P.O Box: 76169133, Kerman, Iran
Full list of author information is available at the end of the article

as age, sex, animal weight, and clinical stage have no robust efficiency for predicting overall survival and disease-free survival (DFS) times [5]. Some cellular proliferation markers such as Ki-67, PCNA, and AgNOR have been evaluated as suitable prognosis predictor. Indeed, Ki-67 and AgNOR have been reported as appropriate prognostic markers in human and canine malignant lymphoma [5, 8, 9], where AgNOR can be utilized for the grading of the canine and human NHL [10, 11].

Molecular phenotyping is a robust method for the definition of tumor subtypes and the detection of prognostic gene genes [12–15]. For instance, the gene expression profile analysis divided human diffuse large-B-cell lymphoma (DLBCL) into 3 distinct subtypes: activated germinal center-like B-cell lymphoma, B-cell lymphoma, and peripheral mediastinal B-cell lymphoma [12]. A similar investigation classified canine malignant lymphoma based on molecular profiling [6]. In different studies, 36 genes have been suggested as prognostic markers for human B-cell lymphoma (majorly DLBCL) (Table 1). To the best of our knowledge, there is limited information on the prognostic efficacy of these important gene markers in canine B-cell lymphoma as an ideal model of human NHL. In the present study, the robustness of these genes for the prediction of DFS in 2 canine B-cell lymphoma microarray datasets was investigated using the univariate/multivariate Cox proportional-hazard model and the Kaplan–Meier analysis. The prognostic efficacy of selected gene(s) in each dataset was validated via the other dataset.

Table 1 List of human B-cell lymphoma prognostic genes used in our study

BCL2 [1–4]	Ki-67 [5]
BCL6 [4, 6, 7]	LMO2 [4, 8]
BCL7A [4]	LRMP [4]
BIRC5 [9]	MYBL1 [4]
CCND1 [10]	MYCN [6]
CCND2 [8, 11]	NPM3 [6]
CD10 [4]	NR4A3 [12]
CD38 [4]	P53 [13]
CD44 [14]	PAX5 [15]
CFLAR [4]	PDE4B [12]
CR2 [4]	PIK3CG [4]
EEF1A1L4 [6]	PLAU [6]
FN1 [6]	PMS1 [4, 11]
HGAL [4, 6]	PRDM1 [11]
HLA-DQA1 [6]	SCYA3 [8, 11]
HLA-DRA [6]	SLA [4]
ICAM1 (CD54) [16]	SLAM [4]
IRF4 [4]	WASPIP [4]

References were provided in Additional file 1

Methods

Microarray expression datasets

Two canine B-cell lymphoma microarray datasets, namely GSE43664 [16] and GSE39365 [6] (platform: GPL3738), were obtained from the GEO database (http://www.ncbi.nlm.nih.gov/geo/). Expression data were downloaded in the CEL file format. The GSE43664 and GSE39365 datasets comprised 58 and 36 samples, respectively, where the GSE43664 samples were solely canine B-cell lymphoma (mainly diffuse large B-cell lymphoma [DLBCL]) and the GSE39365 samples contained both B-cell ($n = 18$) and T-cell lymphoma ($n = 18$). In the GSE39365 dataset, only B-cell lymphoma samples were included in the study. B-cell lymphoma samples in GSE43664 included DLBCL (mainly), MZL, and unknown. Additionally, B-cell lymphoma samples in GSE39365 included DLBCL (mainly), MZL, and BL. The clinical features of the studied cases are summarized in Additional file 1: Table S1 and S2. The data were first converted into expression values and then transformed logarithmically using the Affy package [17] in R environment, version 3.0.2 (http://www.r-project.org/). Survival time, compared using Student's t-test between two datasets (GSE43664: 9.6 ± 8.7 months and GSE39365:11.7 ± 12.1 months), wasn't statistically different ($P = 0.42$).

Extraction of prognostic gene expression values

Thirty-six human-specific genes, presumed as prognostic genes, were tested in the current study (Table 1). The literatures were mined to retrieve papers exploring prognostic genes or gene signatures in human B-cell lymphoma. Public databases (especially PubMed) were screened for papers describing genes predicting survival in human B-cell lymphoma. Finally, 36 genes were extracted from papers, where some of these genes weren't evaluated as a single prognostic gene and proposed as a prognostic gene signature with the other genes. So, to perform a comprehensive assessment, we included all genes in our analysis. The corresponding probe sets of these genes and the related expression value for each probe set were retrieved from both datasets using MATLAB 7.8.0 (R2009a) (MathWorks, Natick, MA).

Survival analysis and external validation

Survival analysis was performed using *Survival* (http://cran.r-project.org/package=survival) and *Survcomp* [18] packages in R environment. The Cox proportional-hazards analysis was used for constructing a model for the prediction of survival. In this analysis, the association between a group of covariates (genes) and the response variable (DFS) was evaluated. Two datasets were employed as training and validation (test) groups, where important prognostic gene(s) was identified in a group (training group) and then validated in the other dataset (validation group). We used an external validation instead of internal validation, as the former is generally more robust to the overfitting problem [19].

First, the univariate Cox analysis was performed and genes with a z score greater than 1.5 or less than -1.5 [13, 20] were selected for the multivariate Cox analysis, where a negative score and a positive score associated with longer and shorter survival respectivley. In the multivariate Cox analysis, statistically significant genes were entered into the analysis and significant covariate(s) was detected at a P-value lower than 0.05. Survival curves were depicted by Kaplan–Meier method and compared using the log-rank test. Furthermore, some clinical prognosis parameters such as animal age, sex, and tumor grade (high or low) (Additional file 1: Table S2) were assessed in the Cox analysis to determine their roles in the prediction model.

Next, the external validation of the resulted prognostic genes was determined. The prognostic gene(s) in each group was tested in the other group via the Kaplan-Meier method and the log-rank test. In addition, the expression of the prognostic genes were compared in human ABC-like (activated B-cell like) and human GCB-like (germinal center B like) groups, because GCB-like and ABC-like cases are associated with better and poorer prognoses, correspondingly [21]. For this analysis, the patients were categorized as GCB-like and ABC-like groups based on 1,180 canine-specific differentially expressed probe sets proposed by Richards et al. (2013) [16]. Grouping was carried out using the hierarchal clustering analysis provided in geWorkbench 2.5.1 package [22]. Subsequently, the expressions of the prognostic genes were compared between the two groups using the Student's t-test analysis provided in geWorkbench 2.5.1 package.

Verification of the results by quantitative real-time PCR (qRT-PCR)

qRT-PCR procedure was performed as previously described [23, 24] on lymph node biopsy samples obtained from 60 dogs with B-cell lymphoma. All applicable international, national, and/or institutional guidelines for the care and use of animals were followed. Biopsy samples were processed using hematoxylin and eosin (H&E) staining method for the routine histopathology evaluation. Samples were diagnosed and subtyped based on the World Health Organization classification of hematopoietic and lymphoid tissues [25]. CD79a and CD3 antibodies (Dako, Denmark) were used for the confirmation of B-cell phenotype. CD79a-positive and CD3-negative samples were selected for subsequent analysis. Because mean survival time of GEO datasets samples that had lower expression (short survival) and higher expression (long survival) values than *CCND1* or *BIRCS5* median value

were 6.9 months and 12.1 months respectively (see results), the selected cases for qRT-PCR included 30 dogs with DFS <7 months and 30 dogs with DFS >12 months. Mean age of the dogs with DFS >12 months and dogs with DFS <7 months were 8.3 years (range: 3-12 years) and 7 years (range: 2-10 years) respectively.

In brief, total RNA was extracted using Tripure isolation reagent (Roche, Germany) according to the manufacturer's protocol. cDNA was synthesized using Maxime RT PreMix Kit (Intron biotechnology, Korea) according to the manufacturer's instructions. The cDNA synthesis reaction was run at 45 °C for 60 min, followed by 95 °C for 5 min. Synthesized cDNA was used for final PCR assay. SYBR green-based quantitative real-time PCR (qRT-PCR) was performed using the Applied Biosystems 7500 Real- Time PCR system. Cycle conditions were 95 °C for 10 minutes, followed by 40 cycles of 95 °C for 15 s, 52 °C for 45 s, and 72 °C for 1 min. Data were analyzed by SDS 2.0 software (Applied Biosystems). Specific primers used for *CCND1* and *BIRCS5* were presented in Additional file 1: Table S3. HPRT was used as the reference gene for normalization of target gene expression. Comparative ΔCT-method was used for calculation of relative expression of the target gene [23]. Data are presented as fold change in gene expression level of the target gene. Fold changes in gene expression was compared between two groups (DFS <7 months vs. DFS >12 months) by Student's t-test. A P value lower than 0.05 was considered significant.

Results

Probe sets corresponding to the prognostic genes were obtained from both datasets and subjected to subsequent survival analysis. Ninety one probe sets corresponding to 36 genes were retrieved from the each datasets. In the univariate analysis, the genes with a z score higher than 1.5 or lower than -1.5 were selected for the multivariate analysis. The results of the univariate analysis are summarized in Table 2. In the 58-sample dataset, *CCND1, CCND2, PAX5, CR2, BCL2L14, LMO2, HLA-DQA1, P53, MYC-N,* and *BIRCS5* had z scores lower than -1.5, which is associated with longer DFS. Conversely, *CD44, PLAU,* and *FN1* had positive z scores (higher than 1.5), which is correlated with shorter DFS. Moreover, in the 18-sample dataset, *CCND1, BIRCS5, MYC-N, LMO2, MYBL1,* and *CD38* had significant negative z scores (lower than -1.5). No genes with a z score higher than 1.5 was detected in the univariate analysis of the GSE39365 dataset (Table 2). Our subsequent multivariate analysis indicated that *CCND1* was a robust predictor in both datasets. Furthermore, *BIRCS5* in the GSE39365 dataset reached a statistically significant level (Table 3).

Appropriate external validation was confirmed by validating the prognostic gene(s) in each group in the other

Table 2 Univariate Cox proportional-hazard analysis of B-cell lymphoma prognostic gene signatures in GSE43664 and GSE39365 datasets

	Coef	Exp (coef)	SE (coef)	z score	P
GSE43664 dataset					
Cfa.21188.1.S1_s_at: (CCND2)	-0.672	0.511	0.207	-3.24	0.0012
Cfa.19972.1.S1_at: (BCL2L14)	-3.44	0.0321	1.26	-2.72	0.0065
CfaAffx.18137.1.S1_at: (CR2)	-0.902	0.406	0.371	-2.43	0.015
CfaAffx.4397.1.S1_x_at: (PAX5)	-1.03	0.357	0.446	-2.31	0.021
Cfa.37.1.S1_at: (BIRC5)	-1.44	0.236	0.627	-2.3	0.021
Cfa.16248.1.S1_at: (CCND1)	-0.505	0.604	0.257	-2.1	0.049
Cfa.16217.1.S1_s_at: (CR2)	-0.527	0.59	0.272	-1.94	0.052
Cfa.182.1.S2_at: (HLA-DQA1)	-0.467	0.627	0.241	-1.93	0.053
Cfa.10937.1.S1_at: (LMO2)	-0.676	0.509	0.354	-1.91	0.056
CfaAffx.6511.1.S1_at: (MYCN)	-1.19	0.304	0.63	-1.89	0.059
Cfa.15639.1.A1_at: (TP53)	-0.373	0.688	0.202	-1.85	0.064
Cfa.5536.1.A1_at: (MYCN)	-0.781	0.458	0.443	-1.76	0.078
CfaAffx.18218.1.S1_at: (CR2)	-0.391	0.677	0.225	-1.74	0.083
CfaAffx.18149.1.S1_s_at: (CR2)	-0.429	0.651	0.248	-1.73	0.083
CfaAffx.18202.1.S1_s_at: (CR2)	-0.454	0.635	0.272	-1.67	0.095
Cfa.19191.1.S1_at: (PDE4B)	-0.857	0.425	0.518	-1.65	0.098
CfaAffx.4400.1.S1_at: (PAX5)	-1.65	0.192	1.05	-1.58	0.11
CfaAffx.11868.1.S1_at: (MYBL1)	-1.21	0.297	0.773	-1.57	0.12
Cfa.3707.1.A1_s_at: (FN1)	0.622	1.86	0.415	1.5	0.13
Cfa.3800.2.S1_at: (CD44)	0.226	1.25	0.14	1.61	0.11
CfaAffx.11235.1.S1_s_at: (CD44)	0.259	1.3	0.142	1.82	0.068
Cfa.127.1.S1_s_at: (PLAU)	0.884	2.42	0.463	1.91	0.057
Cfa.3707.2.S1_at: (FN1)	0.277	1.32	0.129	2.15	0.031
CfaAffx.22155.1.S1_s_at: (FN1)	0.347	1.41	0.154	2.26	0.024
Cfa.3707.3.S1_s_at: (FN1)	0.827	2.29	0.336	2.46	0.014
GSE39365 dataset					
Cfa.15826.1.S1_s_at: (BIRC5)	-0.832	0.435	0.477	-1.74	0.081
Cfa.16248.1.S1_at: (CCND1)	-0.923	0.397	0.54	-1.71	0.088
Cfa.5536.1.A1_at: (MYCN)	-2.44	0.0875	1.44	-1.69	0.091
Cfa.10937.1.S1_at: (LMO2)	-0.825	0.438	0.516	-1.6	0.11
Cfa.3619.1.S1_at: (CD38)	-0.804	0.448	0.512	-1.57	0.12
Cfa.3619.1.S1_s_at: (CD38)	-0.605	0.546	0.39	-1.55	0.12
CfaAffx.11868.1.S1_at: (MYBL1)	-1.76	0.171	1.16	-1.52	0.12
Clinical features (GSE39365 dataset)					
Age at diagnosis (years)	0.0774	1.08	0.0893	0.866	0.39
Sex	0.165	1.18	0.576	0.287	0.77
Grade	-1.04	0.354	0.68	-1.53	0.13

Genes with z score higher than 1.5 or lower than -1.5 were listed. Exp (coef) indicates hazard ratio. Positive and negative z score denotes shorter and longer survival time respectively

group. The correlation between *CCND1* and *BIRCS5* expression and DFS time was tested using the Kaplan-Meier estimator and log-rank test. The patients were divided into high-risk and low-risk groups based on the median of the *CCND1* and *BIRCS5* expression values, and their survival durations were compared using the log-rank test. High-risk and low-risk groups had expression values lower than and higher than the median value

Table 3 Multivariate Cox proportional-hazard analysis of B-cell lymphoma prognostic gene signatures in GSE43664 and GSE39365 datasets

	Coef	Exp (coef)	SE (coef)	z score	P
GSE43664 dataset					
CCND1	-0.72	0.487	0.353	-2.041	0.041
GSE39365 dataset					
BRICS5	-2.322	0.098	0.834	-2.785	0.0054
CCND1	-3.017	0.0489	1.427	-2.114	0.035

Exp (coef) indicates hazard ratio

respectively. The DFS time in the GSE43664 dataset was statistically different in the survival curves constructed based on *CCND1* ($P = 0.007$) and *BIRCS5* ($P = 0.0042$) expressions (Fig. 1 b and c). However, the DFS time in high-risk and low-risk groups of the GSE39365 dataset tended to be significant ($P = 0.058$) (Fig. 2 b). Additionally, the expression levels of *CCND1* and *BIRCS5* were tested in the GCB-like and ABC-like groups. To that end, the samples were first classified into two groups based on 1,180 canine-specific probe sets. Then, the expression level of *CCND1* was compared between the two groups. For the GSE43664 dataset, a clear clustering pattern was reconstructed (Additional file 1: Figure S1),

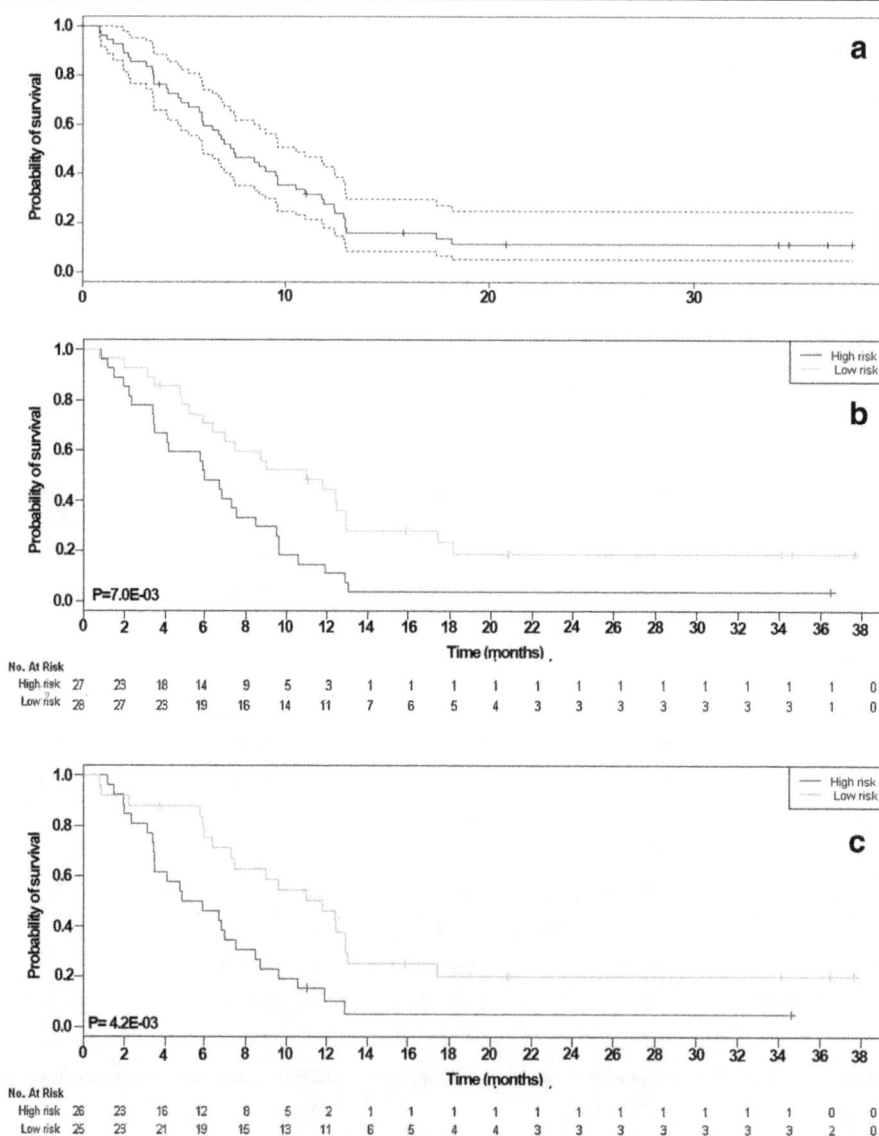

Fig. 1 Survival analysis for evaluation of the correlation between GSE39365 prognostic genes and DFS time in GSE43664 dataset. Panel **a** indicated Kaplan-Meier estimate with 95% confidence bound in GSE43664 dataset. There was significant correlation between DFS with *CCND1* (**b**) ($P = 0.007$) and *BIRCS5* (**c**) ($P = 0.042$). *Green and red lines* indicated samples had higher and lower expression value than median value respectively

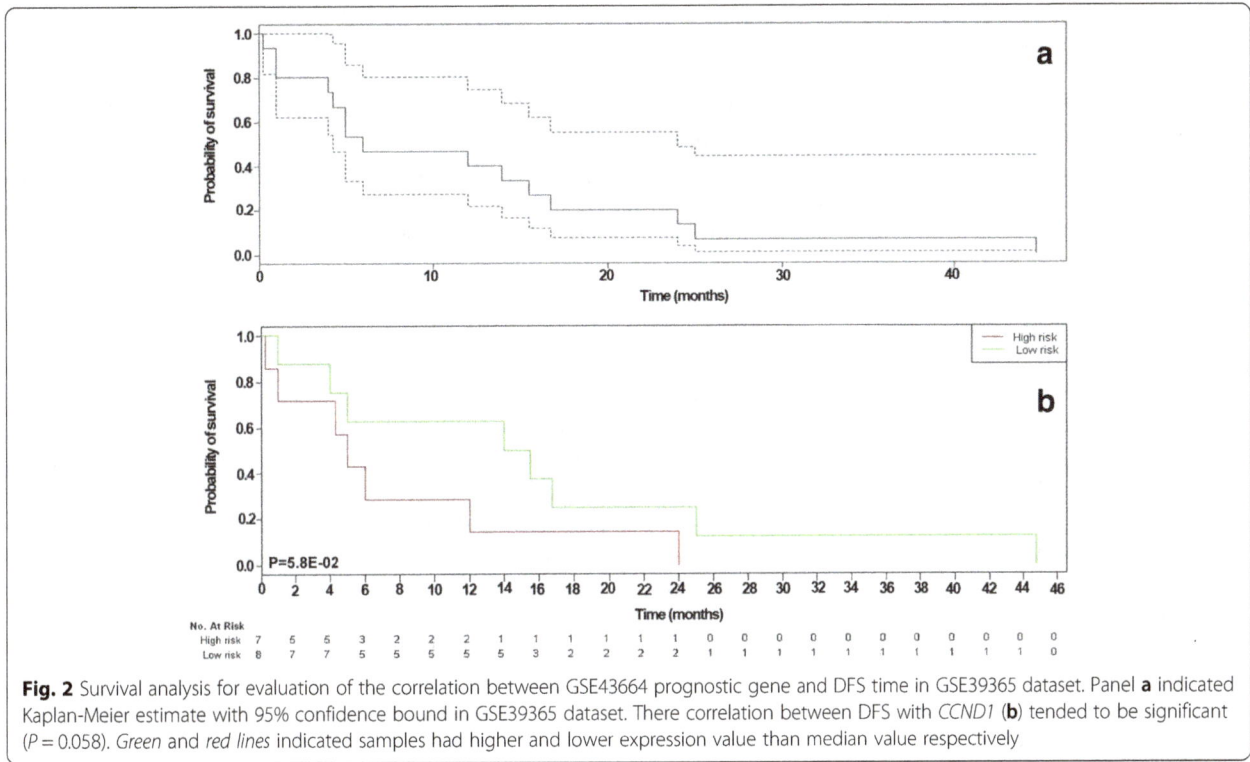

Fig. 2 Survival analysis for evaluation of the correlation between GSE43664 prognostic gene and DFS time in GSE39365 dataset. Panel **a** indicated Kaplan-Meier estimate with 95% confidence bound in GSE39365 dataset. There correlation between DFS with *CCND1* (**b**) tended to be significant ($P = 0.058$). *Green* and *red lines* indicated samples had higher and lower expression value than median value respectively

while the GCB-like and ABC-like groups were not clearly created for the GSE39365 dataset maybe because of its small sample size (Additional file 1: Figure S2). Hence, the T-test analysis was performed only on the GSE43664 dataset and reveled that the differences between *CCND1* expression in the GCB-like (mean ± SD = 8.03 ± 0.86) and ABC-like (mean ± SD = 7.7 ± 0.54) groups tended to be significant ($P = 0.052$) while *BIRCS5* expression in the GCB-like (mean ± SD = 5.32 ± 0.21) and ABC-like (mean ± SD = 5.26 ± 0.23) groups wasn't significant ($P = 0.36$).

qRT-PCR analysis confirmed *CCND1* as final prognostic gene because *CCND1* expression was significantly higher in the dogs with DFS >12 months than the dogs with DFS <7 months while expression level of the *BIRCS5* wasn't significantly different between two groups (Fig. 3).

As was expected in light of our literature review [2, 6], clinical characteristics such as age, sex, and tumor grade were not significant predictor components in canine B-cell lymphoma. More statistical details about the patients' clinical characteristics are summarized in Table 2.

Discussion

Although prognostic gene genes for human NHL and especially DLBCL have been meticulously investigated by various researchers, there is little information on molecular prognostic genes for canine B-cell lymphoma. For example, Rosenwald et al. (2002) [14] proposed germinal-center B-cell, MHC class II, lymph-node, and cell proliferation signatures as a molecular profiling for

predicting progression-free survival after chemotherapy in patients with DLBCL. HLA-DPα, HLA-DQα, HLA-DRα, and HLA-DRβ as members of the MHC class II module; BCL-6 as a member of the germinal-center B-cell module; fibronectin, α-Actinin, connective-tissue growth factor, urokinase plasminogen activator, collagen type IIIα1, and KIAA0233 as members of the lymph-node module; and E21G3, c-myc, and NPM3 as members of the proliferation module constituted the more

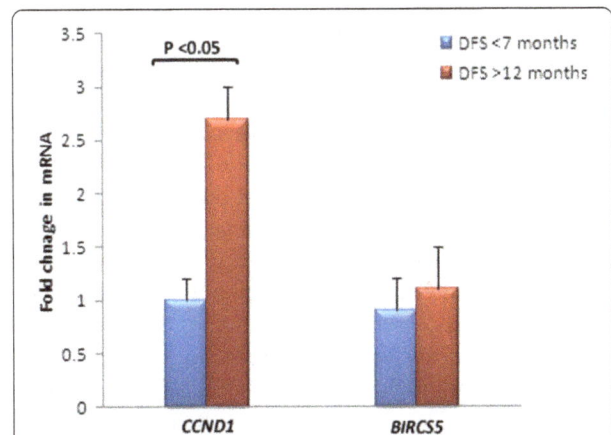

Fig. 3 Quantitative real-time PCR (qRT-PCR) analysis of the prognostic genes. Gene expression level of *CCND1* was significantly higher in patients with long DFS time (>12 months) than ones with short DFS time (<7 months). No significant difference was detected in *BIRCS5* expression level between two groups

prominent elements of prognostic signatures [14]. Furthermore, Lossos et al. (2004) [13] proposed a complex of LMO2, FN1, BCL6, SCYA3, CCND2, and BCL2 as a suitable predictor in patients with DLBCL, independent of the International Prognostic Index (IPI). In addition, the authors reported HGAL and BCL6 as predictors of overall survival, independent of the IPI [26, 27]. A comprehensive list of the prognostic genes in human B-cell lymphoma and related studies is presented in the Materials/Methods (Table 1).

The current study utilized human B-cell lymphoma prognostic genes so as to detect valuable genes that can serve as prognostic predictors in canine B-cell lymphoma. There is currently no counterpart for the IPI as regards canine lymphoma inasmuch as the prognostic efficacy of the IPI is evaluated alongside molecular genes. Among genes analyzed in our investigation, CCND1 was found to be the most appropriate prognostic factor. CCND1 was confirmed in both datasets while BIRCS5 was solely verified in one dataset. Additionally qRT-PCR verified CCND1 prognostic efficacy.

CCND1, encoding cyclin D1 protein, plays a critical role in the cell cycle machinery; i.e. in G1-S transition. The overexpression of CCND1 has been indicated in various human B-cell lymphoma subtypes, including mantle cell lymphoma (MCL) [28, 29], DLBCL [30–32], and plasma cell myeloma [33]. Nevertheless, the overexpression of cyclin D1 is regarded as an unusual characteristic in human DLBCL [34, 35]. In general, cyclin D1 has been proposed as the most critical prognostic gene majorly in MCL [36, 37] and seldom for other human B-cell lymphoma subtypes. In one study, cyclin D1 was verified as an independent prognostic factor from the IPI and 5-year overall survival was significantly higher in cyclin D1-negative MCL than cyclin D1-positive MCL (86% vs. 30%) [37]. Furthermore, the m-RNA level of CCND1 in blood and bone marrow has been proposed as an appropriate prognostic factor in patients with MCL [38]. Cyclin D1 overexpression showed a correlation with longer survival in breast carcinoma [39] and colorectal cancer [40]. The results of our study demonstrate that CCND1 is a favorable potential prognostic predictor for canine B-cell lymphoma. The results of the present study confirm that CCND1 is an important potential prognostic gene in canine B-cell lymphoma (especially DLBCL subtype) and should, accordingly, be considered for further investigation in future studies. There is no significant comparable data about prognostic efficacy of the CCND1 in human DLBCL while studied samples in our study were majorly DLBCL. In an study by lossos et al [13], although univariate Cox proportional-hazard analysis revealed that CCND1 was a genes with negative z score (longer survival), CCND1 didn't reach a significant level for entering final multivariate analysis.

Additionally previous investigation revealed that patients with cyclin-D1+ CD5+ DLBCL tended to be associated with inferior survival, but the correlation was not statistically significant [32]. Discrepancy between prognostic efficacy of the CCND1 in human (especially MCL) and canine B-cell lymphoma can be described in some ways. This discrepancy may stem from the use of different methods for the analysis of CCND1 expression (e.g. imunohistochemistry, Western blotting, or gene expression analysis) [39, 40] or may related to the species-dependent characteristics. Relationship between CCND1 expression and survival time in human MCL was evaluated using immunophenotyping methods [37], while we used a gene expression profiling approach in our study. Additionally, some obvious reverse findings have been found between canine B-cell lymphoma and human counterpart. For example, previous investigation indicated that in contrast to human DLBCL, BCL6 and MUM1/IRF4 rarely expressed in canine B-cell lymphoma [16]. Moreover, an inverse expression pattern for p65 and p52 were found in canine and human DLBCL [41]. Furthermore, some potential confounders such as microsatellite instability (MSI), the CpG island methylator phenotype (CIMP), and BRAF mutation have been suggested as another source of the inconsistent findings regarding association between CCND1 expression and clinical outcome [40]. These genetic aberrations haven't been examined in canine B-cell lymphoma.

Another gene regarded as a prognostic factor in our study was BIRCS5 (survivin), but it wasn't confirmed in final qRT-PCR assay. BIRCS5 is one of the most important inhibitors of apoptosis proteins (IAP) involved in the inhibition of induced cell death in vitro and in vivo [42]. Previous investigations have revealed that overall survival is significantly shorter in patients with high survivin expression in patients with MCL [43] and DLBCL [44]. Analysis has confirmed that survivin can play a role in the prediction of survival independent of the IPI in DLBCL cases [44, 45]. Be that as it may, some authors have indicated that there is no correlation between survivin expression and survival or response to treatment in patients with DLBCL [46]. The overexpression of survivin in other cancers such as colorectal cancer and neuroblastoma is associated with higher proliferation activity and higher relapse rate [47, 48]. In our study, although BIRCS5 was found to be a predictor of DFS in canine B-cell lymphoma in multivariate Cox proportional-hazard analysis, this gene wasn't considered as suitable prognostic factor because its expression level wasn't significantly different between patients with long or short survival time.

Conclusions

To the best of our knowledge, this has been one of the few studies to explore prognostic genes in canine lymphoma using gene expression data analysis. Although microarray data from human cancers are very extensive and informative, microarray data related to animal cancers are rare and incomplete. When mining microarray databases such as GEO and ArrayExpress, there are limited studies exploring canine cancers using gene expression profiling. Similarly, there is same problem with the canine lymphoma. Our mining in the databases provided three datasets (GSE43664, GSE39365, and GSE30881) with ideal sample size on canine B-cell lymphoma, where clinical metadata (including survival time) haven't been provided for GSE30881 dataset. Therefore, we excluded this dataset and used other two datasets. However, to gain more robust and reliable results, both datasets were used as training and validation groups. Although our results may affect by small sample size of a dataset, we hope that with extending larger canine datasets, future studies by our group or other veterinary oncology researchers will provide more remarkable findings. In conclusion, although the results of the present study reveal *CCND1* as a potential prognostic factor in canine B-cell lymphoma, further studies on more extensive gene expression databases are required to clarify other prognostic genes which can be used as robust survival predictors.

Abbreviations
ABC-like: Activated B-cell like; DFS: Disease-free survival; DLBCL: Diffuse large B-cell lymphoma; GCB-like: Germinal center B like; qRT-PCR: Quantitative real-time PCR

Acknowledgments
We wish to thank Mr. Pedram Amouzadeh who assisted in the proof-reading of the manuscript. We also thank Lelia Haghighi for her technical support.

Funding
This study had no funding support.

Authors' contributions
MZA, SA, and KI participated in the study design, performing the experiments, and analysis of the data. MZA and SA wrote the manuscript. All authors read and approved the final manuscript.

Competing interests
The authors declare that they have no competing interest.

Consent for publication
Not applicable.

Author details
[1]Department of Clinical Science, Faculty of Veterinary Medicine, Shahid Bahonar University of Kerman, P.O Box: 76169133, Kerman, Iran. [2]Department of Clinical Science, Faculty of Veterinary Medicine, Islamic Azad University, Garmsar Branch, Garmsar, Iran.

References
1. MacEwen EG. Spontaneous tumors in dogs and cats: models for the study of cancer biology and treatment. Cancer Metastasis Rev. 1990;9(2):125–36.
2. Jacobs RM MJ, Valli VE. Hemolymphatic system. In: Meuten DJ, editor. Tumors in Domestic Animals edn. Iowa: Iowa State Press; 2002. p. 138–43.
3. McCaw DL, Chan AS, Stegner AL, Mooney B, Bryan JN, Turnquist SE, Henry CJ, Alexander H, Alexander S. Proteomics of Canine Lymphoma Identifies Potential Cancer-Specific Protein Markers. Clin Cancer Res. 2007;13(8):2496–503.
4. Vail DM ME, Young KM. Canine lymphoma and lymphoid leukemias. In: Withrow SJ, Vail DM, Page RL, editors. Withrow and MacEwen's Small Animal Clinical Oncology edn. Philadelphia: Elsevier Health Sciences; 2001. p. 558–84.
5. Kiupel M, Teske E, Bostock D. Prognostic factors for treated canine malignant lymphoma. Vet Pathol. 1999;36(4):292–300.
6. Frantz AM, Sarver AL, Ito D, Phang TL, Karimpour-Fard A, Scott MC, Valli VEO, Lindblad-Toh K, Burgess KE, Husbands BD, et al. Molecular profiling reveals prognostically significant subtypes of canine lymphoma. Vet Pathol. 2013;50(4):693–703.
7. Teske E, van Heerde P, Rutteman GR, Kurzman ID, Moore PF, MacEwen EG. Prognostic factors for treatment of malignant lymphoma in dogs. J Am Vet Med Assoc. 1994;205(12):1722–8.
8. Löhr CV, Teifke JP, Failing K, Weiss E. Characterization of the proliferation state in canine mammary tumors by the standardized AgNOR method with postfixation and immunohistologic detection of Ki-67 and PCNA. Vet Pathol. 1997;34(3):212–21.
9. Rmi J, Pg M, Crocker J, Mj L. Sequential demonstration of nucleolar organizer regions and Ki67 immunolabelling in non-Hodgkin's lymphomas. Clinical & Laboratory Haematology. 1990;12(4):395–9.
10. Yekeler H, Ozercan MR, Yumbul AZ, Ağan M, Ozercan IH. Nucleolar organizer regions in lymphomas: a quantitative study. Pathologica. 1993;85(1097):353–60.
11. Vail DM, Kisseberth WC, Obradovich JE, Moore FM, London CA, MacEwen EG, Ritter MA. Assessment of potential doubling time (Tpot), argyrophilic nucleolar organizer regions (AgNOR), and proliferating cell nuclear antigen (PCNA) as predictors of therapy response in canine non-Hodgkin's lymphoma. Exp Hematol. 1996;24(7):807–15.
12. Alizadeh AA, Eisen MB, Davis RE, Ma C, Lossos IS, Rosenwald A, Boldrick JC, Sabet H, Tran T, Yu X, et al. Distinct types of diffuse large B-cell lymphoma identified by gene expression profiling. Nature. 2000;403(6769):503–11.
13. Lossos IS, Czerwinski DK, Alizadeh AA, Wechser MA, Tibshirani R, Botstein D, Levy R. Prediction of survival in diffuse large-B-cell lymphoma based on the expression of six genes. N Engl J Med. 2004;350(18):1828–37.
14. Rosenwald A, Wright G, Chan WC, Connors JM, Campo E, Fisher RI, Gascoyne RD, Muller-Hermelink HK, Smeland EB, Giltnane JM, et al. The use of molecular profiling to predict survival after chemotherapy for diffuse large-B-cell lymphoma. N Engl J Med. 2002;346(25):1937–47.
15. Shipp MA, Ross KN, Tamayo P, Weng AP, Kutok JL, Aguiar RCT, Gaasenbeek M, Angelo M, Reich M, Pinkus GS, et al. Diffuse large B-cell lymphoma outcome prediction by gene-expression profiling and supervised machine learning. Nat Med. 2002;8(1):68–74.
16. Richards KL, Motsinger-Reif AA, Chen H-W, Fedoriw Y, Fan C, Nielsen DM, Small GW, Thomas R, Smith C, Dave SS, et al. Gene profiling of canine B-cell lymphoma reveals germinal center and postgerminal center subtypes with different survival times, modeling human DLBCL. Cancer Res. 2013;73(16):5029–39.
17. Gautier L, Cope L, Bolstad BM, Irizarry RA. affy–analysis of Affymetrix GeneChip data at the probe level. Bioinformatics. 2004;20(3):307–15.
18. Schroder MS, Culhane AC, Quackenbush J, Haibe-Kains B. survcomp: an R/Bioconductor package for performance assessment and comparison of survival models. Bioinformatics. 2011;27(22):3206–8.
19. Simon R. Roadmap for developing and validating therapeutically relevant genomic classifiers. J Clin Oncol. 2005;23(29):7332–41.
20. Schetter AJ, Nguyen GH, Bowman ED, Mathé EA, Yuen ST, Hawkes JE, Croce CM, Leung SY, Harris CC. Association of inflammation-related and microRNA gene expression with cancer-specific mortality of colon adenocarcinoma. Clin Cancer Res. 2009;15(18):5878–87.
21. Mey U, Hitz F, Lohri A, Pederiva S, Taverna C, Tzankov A, Meier O, Yeow K, Renner C. Diagnosis and treatment of diffuse large B-cell lymphoma. Swiss Med Wkly. 2012;142.
22. Floratos A, Smith K, Ji Z, Watkinson J, Califano A. geWorkbench: an open source platform for integrative genomics. Bioinformatics. 2010;26(14):1779–80.

23. Livak KJ, Schmittgen TD. Analysis of relative gene expression data using real-time quantitative PCR and the 2(-Delta Delta C(T)) Method. Methods. 2001;25(4):402–8.

24. Klopfleisch R, Lenze D, Hummel M, Gruber AD. Metastatic canine mammary carcinomas can be identified by a gene expression profile that partly overlaps with human breast cancer profiles. BMC Cancer. 2010;10(1):618.

25. Swerdlow S, Campo E, Harris NL, Jaffe ES, Pileri SA, Stein H, Thiele J, Vardiman JW. WHO Classification of Tumours of Haematopoietic and Lymphoid Tissue, 4 edition edn. Lyon: World Health Organization; 2008.

26. Lossos IS, Alizadeh AA, Rajapaksa R, Tibshirani R, Levy R. HGAL is a novel interleukin-4-inducible gene that strongly predicts survival in diffuse large B-cell lymphoma. Blood. 2003;101(2):433–40.

27. Lossos IS, Jones CD, Warnke R, Natkunam Y, Kaizer H, Zehnder JL, Tibshirani R, Levy R. Expression of a single gene, BCL-6, strongly predicts survival in patients with diffuse large B-cell lymphoma. Blood. 2001;98(4):945–51.

28. de Boer CJ, van Krieken JH, Kluin-Nelemans HC, Kluin PM, Schuuring E. Cyclin D1 messenger RNA overexpression as a marker for mantle cell lymphoma. Oncogene. 1995;10(9):1833–40.

29. Gladkikh A, Potashnikova D, Korneva E, Khudoleeva O, Vorobjev I. Cyclin D1 expression in B-cell lymphomas. Exp Hematol. 2010;38(11):1047–57.

30. Vela-Chávez T, Adam P, Kremer M, Bink K, Bacon CM, Menon G, Ferry JA, Fend F, Jaffe ES, Quintanilla-Martínez L. Cyclin D1 positive diffuse large B-cell lymphoma is a post-germinal center-type lymphoma without alterations in the CCND1 gene locus. Leuk Lymphoma. 2011;52(3):458–66.

31. Hsiao S-C, Cortada IR, Colomo L, Ye H, Liu H, Kuo S-Y, Lin S-H, Chang S-T, Kuo TU, Campo E, et al. SOX11 is useful in differentiating cyclin D1-positive diffuse large B-cell lymphoma from mantle cell lymphoma. Histopathology. 2012;61(4):685–93.

32. Zhang A, Ohshima K, Sato K, Kanda M, Suzumiya J, Shimazaki K, Kawasaki C, Kikuchi M. Prognostic clinicopathologic factors, including immunologic expression in diffuse large B-cell lymphomas. Pathol Int. 1999;49(12):1043–52.

33. Troussard X, Avet-Loiseau H, Macro M, Mellerin MP, Malet M, Roussel M, Sola B. Cyclin D1 expression in patients with multiple myeloma. Hematol J. 2000;1(3):181–5.

34. Juskevicius D, Ruiz C, Dirnhofer S, Tzankov A. Clinical, morphologic, phenotypic, and genetic evidence of cyclin D1-positive diffuse large B-cell lymphomas with CYCLIN D1 gene rearrangements. Am J Surg Pathol. 2014;38(5):719–27.

35. Ok CY, Xu-Monette ZY, Tzankov A, O'Malley DP, Montes-Moreno S, Visco C, Møller MB, Dybkaer K, Orazi A, Zu Y, et al. Prevalence and clinical implications of cyclin D1 expression in diffuse large B-cell lymphoma (DLBCL) treated with immunochemotherapy: a report from the International DLBCL Rituximab-CHOP Consortium Program. Cancer. 2014;120(12):1818–29.

36. Baldin V, Lukas J, Marcote MJ, Pagano M, Draetta G. Cyclin D1 is a nuclear protein required for cell cycle progression in G1. Genes Dev. 1993;7(5):812–21.

37. Yatabe Y, Suzuki R, Tobinai K, Matsuno Y, Ichinohasama R, Okamoto M, Yamaguchi M, Tamaru J, Uike N, Hashimoto Y, et al. Significance of cyclin D1 overexpression for the diagnosis of mantle cell lymphoma: a clinicopathologic comparison of cyclin D1-positive MCL and cyclin D1-negative MCL-like B-cell lymphoma. Blood. 2000;95(7):2253–61.

38. Siddon AJ, Torres R, Rinder HM, Smith BR, Howe JG, Tormey CA. Normalized CCND1 expression has prognostic value in mantle cell lymphoma. Br J Haematol. 2012;158(4):551–3.

39. Reis-Filho JS, Savage K, Lambros MBK, James M, Steele D, Jones RL, Dowsett M. Cyclin D1 protein overexpression and CCND1 amplification in breast carcinomas: an immunohistochemical and chromogenic in situ hybridisation analysis. Mod Pathol. 2006;19(7):999–1009.

40. Ogino S, Nosho K, Irahara N, Kure S, Shima K, Baba Y, Toyoda S, Chen L, Giovannucci EL, Meyerhardt JA, et al. A cohort study of cyclin D1 expression and prognosis in 602 colon cancer cases. Clin Cancer Res. 2009;15(13):4431–8.

41. Mudaliar MAV, Haggart RD, Miele G, Sellar G, Tan KAL, Goodlad JR, Milne E, Vail DM, Kurzman I, Crowther D et al. Comparative gene expression profiling identifies common molecular signatures of NF-κB activation in canine and human diffuse large B cell lymphoma (DLBCL). PLoS ONE. 2013;8(9):e72591.

42. Altieri DC. Validating survivin as a cancer therapeutic target. Nat Rev Cancer. 2003;3(1):46–54.

43. Martinez A, Bellosillo B, Bosch F, Ferrer A, Marcé S, Villamor N, Ott G, Montserrat E, Campo E, Colomer D. Nuclear Survivin Expression in Mantle Cell Lymphoma Is Associated with Cell Proliferation and Survival. Am J Pathol. 2004;164(2):501–10.

44. Adida C, Haioun C, Gaulard P, Lepage E, Morel P, Briere J, Dombret H, Reyes F, Diebold J, Gisselbrecht C, et al. Prognostic significance of survivin expression in diffuse large B-cell lymphomas. Blood. 2000;96(5):1921–5.

45. Markovic O, Marisavljevic D, Cemerikic-Martinovic V, Martinovic T, Filipovic B, Stanisavljevic D, Zivković R, Hajder J, Stanisavljevic N, Mihaljevic B. Survivin expression in patients with newly diagnosed nodal diffuse large B cell lymphoma (DLBCL). Med Oncol. 2012;29(5):3515–21.

46. Mitrović Z, Ilić I, Aurer I, Kinda SB, Radman I, Dotlić S, Ajduković R, Labar B. Prognostic significance of survivin and caspase-3 immunohistochemical expression in patients with diffuse large B-cell lymphoma treated with rituximab and CHOP. Pathol Oncol Res. 2011;17(2):243–7.

47. Islam A, Kageyama H, Takada N, Kawamoto T, Takayasu H, Isogai E, Ohira M, Hashizume K, Kobayashi H, Kaneko Y, et al. High expression of Survivin, mapped to 17q25, is significantly associated with poor prognostic factors and promotes cell survival in human neuroblastoma. Oncogene. 2000;19(5):617–23.

48. Kawasaki H, Altieri DC, Lu CD, Toyoda M, Tenjo T, Tanigawa N. Inhibition of apoptosis by survivin predicts shorter survival rates in colorectal cancer. Cancer Res. 1998;58(22):5071–4.

Expression profiles of immune mediators in feline Coronavirus-infected cells and clinical samples of feline Coronavirus-positive cats

Nikoo Safi[1,3], Amin Haghani[1,3], Shing Wei Ng[1], Gayathri Thevi Selvarajah[2], Farina Mustaffa-Kamal[2*] and Abdul Rahman Omar[1,2]

Abstract

Background: There are two biotypes of feline coronavirus (FCoV): the self-limiting feline enteric coronavirus (FECV) and the feline infectious peritonitis virus (FIPV), which causes feline infectious peritonitis (FIP), a fatal disease associated with cats living in multi-cat environments. This study provides an insight on the various immune mediators detected in FCoV-positive cats which may be responsible for the development of FIP.

Results: In this study, using real-time PCR and multiplex bead-based immunoassay, the expression profiles of several immune mediators were examined in Crandell-Reese feline kidney (CRFK) cells infected with the feline coronavirus (FCoV) strain FIPV 79–1146 and in samples obtained from FCoV-positive cats. CRFK cells infected with FIPV 79–1146 showed an increase in the expression of interferon-related genes and pro-inflammatory cytokines such as MX1, viperin, CXCL10, CCL8, RANTES, KC, MCP1, and IL8. In addition, an increase in the expression of the above cytokines as well as GM-CSF and IFNγ was also detected in the PBMC, serum, and peritoneal effusions of FCoV-positive cats. Although the expression of MX1 and viperin genes was variable between cats, the expression of these two genes was relatively higher in cats having peritoneal effusion compared to cats without clinically obvious effusion. Higher viral load was also detected in the supernatant of peritoneal effusions compared to in the plasma of FCoV-positive cats. As expected, the secretion of IL1β, IL6 and TNFα was readily detected in the supernatant of peritoneal effusions of the FCoV-positive cats.

Conclusions: This study has identified various pro-inflammatory cytokines and interferon-related genes such as MX1, viperin, CXCL10, CCL8, RANTES, KC, MCP1, IL8, GM-CSF and IFNγ in FCoV-positive cats. With the exception of MX1 and viperin, no distinct pattern of immune mediators was observed that distinguished between FCoV-positive cats with and without peritoneal effusion. Further studies based on definitive diagnosis of FIP need to be performed to confirm the clinical importance of this study.

Keywords: Feline Coronavirus, Cytokine, Immune-mediators

Background

Feline coronavirus (FCoV) can be divided into two biotypes: the ubiquitous feline enteric coronavirus (FECV) which often causes self-limiting diarrhea, and the feline infectious peritonitis virus (FIPV), the mutated form which causes fatal disease in cats [1, 2]. The widely accepted 'internal mutation' theory describes that mutations in FECV give rise to FIP de novo. In addition, it was suggested that these mutations occur in the monocytes, rather than the intestinal epithelial cells where the FECV first enters the host [3, 4]. FCoV travels to organs and tissues through monocyte-associated viremia where it is later disseminated in the endothelial venules of the serosa, omentum, pleura, meninges and uveal tract (reviewed in [1, 2]).

Currently, there are no specific markers to distinguish the two biotypes, thus making the diagnosis of feline infectious peritonitis (FIP) difficult. Although several studies have reported several point mutations in the S gene that are associated with occurrence of FIPV, it

* Correspondence: farina@upm.edu.my
[2]Faculty of Veterinary Medicine, Universiti Putra Malaysia, Serdang, Selangor, Malaysia

remains unclear whether the mutations contributed solely to the development of FIP [5–7]. Therefore, ante-mortem confirmation of FIP remains a challenging task in clinical research of FIP.

Information on the immunopathogenesis and the role of cytokines, and immune mediators in FCoV infection are relatively sparse. Although it is generally known that FECV causes self-limiting disease, cats can become persistent shedders contributing to the transmission of the disease (reviewed in [1, 2]). However, only approximately 5% of cats harboring FECV actually develop FIP [1, 8]. The exact nature of this immunity is still unknown although the development of FIP has been postulated to correlate with the magnitude of immune responses, as cats with robust cell-mediated immune (CMI) response have been found to resist the disease [9]. In contrast, humoral response does not seem to be beneficial and could lead to the dissemination of the virus through complement activation via formation of immune complexes and vasculitis associated with type III hypersensitivity (reviewed in [1, 2]). This would then lead to effusive FIP (wet form), the most commonly reported form of FIP due to the obvious sign of peritoneal effusion. The non-effusive form of FIP is associated with partial CMI response in the individual cat to contain the virus leading to the formation of granulomas containing macrophages, which could then be replaced by B cells and plasma cells [10, 11].

To date, there are no specific immune markers that could distinguish FECV from FIPV infections. However, the observed cytokine patterns are different between asymptomatic FCoV-infected cats and those with clinical signs of FIP [12]. Asymptomatic FCoV-infected cats generally show higher IL10 in the spleen, suggesting the ability to control excessive inflammation triggered by macrophages. Furthermore, lymphocyte depletion has been indicated as one of the hallmarks of FIP and postulated to be induced by excessive production of TNFα [13–15]. In contrast, high IFN γ and IL 1β production has been associated with protection against FIP [16]. Increase in Th1-like cytokines such as IL12/p40 and IFNγ, which were associated with the decrease of IL4 in the lymphoid tissue, has been observed in cats experimentally infected with FIPV [13]. Furthermore, previous studies showed deregulation of different mediators, illustrated by the upregulation of pro-inflammatory cytokines such as IL1β, IL6, TNFα, MIP1α, RANTES, and IFNγ in peritoneal effusions and serum samples of FIP clinical cases [17–19].

Recently, we used a transcriptomic approach by next-generation sequencing of RNA from Crandell-Reese feline kidney (CRFK) cells infected with the FCoV strain FIPV 79–1146 to elucidate the complex interaction between the virus and host cells in vitro [20, 21]. Results revealed that, during the first 3 h of infection, at least 96

transcripts associated with immune responses (e.g. ISGs, MX1, RSAD2, A3C, ID1, CRIP1, TRIM25 and MDA5), apoptosis (ID1, ATF3, TNFα, and RNF7), and pro-inflammatory responses (e.g. PD-L1, CCL8, CXCL10 and CCL17) were downregulated. Only a few genes, namely PD-1, PD-L1 and A3H, has been previously characterized in a study on FCoV-infected CRFK cells and expression profiles in peripheral blood mononuclear cells (PBMC) of cats diagnosed with FIP [20]. Characterization of additional immune mediators that modulate innate and acquired immune responses will increase our understanding of their involvement during FIPV infection. The objective of this study was to investigate the immune mediator profiles in CRFK-infected cells and FCoV-positive cats. Both gene and protein expression profiles were determined by quantitative real-time PCR (qPCR) and multiplex bead-based assays.

Methods
In vitro analysis of FCoV-infected cells
TCID50 of the FCoV strain FIPV 79–1146 (ATCC® VR2202) [22] was determined using endpoint dilution assay. Virus infectivity was confirmed by RT-PCR (Bioline, UK) detecting the FCoV conserved 3′ untranslated region (3′-UTR) [23]. To prepare a sufficient amount of infected cells at different time points, two confluent 75 cm^2 flasks of CRFK cells (ATCC® CCL-94™) were inoculated at each time point with 3 ml TCID$_{50}$/ml (MOI = 0.1) of FIPV 79–1146 and the virus inoculum was left in the culture. At 3, 12, 24, 48 and 72 h post-inoculation (hpi), the cells were trypsinized and cell pellets were collected upon centrifugation. The uninfected flask was designated as 0 hpi. The cell pellets were stored at –80 °C until further use for virus and immune mediator detection by real-time PCR and multiplex bead-based immunoassay.

Selection criteria for FCoV-positive cats
Before performing the in vivo phase of the study, approval for handling and sampling cats was obtained from the Institutional Animal Care and Use Committee (IACUC), Faculty of Veterinary Medicine, Universiti Putra Malaysia (UPM) with the reference number UPM/ IACUC/AUP-R040/2014. The status of FCoV infection was evaluated in cats that were presented to the University Veterinary Hospital (UVH), UPM, using Biogal's Immunocomb Antibody Test Kit (Biogal-Galed Laboratories, Israel) to determine the antibody titer, followed by reverse transcriptase quantitative PCR (RT-qPCR) to detect the presence of FCoV in the serum [23]. Combscale S value was used as a colorimetric indicator for the determination of anti-FCoV antibody titer, where cats with antibody titers ≥ S2+ were chosen for further analysis [24]. In addition, cats were also screened serologically for Feline Immunodeficiency Virus (FIV) and Feline Leukemia Virus

(FELV) using the SNAP FIV/FELV Combo test (IDEXX Laboratories, USA) according to the manufacturer's protocol. Cats with high antibody levels against FCoV (titer ≥ S2+) and that are seronegative for FIV and FELV were selected and further underwent hematology evaluation. In addition to that, the presence or absence of peritoneal effusion was also evaluated in these selected cats. Post-mortem examination and follow-up analysis were not carried out to arrive at definitive diagnosis of FIP. Healthy seronegative FIV/FELV cats with absence of antibody titer against FCoV were considered as negative control cats.

Blood collection for preparation of PBMC and plasma

A total of 2.5 ml blood was collected from FCoV antibody titer ≥ S2+, FIV- and FELV- cats. The collected blood samples were immediately divided into two tubes for different purposes. First, 0.5 ml of blood was stored in clot activator tubes (BD Vacutainer® Tubes with BD hemoguard closure, USA) on ice and kept at 4 °C for serum separation. The remainder of the blood was transferred into EDTA tubes (BD Vacutainer® Tubes with BD hemoguard closure, USA) for PBMC isolation and plasma collection. The collected serum was stored at −80 °C for multiplex bead-based immunoassay. Isolation of PBMC was performed using Ficoll-Paque PLUS (GE Healthcare Life Science, USA) following the steps provided by the manufacturer. Plasma and PBMC were collected separately and stored at −80 °C until further use in real-time PCR for measuring viral load and mRNA expression of immune-related genes.

Peritoneal effusion

Peritoneal effusion (PE) samples were collected from FCoV-positive cats and centrifuged at 400×g for 10 min at 4 °C. The obtained cell pellets were used for detecting expression of immune-related genes using real-time PCR, whereas the supernatants were used for virus detection using RT-qPCR and for measuring cytokine and chemokine levels using multiplex bead-based immunoassay.

RNA extraction

Cellular RNA was extracted from the CRFK, PBMC and PE cells using the RNeasy Mini Kit, which includes DNase treatment (Qiagen, Germany), following the protocol supplied by the manufacturer. Viral RNA was extracted from the cell culture pellet, plasma, and supernatant of the PE (PES) using the Viral Nucleic Acid Extraction Kit 2 (Geneaid, Taiwan) according to the manufacturer's instructions. The concentration and quality of the extracted RNA were analyzed using a BioSpectrometer (Eppendorf, Germany). The extracted RNA samples (100 ng/μl) were used immediately to synthesize cDNA or kept at −80 °C for future usage.

Detection of viral load by SYBR green-based real-time PCR

cDNA was synthesized using the SensiFAST™ cDNA Kit (Bioline, UK), as instructed by the manufacturer. Virus quantification was performed using SYBR Green-based real-time PCR as described previously with a slight modification [25]. Briefly, quantitative real-time PCR (qPCR) was performed in a 20 μl reaction consisting of 1 μl cDNA, 1 μl forward primer (1 μmol), 1 μl reverse primer (1 μmol), 7 μl nuclease-free water and 10 μl 2× SensiFAST SYBR® No-ROX mix (Bioline, UK). The qPCR reaction was performed using the CFX96 Touch TM Real-Time PCR Detection System (Bio-Rad, USA) with the following cycling conditions: one cycle at 95 °C for PCR activation and 40 cycles of denaturation at 95 °C for 5 s, annealing at 60 °C for 10 s, and extension at 70 °C for 20 s. Detection of viral load was done by absolute quantification based on a standard curve generated from the serial dilution of a cDNA template. Viral load was expressed as viral copy number following a formula described previously [26].

Detection of immune-related mRNA expression by TaqMan-based real-time PCR

The expression of five immune-related genes, namely CCL8 (MCP2), viperin (RSAD2), CXCL10, MX1, and CCL17, and one reference gene (GAPDH) was measured by TaqMan-based real-time PCR (qPCR). The forward primers, reverse primers and TaqMan MGB probes were designed based on the *Felis catus* genome sequence [27]. The sequences of the primers and probes were designed using the CLC genomic workbench software, while primer characteristics were analyzed using Primer3 (http://bioinfo.ut.ee/primer3-0.4.0/) and Basic Local Alignment Search Tool (BLAST) to confirm alignment with more than 80% of the related gene in the *Felis catus* genome (Applied Biosystem, USA) (Table 1). cDNA was prepared using the Tetro cDNA Synthesis Kit (Bioline, UK) according to the manufacturer's protocol with a slight modification, in which specific forward and reverse primers for each gene were used instead of random hexamers. The RNA extracted from FIPV-infected CRFK cells at 48 hpi was used to optimize the real-time PCR assay before the assay was used to measure expression in the clinical samples obtained from FCoV-positive cats. Using serially diluted cDNA of each gene, the designed primer sets produced specific amplification with high PCR efficiency. Furthermore, primers for each gene were designed spanning two different exons to ensure specificity.

qPCR was performed using the TaqMan Fast Advanced Master Mix (Life Technologies®, Applied Biosystems,

Table 1 TaqMan primers, MGB probes and accession numbers of the analyzed immune-related genes

Gene	Primers sequences	MGB Probe	Accession number	Annealing temperature (°C)
CCL8	117CTTGCTCAGCCAGGTTCAGTT137 183GGATCTTCCCTTTGACCACACT162	6FAMCCATCCCAATTACCTGCTMGBNFQ	XM_003996558	66
Viperin	219CCCCCACCAGCGTCAAC235 281GGAAGCAGAAGCCACACTTGT261	6FAMACCACTTCACCCGCCAGMGBNFQ	XM_003984516	60
CXCL10	332ACACAGAAGCATAATCACCGTACTG356 399GGGAAATGATGGCAGAGGTAGT378	6FAMCAAAGATGGACCAGAAAGMGBNFQ	XM_003985274	60
MX1	469CAGGACTTTGAGACGGAGATTTC491 535CATTCTGGGCTGTATTGATTGC514	6FAMCCCTTCGGAGGTGGAMGBNFQ	XM_006935851	60
CCL17	119GGGCCATCCCTCTCAGAAG137 189CACTATGGCGTCTTTGGAACACT167	6FAMTGACAGGGTGGTACAGGAMGBNFQ	NM_001009849	60
GAPDH[a]	71GTCCCCGAGACACGATGGT89 130CCAGGCGCCCAATACG115	6FAMAAGGTCGGAGTCAACGGMGBNFQ	XM_006933438	57

Note: [a]Reference gene

USA) according to the manufacturer's protocol. 20 μl reactions were prepared as follows: 1 μl cDNA template, 0.5 μl forward primer (450 ηM), 0.5 μl reverse primer (450 ηM), 1 μl probe (250 ηM), 7 μl nuclease-free water and 10 μl of Fast Advanced Master Mix. The Taqman Fast Advanced Master Mix consisted of AmpliTaq Fast DNA Polymerase, Uracil-N-glycosylase (UNG), dNTPs with dUTP, ROX dye, and optimized buffer components. RT-qPCR was performed on the CFX96 Touch TM Real-Time PCR Detection System (Bio-Rad, USA) with the following steps: initial UNG incubation at 50 °C for 2 min and PCR activation at 95 °C for 20 s, followed by 40 cycles of denaturation at 95 °C for 5 s, annealing at optimized temperature for 10 s (Table 1), and extension at 72 °C for 20 s. The PCR efficiency of GAPDH, CXCL10, MX-1, viperin, CCL17 and CCL8 was 100, 99, 101, 102, 100 and 100%, respectively. For data interpretation, relative expression analysis ($\Delta\Delta Cq$) followed by analysis of variance (ANOVA) ($p < 0.05$) were carried out to determine the expression changes of target genes across different time points. Relative expression of the different immune-related genes were normalized to GAPDH and the negative controls.

Detection of immune-related protein expression by multiplex bead-based immunoassay

Measurement of 19 different immune-related protein expression was performed using the feline cytokines/chemokine magnetic bead-based panel immunoassay, FCYTOMAG-20 K FCYTMAG-20 K-PMX (MILLIPLEX MAP Kit, EMD Millipore Corporation, USA) following the manufacturer's instructions. The assay's principle of quantitative analysis was based on the standard provided in the kit. The standard was a mixture of all immune-related proteins at certain concentrations prepared by dilution as described by the kit. Hence, the concentrations of immune-related proteins in the samples were measured using the standard curve generated by the

standard. The prepared incubated plates (containing samples, standard and quality controls) were read on a Luminex analyzer (MAGPIX). Data obtained from the analyzer were analyzed by the MILLIPLEX analyst v5.1 software using five parameters logistic regression (EMD Millipore).

Statistical analysis

Data generated from this study were represented as means ± standard error of the mean (SEM). Statistical package for the social sciences (SPSS) version 22 was used to perform factorial analysis of variance (ANOVA) at 0.05 levels of significance for both the in vitro and in vivo experiments. Duncan test was used for post hoc analysis between the groups.

Results

Detection of viral load

Viral load in the infected cells was detected based on the 3' UTR region of FIPV using SYBR green-based real-time PCR. An increase in viral load was detected at different time points, with the peak viral load of $10^{12.54}$ occurring at 48 hpi, while the lowest viral load was detected at 3 hpi (Table 2). Total RNA obtained from the CRFK cells at 72 hpi was used to optimize the real-time PCR. The real-time PCR assay has a PCR efficiency of 100%.

Expression profiles of immune-related genes in FIPV 79–1146-infected cells

All the analyzed immune-related genes showed significant ($p < 0.05$) changes in expression levels at different time points following infection with FCoV strain FIPV 79–1146. These genes were selected based on transcriptome data from our previous study on CRFK cells infected with FIPV 79–1146 [14]. In this study, we confirmed the upregulation of these genes at 3 hpi using Taqman real-time PCR. CCL8 and MX1 showed peak expression levels at 48 hpi, while CXCL10 and viperin showed the highest

Table 2 Intracellular FCoV load in CRFK cells at different time points post infection

Time points (hpi)	FCoV copy number [Mean ± SEM (log10)]
	Intracellular
0[a]	-
3[b]	5.22 ± 0.12
12[d]	10.28 ± 0.06
24[c]	6.33 ± 0.02
48[f]	12.54 ± 0.34
72[e]	11.83 ± 0.05

Note: Different alphabets indicate significant difference ($p < 0.05$) following Duncan post hoc analysis of three replicates from three independent experiments

expression at 72 hpi (Table 3). Although the expression of viperin was upregulated at 48 and 72 hpi, its expression was downregulated at 3 and 12 hpi (Table 3).

Detection of immune-related proteins in FIPV 79–1146-infected CRFK cells

A total of 19 different immune-related proteins were analyzed by a bead-based multiplex immunoassay at different time points, following infection with FIPV 79–1146. The panel of proteins was chosen since it comprised of mediators with known functions in antiviral immunity, modulation of pro-inflammatory responses and regulation of viral-induced apoptosis. Out of the 19 immune-related proteins, only IL8 (CXCL8), KC (CXCL1), RANTES (CCL5) and MCP1 (CCL2) were detected in the CRFK-infected cells (Table 4). We were unable to detect the expression of other proteins, most likely due to the non-hematopoietic origin of CRFK cells whereby they did not secrete the proteins and/or the expression levels were too low beyond the detection limit of the assay.

FIPV infection of CRFK cells caused a significant modulation in the expression of the detectable cytokines, with peak expression detected at 48 hpi (CCL2 and CCL5) or 72 hpi (CXCL1 and CXCL8). However, CXCL8 and CCL5 were downregulated at 3 hpi ($p > 0.05$). CCL2

showed the least changes in expression compared to other cytokines following FIPV 79–1146 infection.

Detection of immune-related protein expression in FCoV-positive cats
Clinical features of the cats

The sampling of FCoV-positive cats was carried out at the University Veterinary Hospital-Universiti Putra Malaysia (UVH-UPM) over 1 year. Out of 150 cats, a total of 15 cats of different sex, age and breed that tested positive for high ($\geq$ S + 2) FCoV antibody titer and FCoV RNA by RT-PCR but negative for FELV and FIV antibodies were considered for this study (Table 5). In addition, among the 15 FCoV-positive cats, nine cats were presented with peritoneal effusions, hence they were categorized into the effusive cohort. The remaining six cats were either asymptomatic (cat 6, 14 and 15) or having signs associated with non-effusive FIP (cat 2, 3 and 16) (Table 5).

Hematology examination of the nine cats with effusions showed evidence of thrombocytopenia, hyperbilirubinemia, hyperglobulinemia and hypoalbuminemia, with three of these cats also having lymphopenia and icterus. In addition, the cats had albumin/globulin (A: G) ratios of between 0.3–0.6. Cat 1 represents three healthy FCoV-negative cats aged 2–4 years that also tested negative for FIV and FELV antibodies.

Detection of FCoV load in FCoV-seropositive cats

FCoV was quantified by RT-qPCR in blood plasma and supernatant of the peritoneal effusion (PES) taken from the FCoV-seropositive cats. All of the cats, except for the FCoV-seronegative cats, had positive viral load in the plasma and PES (Table 6). Furthermore, the level of viral load in the PES was significantly higher ($p < 0.05$) than in the plasma for the majority of the cats (Table 6). Only two cats (cats 10 and 11) exhibited higher viral load in the plasma. Almost all cats with peritoneal effusions had higher plasma viral load ($p < 0.05$) compared to cats without peritoneal effusion.

Table 3 Relative expression of immune-related genes following FIPV 79–1146 infection of CRFK cells

Time points (hpi)	CCL8 (MCP2)	CXCL10 (IP10)	CCL17	MX1	Viperin (RSAD2)
0	1 ± 0[a]	1 ± 0[a]	1 ± 0[a]	1 ± 0[a]	1 ± 0[c]
3	21.67 ± 0.57[d]	13,341.2 ± 197.75[c]	39.68 ± 1.61[e]	4.49 ± 0.62[c]	−13.04 ± 0[a]
12	3.41 ± 0.07[b]	8712.95 ± 343.29[b]	3.56 ± 0[b]	9.16 ± 1.27[d]	−7.82 ± 0.02[b]
24	4.92 ± 0.04[c]	1,835,241.44 ± 7662.16[d]	22.87 ± 0.69[d]	2.69 ± 0.11[b]	5.72 ± 0.03[d]
48	40,322.18 ± 14.38[f]	8,569,241.92 ± 44,483.37[e]	39.86 ± 0.6[e]	900.72 ± 4.25[f]	353.53 ± 1.82[e]
72	21,651.02 ± 510.17[e]	8,776,535.79 ± 30,986.02[e]	8.51 ± 0.44[c]	517.06 ± 5.38[e]	583.3 ± 9.86[f]

Note: Data are presented as means ± SEM of three replicates from two independent experiments. Different alphabets above the data indicate significant difference following Duncan post hoc comparison of each column ($p < 0.05$). Relative expression (ΔΔCq) was calculated by normalizing with the reference gene (GAPDH) and the negative controls

Table 4 Measurement of immune-related protein concentrations (pg/ml) in FIPV 79–1146-infected CRFK cells at different time points

Time points (hpi)	CXCL8 (IL8)	CXCL1 (KC)	CCL5 (RANTES)	CCL2 (MCP1)
0	465.33 ± 2.14[b]	9.23 ± 0.02[a]	22.63 ± 0.27[c]	913.03 ± 0.005[a]
3	166.75 ± 25.74[a]	28.55 ± 9.21[b]	8.35 ± 0.004[a]	960.84 ± 0.005[b]
12	444.32 ± 3.03[b]	8.32 ± 0.01[a]	31.18 ± 0.61[d]	923.22 ± 0.004[a]
24	1564.5 ± 45[c]	151.55 ± 9.98[c]	16.75 ± 0.73[b]	994.92 ± 7.38[b]
48	1499.5 ± 82.34[c]	119.02 ± 12.54[c]	2470 ± 114.67[f]	1068.5 ± 41.67[c]
72	2551 ± 93.33[d]	334.83 ± 9.49[d]	126.6 ± 2.4[e]	1050 ± 0.001[c]

Note: Data are represented as means ± SEM of three replicates from two independent experiments. Different alphabets above the data indicate significant difference following Duncan post hoc comparison of each column ($p < 0.05$). Peak expression levels of the cytokines were detected at 48 and/or 72 hpi

Expression profiles of immune-related genes in PBMC

The expression profiles of five immune-related genes, which were analyzed following in vitro infection of CRFK cells, were also analyzed in the PBMC and PE cells isolated from the FCoV-positive cats. In addition to normalization to GAPDH, the relative expression of the immune-related genes were normalized to the negative controls. As shown in Table 7, expression of all the genes except for CCL17 were detected in the PBMC of the sampled cats. However, gene expression levels varied among the cats. Most of the cats did not express or expressed very low levels of CCL8 and CXCL10 compared to healthy cats, except for cats 2, 3 and 5.

The expression of MX1 was detected in all FCoV-seropositive cats but not in healthy cats, and higher expression levels were detected in FCoV-positive cats with effusions (Table 7). Although viperin functions as an IFN-induced antiviral protein, similar to MX1, different patterns of viperin expression was observed. In addition, five out of six cats without signs of effusion showed downregulation of viperin compared to control cats (Table 7). Nevertheless, in cats with effusions, expression of viperin showed a trend similar that of MX1. In addition, a majority of the FCoV-positive cats with effusions showed markedly elevated expression levels of MX1 and viperin. As expected, the FCoV-negative cats did not express any of the analyzed immune-related genes, except for viperin.

Expression profiles of immune-related genes in peritoneal effusion cells

No distinct expression pattern was observed in the cellular component of PE collected from FCoV-positive cats (Table 8). However, high expression of CCL17 was detected in PE samples from three out of eight FCoV-

Table 5 Demographic and clinical features of the cats considered for this study

ID	Age	Sex	Breed	FCoV titer	FELV /FIV titer	Body temperature °C	Peritoneal effusion	A:G ratio
1	2–4 years	F	DSH	0	–	–	–	NA
2	1 year	M	Persian	S2+	–	N/A	–	0.6
3	7 months	M	Persian	S3+	–	N/A	–	NA
6	8 months	F	DSH	S5+	–	N/A	–	NA
14	2 years	M	DSH	S5+	–	N/A	–	NA
15	2 years	F	DSH	S5+	–	N/A	–	NA
16	8 months	F	Persian	S5+	–	37.9	–	0.3
4	2 years	M	DSH	S3+	–	N/A	+	NA
7	7 months	M	Maine coon	S5+	–	37.3	+	0.3
8	9 months	M	DSH	S4+	–	39.2	+	0.4
9	3 years	M	DSH	S5+	–	38.6	+	0.6
5	2 years	M	DSH	S5+	–	39.8	+	0.3
10	8 months	M	DSH	S5+	–	N/A	+	0.3
11	10 months	M	Maine coon	S4+	–	40.5	+	0.3
12	1 year	M	Maine coon	S4+	–	38.3	+	0.5
13	11 months	M	Persian	S5+	–	40.0	+	0.4

Note: NA not available, DSH Domestic short hair, A:G Albumin/Globulin, F Female, M Male, FCoV scoring of S2+ titer low positive reaction, ≥S3+ titer positive reaction, ≥S5+ titer high positive reaction

Table 6 Detection of FCoV load in plasma and supernatant of peritoneal effusion

Cat status	Cat ID	FCoV copy number [Mean ± SEM (log10)]	
		Plasma	PES
Negative controls	1[*]	-[a]	-
Non effusive	2	9.6 ± 0.05[b]	-
	3	10.73 ± 0.06[cdefg]	-
	6	10.41 ± 0.82[cde]	-
	14	10.25 ± 0.17[c]	-
	15	10.53 ± 0.01[cde]	-
	16	10.92 ± 0.34[cdefgh]	-
Effusive	4	11.06 ± 0.28[efghi]	N/A
	7	11.31 ± 0.33[ghi]	14.16 ± 0.05[l]
	8	10.74 ± 0.09[cdefg]	13.01 ± 0.04[k]
	9	11.72 ± 0.06[ij]	12.13 ± 0.18[j]
	5	11.28 ± 0.31[fghi]	13.21 ± 0.05[k]
	10	12.13 ± 0.35[j]	10.6 ± 0.65[cdef]
	11	10.99 ± 0.07[defgh]	10.31 ± 0.09[cd]
	12	11.57 ± 0.28[hij]	11.69 ± 0.19[ij]
	13	10.78 ± 0.74[cdefg]	12.02 ± 0.05[j]

N/A not available, *PES* supernatant of peritoneal effusion
[*]Cat 1 represents three healthy cats as negative controls
Note: Data are presented as means ± SEM of three replicates. Different alphabets denote significant difference ($p < 0.05$) following Duncan post hoc analysis

positive cats with effusions. Meanwhile, cat 8, which showed the highest expression of CCL17, also exhibited the highest expression of MX1 and viperin as well. In addition, most of the cats that expressed MX1 also expressed viperin and CXCL10, suggesting the involvement of interferon-induced antiviral proteins; however, their expression levels varied significantly among different cats.

Expression profiles of immune-related proteins in serum and peritoneal effusion supernatant

MILLIPLEX analysis of the serum and PES from the FCoV-positive cats revealed that all 19 immune-related proteins were detectable (Tables 9 and 10). However, no clear pattern was observed between the different levels of cytokines in cats with or without the presence of peritoneal effusions. Nevertheless, the expression of the immune-related proteins was higher in PES than in serum.

Although no common pattern of expression was seen among the FCoV-positive cats, detected levels of the different immune-related proteins in serum were higher in cats with peritoneal effusions compared to non-effusive FCoV-positive cats. The expression of pro-inflammatory cytokines and chemokines, such as GM-CSF, IFNγ, IL8, KC, RANTES, and MCP1, was readily detected in the serum of FCoV-positive cats (Table 9). The expression of IL1β and IL6 was not detected in the serum of the majority of the cats; however, these cytokines were detected in

Table 7 Relative expression profiles of immune-related genes in PBMC of FCoV-positive cats

Cat status	Cat ID	CCL8 (MCP2)	CXCL10 (IP10)	MX1	Viperin (RSAD2)
Negative	1[*]	ND	ND	ND	1 ± 0[bc]
Non-effusive	2	ND	18.67 ± 0.33[b]	6.79 ± 1.8[e]	−1.88 ± 0.27[bc]
	3	16.32 ± 5.48[c]	ND	0.91 ± 0.1[cd]	ND
	6	ND	ND	0.03 ± 0[a]	−86.21 ± 0.01[a]
	14	0.42 ± 0.02[a]	ND	1.45 ± 0.36[d]	−28.01 ± 0.02[b]
	15	ND	ND	0.58 ± 0.04[c]	−94.34 ± 0.01[a]
	16	ND	ND	0.32 ± 0.07[b]	−39.84 ± 0.02[b]
Effusive	4	ND	ND	0.05 ± 0[a]	ND
	7	0.1 ± 0.05[a]	0.23 ± 0.22[a]	13.62 ± 5.07[fg]	4.87 ± 1.39[cd]
	8	ND	ND	3773.07 ± 67.71[j]	437.28 ± 31.23[f]
	9	ND	ND	7309.7 ± 52.55[k]	50.48 ± 3.44[e]
	5	1.08 ± 0.38[b]	19.17 ± 0[c]	19.14 ± 0.02[gh]	4.95 ± 0.31[cd]
	10	ND	ND	56.48 ± 13.47[i]	7.91 ± 5.25[de]
	11	ND	ND	6.79 ± 0.74[ef]	−3.35 ± 0.17[c]
	12	ND	ND	16.37 ± 5.13[g]	1.83 ± 0.45[bcd]
	13	ND	ND	26.9 ± 1.61[h]	10.16 ± 1.08[de]

ND Not detected
[*]Average expression of three healthy cats as negative controls. Relative expression (ΔΔCq) was calculated by normalizing to the reference gene (GAPDH) and negative controls
Note: Data are presented as means ± SEM of three replicates. Different alphabets indicate significant difference following Duncan post hoc comparison of each column ($p < 0.05$)

Table 8 Relative expression profiles of immune-related genes in cells from peritoneal effusion

Cat ID	CCL8 (MCP2)	CXCL10 (IP10)	CCL17	MX1	Viperin (RSAD2)
7	1.77 ± 0.29^d	2.14 ± 0^e	0.37 ± 0.19^{bc}	1.65 ± 0.09^c	2.14 ± 0^e
8	0.29 ± 0.06^b	0.57 ± 0.2^{bc}	18.95 ± 16.6^{cd}	11.24 ± 0.82^e	13.31 ± 1.98^f
9	0.46 ± 0.04^{bc}	0.36 ± 0.1^b	12.69 ± 6.01^d	0.58 ± 0.02^b	0.03 ± 0^a
5	0.12 ± 0.02^a	0.06 ± 0.01^a	0.37 ± 0.18^{cd}	0.61 ± 0.03^b	0.34 ± 0.02^b
10	1.43 ± 0.11^d	0.64 ± 0.1^{bcd}	0 ± 0^a	1.36 ± 0.1^c	0.79 ± 0.12^c
11	0.1 ± 0.04^a	0.85 ± 0.07^{cd}	9.18 ± 3.87^d	0.21 ± 0.03^a	1.15 ± 0.13^d
12	4.62 ± 0.08^e	2.21 ± 0.38^e	0.03 ± 0.03^{ab}	4.7 ± 0^d	1.97 ± 0.34^e
13	0.79 ± 0.1^c	1.04 ± 0.14^d	1.83 ± 1.17^{cd}	0.51 ± 0.05^b	0.97 ± 0.07^{cd}

Note: Data are presented as means ± SEM of three replicates. Different alphabets indicate significantly different groupings following Duncan post hoc comparison of each column ($p < 0.05$). Relative expression ($\Delta\Delta Cq$) was calculated by normalizing to the reference gene (GAPDH) and negative controls

the PES of cats with peritoneal effusions (Table 10). TNFα production was detected in both FCoV-positive and negative cohorts. The production of this cytokine in the control cats could be due to an inflammatory process unrelated to FCoV infection, such as physiological stress [28]. In addition, the pro-inflammatory cytokine IL-18 was not consistently detected in both serum and PES. Unlike other immune-related proteins, serum levels of stem cell factor (SCF) were lower in the FCoV-positive cats compared to the control cats (Table 9).

Discussion

Feline infectious peritonitis (FIP) is one of the leading causes of death among young cats [1]. Since FIP is an immune-mediated viral disease, studies using immunological approaches are crucial for a better understanding of the illness, particularly by using clinical samples of FIP cases before further studies utilizing experimental infection in cats could be justified. Detection of FCoV antigen in affected tissues by immunohistochemistry remains the gold standard in the confirmation of FIP [2].

One of the limitations of this study is that definitive confirmation of FIP was not made due to the unavailability of post-mortem samples. Therefore, the cats were selected based on their FCoV antibody and antigen status. In addition, the selected FCoV-positive cats were grouped according to the presence of peritoneal effusions at the time of clinical evaluation. Although we could not confirm the status of FIP in these cats, this study provides a preliminary examination on the array of immune mediators that may be involved in the development of FIP. In this study, more than 20 immune mediators were characterized following FIPV 79–1146 infection of CRFK cells and in FCoV-positive cats. Different expression profiles of immune mediators were detected in FIPV 79–1146-infected CRFK cells and those from FCoV-positive cats. Furthermore, the CRFK cells were used to optimize the real-time PCR detection of the different immune-related genes and to detect interferon-related genes during viral infection.

Based on an NGS transcriptomic study, we showed that pro-inflammatory and interferon-related genes, namely CCL8 (MCP2), CXCL10 (IP10), CCL17, MX1 and viperin (RSAD2), were upregulated in FIPV 79–1146-infected CRFK cells [14]. In this study, we confirmed the upregulation of these genes using Taqman real-time PCR (Table 2); however, detected levels of expression varied, which could be due to the differences in the sensitivity of these different platforms. One of the genes of interest that was highly upregulated and associated with an increase in viral load is MX1, an interferon-induced GTP-binding protein. Previous studies have shown that MX1 is an interferon-inducible protein found in humans and various animals that mediates resistance against RNA viruses [29]. In this study, we showed that mRNA expression of MX1 was significantly upregulated at 48 and 72 hpi and found to be correlated with the viral load at 48 hpi (Tables 2 and 3). Previous studies have also shown that the antiviral role of this gene is related to IFNα and β (IFN type 1) induction and GTPase pathways [19]. Similar to MX1, RSAD2, which is also known as viperin, is a gene that encodes for an IFN-induced antiviral protein [30]. However, unlike MX1, which is activated by type I IFN, viperin is induced by different types of IFN [31, 32]. In fact, the expression of viperin can be induced by double-stranded RNA analogs such as poly I:C, lipopolysaccharides and by infection with a broad range of both RNA and DNA viruses, indicating the diverse role of viperin during infection [31, 32]. The importance of this finding is not clear; nevertheless, studies have shown that viruses such as Japanese Encephalitis Virus (JEV) [33] and Dengue Virus type 2 (DENV-2) [34] can downregulate antiviral innate immune responses such as viperin and other IFN-inducible protein expression [31, 32]. Further studies are required to measure type I IFN levels in cats with FIP.

The clinical relevance of the observed variations in MX1 and viperin expression to the development of FIP is unknown. However, a study has shown that expression of viperin is crucial for optimal Th2 cell

Table 9 Concentrations (pg/ml) of immune-related proteins in the serum of FCoV-positive cats

FIP Form	ID	Fas	Flt-3IL	GM-CSF	IFNγ	IL1β	IL2	PDGF-BB	IL12/p40	IL13	IL4	IL6	IL8	KC	SDF1	RANTES	SCF	MCP1	TNFα	IL18
NC	1[a]	<8.3 ± 0	45.3 ± 1.4	8.3 ± 0.1	12.3 ± 0	<17.3 ± 0	19.1 ± 0.2	300.1 ± 4.0	194.3 ± 5.3	5.6 ± 0	106.5 ± 1.7	<36.3 ± 0	13.0 ± 0.2	3.7 ± 0.2	92 ± 1.4	8.4 ± 0.2	118.3 ± 2.5	845.5 ± 0	115 ± 1.7	<71.2 ± 0
Dry	2	<8.3 ± 0	13.5 ± 0.2	7.6 ± 0.3	16.4 ± 0.2	<17.3 ± 0	17.1 ± 0.5	297.5 ± 4.5	1269 ± 11.6	5.9 ± 0.2	124.7 ± 1.4	<36.3 ± 0	32.6 ± 0.2	25.6 ± 0.9	64.8 ± 1	19.8 ± 0.1	49.0 ± 0.3	958 ± 12.5	65.0 ± 1.3	<71.2 ± 0
	3	9.8 ± 0.13	54.7 ± 1.7	15.0 ± 0.2	47.5 ± 0.4	<17.3 ± 0	17.8 ± 0.9	333.2 ± 0	268.5 ± 6.5	8.5 ± 0.1	287.4 ± 2.8	<36.3 ± 0	22.7 ± 0.5	25.7 ± 0.5	97.9 ± 0	19.3 ± 0.6	65.7 ± 2	1890 ± 0	152.3 ± 7.1	151.4 ± 9.8
	6	10.7 ± 0.1	24.9 ± 0.7	24.3 ± 0.1	39.2 ± 0.7	19 ± 0.94	24.8 ± 0	363.5 ± 3.3	147.6 ± 1.8	13.3 ± 0.4	323.2 ± 12.4	<36.3 ± 0	28.0 ± 0.6	22.8 ± 1.0	117.7 ± 0	8.6 ± 0.3	73.2 ± 2.3	1738 ± 41	104.28 ± 2	477.9 ± 5.7
Wet	7	9.1 ± 0.3	27.3 ± 2.4	15.2 ± 0.5	43.2 ± 2.5	<17.3 ± 0	17.8 ± 0.9	319.3 ± 8.1	543.9 ± 40.5	8.2 ± 0.3	117.3 ± 2.9	<36.3 ± 0	17.8 ± 1.6	3.3 ± 0.5	96.4 ± 2.6	16.8 ± 1.7	39.2 ± 3.7	914 ± 12.9	59.3 ± 2	<71.2 ± 0
	8	8.9 ± 0.1	14.1 ± 0.1	27.0 ± 0.3	14.2 ± 0.2	<17.3 ± 0	17.9 ± 0	339.6 ± 3.7	237.5 ± 0.5	6.2 ± 0	107.4 ± 2.9	<36.3 ± 0	19 ± 0.2	27.6 ± 0.7	85.9 ± 1.8	9.0 ± 0.2		<32.5 ± 0	868.6 ± 13.4	55 ± 0.5
																			<71.2 ± 0	9
		9.2 ± 0	39.5 ± 1.1	20.2 ± 0.1	61.9 ± 1.4	<17.3 ± 0	20.8 ± 0	332.8 ± 7.6	958.2 ± 36.8	7.8 ± 0	166.5 ± 0	<36.3 ± 0	16.0 ± 0.3	45.3 ± 1.9	84.3 ± 0.9	11.7 ± 0.3	39.5 ± 0.9	914.1 ± 12.9	66.3 ± 0	<71.2 ± 0
	5	11.5 ± 0.1	56.4 ± 0.1	16.2 ± 0.3	21.9 ± 0	<17.3 ± 0	22.9 ± 0.4	333.2 ± 0	2923.5 ± 70.7	7.1 ± 0.1	139.5 ± 1.4	<36.3 ± 0	28.9 ± 0.5	4.1 ± 0.1	90.5 ± 0.9	14.3 ± 0.1	46.6 ± 0.2	979.6 ± 0	88.8 ± 0	<71.2 ± 0
	10	13.5 ± 0.3	44.2 ± 0.8	13.8 ± 0.2	85.6 ± 2.5	32.6 ± 0.3	22.2 ± 0	305.3 ± 0	564.8 ± 5.3	10.4 ± 0.2	420.4 ± 10.9	116.7 ± 7.1	29.3 ± 0.2	3.3 ± 0.2	90.4 ± 4.4	22.8 ± 0.3	76.5 ± 1.5	2379 ± 13.3	158.2 ± 6.1	<71.2 ± 0
	11	12.6 ± 0	29.7 ± 0.9	19.1 ± 0.1	28.3 ± 1.2	<17.3 ± 0	26.0 ± 0	385.2 ± 3.0	1131 ± 17.3	11.2 ± 0.2	187.2 ± 6.3	<36.3 ± 0	37.6 ± 0.2	184.2 ± 7.0	189.3 ± 2.6	35.4 ± 0.6	69.2 ± 1.9	1082 ± 11.6	100 ± 2.5	96 ± 3.9
	12	12.2 ± 0	49.8 ± 1.7	11.1 ± 0.6	36.2 2.5	51.5 ± 6.9	95.3 ± 33.3	418.6 ± 5.2	655.1 ± 8.6	9.1 ± 0.3	294.4 ± 31.8	328.1 ± 56.2	28.9 ± 0.4	39.7 ± 34.8	303.9 ± 25.0	37.7 ± 0.4	48.9 ± 1.9	1370 ± 48.5	403.5 ± 40.6	522 ± 160.3

Note: Each sample was analyzed in three replicates and the data are expressed as means ± SEM
[a]Averaged concentrations from three healthy cats as negative controls (NC)

Table 10 Concentrations (pg/ml) of immune-related proteins in the PES of FCoV-positive cats

Cat ID	Fas	Flt-3lL	GM-CSF	IFNγ	IL1β	IL2	PDGF-BB	IL12/p40	IL13	IL4	IL6	IL8	KC	SDF1	RANTES	SCF	MCP1	TNFα	IL18
7	12.8 ± 0.4	226.1 ± 15.6	18.1 ± 0.4	5157 ± 503.5	54.2 ± 0.7	22.9 ± 0.4	357.5 ± 6.7	1033.6 ± 89.7	7.0 ± 0.2	125.9 ± 6.4	1123 ± 67.6	60.9 ± 5.5	4.9 ± 0.4	225.5 ± 3.1	650.5 ± 55.9	90.5 ± 3.1	968.7 ± 18.7	181.4 ± 2.4	<71.2 ± 0
8	9.6 ± 0	15.5 ± 0.5	23.8 ± 0.7	60.9 ± 1.2	82.7 ± 2.3	19.4 ± 0	319.7 ± 0	1040.9 ± 56.1	6.0 ± 0.1	109.9 ± 1.4	424.0 ± 11.4	308.3 ± 10.8	7.6 ± 0.6	220.7 ± 4	34.1 ± 1.5	44.0 ± 0.6	868.6 ± 13.4	56.7 ± 0.5	<71.2 ± 0
9	11.5 ± 0.4	218.3 ± 7.4	20.6 ± 0.3	5595 ± 250.6	54.8 ± 2.2	20.1 ± 0.4	345.5 ± 7.1	1598.5 ± 66.7	7.5 ± 0.2	149.3 ± 4.3			2998.5 ± 90.9	96.8 ± 3.3	12.1 ± 0.6		368.2 ± 14.3	180.1 ± 8.4	92.1 ± 2.9
															968.7 ± 18.7		234.9 ± 9.1	<71.2 ± 0	
5	10.0 ± 0.3	159.1 ± 6.2	17.4 ± 0.2	21.5 ± 1.1	21.3 ± 1	21.5 ± 0.4	319.7 ± 0	690.7 ± 29.7	7.0 ± 0.2	112.3 ± 2.9	96.2 ± 14.9	76.2 ± 3.3	4.1 ± 0.4	314.4 ± 4.6	27.2 ± 1.1	36.9 ± 1.7	868.6 ± 13.4	67.2 ± 1.5	<71.2 ± 0
10	11.1 ± 0.1	113.5 ± 1	15.9 ± 0.1	1072.5 ± 19.9	43.6 ± 0.5	20.1 ± 0.4	333.2 ± 0	908.8 ± 6.1	8.9 ± 0.1	382.6 ± 2.7	714.5 ± 1.4	86.8 ± 0.6	1.6 ± 0.1	372.4 ± 7.9	83.3 ± 0.7	82.8 ± 1	2228.5 ± 6.6	183.1 ± 0.5	<71.2 ± 0
12	13.7 ± 0.1	121.7 ± 4.4	10.3 ± 0.1	170.0 ± 3.1			128.8 ± 5.7	201.2 ± 8.2	380 ± 0	582.9 ± 8.6	10.8 ± 0	523.8 ± 8.1	1302 ± 61.2	46.7 ± 1.5	22.0 ± 0.8	1679 ± 66.4	64.6 ± 2.3	52.4 ± 0.6	
			1371.5 ± 9.5	988.1 ± 41.5			1412.5 ± 58.6												
13	25.0 ± 0.1	133.6 ± 0.6	11.7 ± 0	1888.5 ± 22.8			242.3 ± 1.8	45.2 ± 0.2		521.1 ± 3.5			3708.5 ± 11.3	13.4 ± 0.2	2000.5 ± 2.6		6736.5 ± 13	303.6 ± 3.6	3.4 ± 0.1
														206.1 ± 0.6	411.6 ± 5.3	36.6 ± 0.4	1268.5 ± 10.1	942.7 ± 10.9	194.0 ± 1.9

Note: Each sample was analyzed in three replicates and the data are expressed as means ± SEM

response in mice [35]. Hence, it is essential to further evaluate the importance of this finding in FIP cats. Earlier studies have proposed that the fundamental difference in the immune profiles of dry and wet forms of FIP is based on the predominant T cell responses. Cats with the dry form of FIP have a higher number of Th1 cells for the induction of CMI response, while cats with the wet form of FIP generally showed Th2-type response that leads to humoral immune response [13, 19].

The majority of FIP cases involve the presence of abdominal effusion, which was observed in eight out of 15 FCoV-positive cats sampled in this study [2]. Based on the pathogenesis of FIP, the accumulation of fluids in the peritoneal cavity of these cats is most probably due to the accumulation of the infected macrophages in the inter-venular space and venule walls [1, 10]. Activated and FCoV-infected monocytes can induce phlebitis through the paracrine and autocrine action of CD18, IL-1β and TNFα [11]. In addition, higher secretion of vascular endothelial growth factor (VEGF) has been associated with an increased production of effusion in cats with FIP [36]. Also, studies have shown that PE of cats diagnosed with FIP consisted primarily of macrophages and neutrophils with a low number of lymphocytes [37]. This study is in agreement with another study that reported a higher viral load in the supernatants of PE compared to those derived from the blood component of affected cats (Table 6) [15]. In addition, as expected, this study detected high expression of pro-inflammatory cytokines and chemokines, namely GM-CSF, IFNγ, IL8, KC, RANTES and MCP1, which are secreted mainly by monocytes/macrophages. The detection of CCL17 in the cell component of PE but not in PBMC indicated the inflammatory nature of the activated cells such as macrophages and dendritic cells (DC) present in the PE which may play an important role in the activation of Th2 cells [38, 39]. Furthermore, the lack of CCL17 expression, a chemokine that is primarily expressed in Th2 cells of cats with allergic inflammation [40], in the PBMC of the cats sampled in this study suggests a local rather than systemic response to the virus as also observed in other studies [17, 41, 42]. Further studies are warranted to confirm the expression of CCL17 by the activated cells from the PE of FIP cats. In addition, the downregulation of SCF (Table 9) is probably associated with the reduction of DC in cats with FIP, since SCF and Flt-3 L are important cytokines for the ex vivo propagation of human and mice DC [43, 44]. It was known that DC could be infected by FCoV; however, the role of SCF and Flt-3 L in FIPV infection warrants further examination [45].

In this study, the immune mediator protein levels vary between individual cats within the different cohorts (Tables 9 and 10). These findings were expected as biological individual variation could occur and has been observed in several other natural and experimental FIPV infections [12, 19]. Nevertheless, the expression of pro-inflammatory cytokines, namely IL1β and IL6, was more readily detected in the PES rather than the serum of the cats diagnosed with FIP. This finding is in agreement with previous studies that showed IL1 and IL6 can be detected in the serum and PE of FIP cases but not in those of healthy cats [18]. Besides, previous studies have shown that IL1β is related to CNS involvement and can only be detected in the inflammatory cells in the brain [19]. In this study, we found that IL-18, a pro-inflammatory cytokine in the IL-1 family that plays a major role in the activation of NK and T cells [46], was not readily detected in both serum and PES. The upregulation of TNFα protein in the serum and PES of some of the cats was in line with findings by previous studies that detected an increase in TNFα mRNA in abdominal effusions and PBMC of FIP-positive cats [14]. In addition, it has been suggested that this cytokine is responsible for T cell apoptosis [14, 21]. Hence, the role of these cytokines in FCoV-positive cats requires further evaluation. Interestingly, most of the FCoV-positive cats in this study have increased Fas serum levels, which may suggest a possible role of Fas in T cell apoptosis observed in FIP, as apoptosis can be induced by overexpression of Fas during viral infection [47].

Conclusions

In conclusion, this study has established some insights on the different expression of immune mediators in FCoV-positive cats, where several immune mediators including pro-inflammatory cytokines, Th1-like cytokines, and IFN-related antiviral proteins were found to be highly expressed. In addition, no clear indication of Th1 and Th2 imbalance was detected in the various samples analyzed in this study. However, in general, MX1, viperin, CXCL10, CCL8, RANTES, KC, MCP1, IL8, GM-CSF and IFNγ were readily detected in FCoV-positive cats whereby MX1 and viperin expression was higher in FCoV-positive cats with peritoneal effusions. Future studies on FIP confirmed cases need to be carried out to further establish the importance of the different immune mediators in the development of FIP.

Abbreviations

3'UTR: 3' untranslated region; BLAST: Basic local alignment search tool; CMI: Cell-mediated immunity; CRFK: Crandell-Reese feline kidney; DC: Dendritic cell; FCoV: Feline coronavirus; FELV: Feline leukemia virus; FIP: Feline infectious peritonitis; FIPV: Feline infectious peritonitis virus;

FIV: Feline immunodeficiency virus; hpi: Hours post inoculation; IACUC: Institutional animal care and use committee; NGS: Next-generation sequencing; PBMC: Peripheral blood mononuclear cell; PE: Peritoneal effusion; PES: Peritoneal effusion supernatant; qRT-PCR: Quantitative reverse transcriptase polymerase chain reaction; SARS: Severe acute respiratory syndrome; SPF: Specific-pathogen-free; SPSS: Statistical package for the social sciences; $TCID_{50}$: Tissue culture infectious dose 50; UNG: Uracil-N-glycosylase

Acknowledgements

The authors would like to thank Dr. Tan Sheau Wei for her technical assistance in the RT-qPCR analysis of the samples.

Funding

This study was supported by a PRGS Grant No: 5530600 from the Ministry of Education, Malaysia. The funding body has no specific role in the study design, data collection and analysis, decision to publish, or preparation of the manuscript.

Authors' contributions

NS and ARO co-defined the research theme. NS and AH designed and carried out the laboratory experiments, analyzed and interpreted the data and drafted the manuscript. SWN, GTS and FMK contributed at different stages of the experiments, depending on the fields of expertise. NS, AH ARO and FMK revised the paper critically for important intellectual content. All authors have seen and approved the manuscript.

Competing interests

The authors declare that they have no competing interests.

Consent for publication

Not applicable.

Author details

[1]Institute of Bioscience, Universiti Putra Malaysia, Serdang, Selangor, Malaysia. [2]Faculty of Veterinary Medicine, Universiti Putra Malaysia, Serdang, Selangor, Malaysia. [3]Leonard Davis School of Gerontology, University of Southern California, Los Angeles, CA, USA.

References

1. Pedersen NC. A review of feline infectious peritonitis virus infection: 1963-2008. J Feline Med Surg. 2009;11(4):225–58.
2. Kipar A, Meli ML. Feline infectious peritonitis: still an enigma? Vet Pathol. 2014;51(2):505–26.
3. Kipar A, Meli ML, Baptiste KE, Bowker LJ, Lutz H. Sites of feline coronavirus persistence in healthy cats. J Gen Virol. 2010;91(Pt 7):1698–707.
4. Pedersen NC, Liu H, Scarlett J, Leutenegger CM, Golovko L, Kennedy H, Kamal FM. Feline infectious peritonitis: role of the feline coronavirus 3c gene in intestinal tropism and pathogenicity based upon isolates from resident and adopted shelter cats. Virus Res. 2012;165(1):17–28.
5. Chang HW, Egberink HF, Halpin R. Spike protein fusion peptide and feline coronavirus virulence. Emerg Infect Dis. 2012;18:1089.
6. Lewis CS, Porter E, Matthews D, Kipar A, Tasker S, Helps CR, Siddell SG. Genotyping coronaviruses associated with feline infectious peritonitis. J Gen Virol. 2015;96(Pt 6):1358–68.
7. Bank-Wolf BR, Stallkamp I, Wiese S, Moritz A, Tekes G, Thiel HJ. Mutations of 3c and spike protein genes correlate with the occurrence of feline infectious peritonitis. Vet Microbiol. 2014;173(3–4):177–88.
8. Chang HW, Egberink HF, Rottier PJ. Sequence analysis of feline coronaviruses and the circulating virulent/avirulent theory. Emerg Infect Dis. 2011;17(4):744–6.
9. de Groot-Mijnes JD, van Dun JM, van der Most RG, de Groot RJ. Natural history of a recurrent feline coronavirus infection and the role of cellular immunity in survival and disease. J Virol. 2005;79(2):1036–44.
10. Kipar A, Bellmann S, Kremendahl J, Kohler K, Reinacher M. Cellular composition, coronavirus antigen expression and production of specific antibodies in lesions in feline infectious peritonitis. Vet Immunol Immunopathol. 1998;65(2–4):243–57.
11. Kipar A, May H, Menger S, Weber M, Leukert W, Reinacher M. Morphologic features and development of granulomatous vasculitis in feline infectious peritonitis. Vet Pathol. 2005;42(3):321–30.
12. Kipar A, Meli ML, Failing K, Euler T, Gomes-Keller MA, Schwartz D, Lutz H, Reinacher M. Natural feline coronavirus infection: differences in cytokine patterns in association with the outcome of infection. Vet Immunol Immunopathol. 2006;112(3–4):141–55.
13. Dean GA, Olivry T, Stanton C, Pedersen NC. In vivo cytokine response to experimental feline infectious peritonitis virus infection. Vet Microbiol. 2003;97(1–2):1–12.
14. Takano T, Hohdatsu T, Hashida Y, Kaneko Y, Tanabe M, Koyama H. A "possible" involvement of TNF-alpha in apoptosis induction in peripheral blood lymphocytes of cats with feline infectious peritonitis. Vet Microbiol. 2007;119(2–4):121–31.
15. Pedersen NC, Eckstrand C, Liu H, Leutenegger C, Murphy B. Levels of feline infectious peritonitis virus in blood, effusions, and various tissues and the role of lymphopenia in disease outcome following experimental infection. Vet Microbiol. 2015;175(2–4):157–66.
16. Gelain ME, Meli M, Paltrinieri S. Whole blood cytokine profiles in cats infected by feline coronavirus and healthy non-FCoV infected specific pathogen-free cats. J Feline Med Surg. 2006;8(6):389–99.
17. Goitsuka R, Furusawa S, Mizoguchi M, Hasegawa A. Detection of interleukin 1 in ascites from cats with feline infectious peritonitis. J Vet Med Sci. 1991;53(3):487–9.
18. Goitsuka R, Ohashi T, Ono K, Yasukawa K, Koishibara Y, Fukui H, Ohsugi Y, Hasegawa A. IL-6 activity in feline infectious peritonitis. J Immunol. 1990;144(7):2599–603.
19. Foley JE, Rand C, Leutenegger C. Inflammation and changes in cytokine levels in neurological feline infectious peritonitis. J Feline Med Surg. 2003;5(6):313–22.
20. Harun MS, Kuan CO, Selvarajah GT, Wei TS, Arshad SS, Hair Bejo M, Omar AR. Transcriptional profiling of feline infectious peritonitis virus infection in CRFK cells and in PBMCs from FIP diagnosed cats. Virol J. 2013;10(1):329.
21. Shuid AN, Safi N, Haghani A, Mehrbod P, Haron MS, Tan SW, Omar AR. Apoptosis transcriptional mechanism of feline infectious peritonitis virus infected cells. Apoptosis. 2015;20(11):1457–70.
22. Herrewegh AA, Smeenk I, Horzinek MC, Rottier PJ, de Groot RJ. Feline coronavirus type II strains 79-1683 and 79-1146 originate from a double recombination between feline coronavirus type I and canine coronavirus. J Virol. 1998;72(5):4508–14.
23. Herrewegh AA, de Groot RJ, Cepica A, Egberink HF, Horzinek MC, Rottier PJ. Detection of feline coronavirus RNA in feces, tissues, and body fluids of naturally infected cats by reverse transcriptase PCR. J Clin Microbiol. 1995;33(3):684–9.
24. Addie D. The diagnosis and prevention of FIP and recent research into feline coronavirus shedding. In: Proceedings of the 8th annual congress of the European Society of Veterinary Internal Medicine, Vienna, Austria: 1998; 1998. p. 110–7.
25. Choong OK, Mehrbod P, Tejo BA, Omar AR. In vitro antiviral activity of circular triple helix forming oligonucleotide RNA towards feline infectious peritonitis virus replication. Biomed Res Int. 2014;2014:654712.
26. Hockett RD, Kilby JM, Derdeyn CA, Saag MS, Sillers M, Squires K, Chiz S, Nowak MA, Shaw GM, Bucy RP. Constant mean viral copy number per infected cell in tissues regardless of high, low, or undetectable plasma HIV RNA. J Exp Med. 1999;189(10):1545–54.
27. Pontius JU, Mullikin JC, Smith DR, Agencourt Sequencing T, Lindblad-Toh K, Gnerre S, Clamp M, Chang J, Stephens R, Neelam B, et al. Initial sequence and comparative analysis of the cat genome. Genome Res. 2007;17(11):1675–89.
28. Himmerich H, Fischer J, Bauer K, Kirkby KC, Sack U, Krugel U. Stress-induced cytokine changes in rats. Eur Cytokine Netw. 2013;24(2):97–103.
29. Sadler AJ, Williams BR. Interferon-inducible antiviral effectors. Nat Rev Immunol. 2008;8(7):559–68.

Expression profiles of immune mediators in feline Coronavirus-infected cells and clinical samples of feline...

207

30. Fitzgerald KA. The interferon inducible gene: Viperin. J Interferon Cytokine Res. 2011;31(1):131–5.

31. Duschene KS, Broderick JB. Viperin: a radical response to viral infection. Biomol Concepts. 2012;3(3):255–66.

32. Wong MT, Chen SS: Emerging roles of interferon-stimulated genes in the innate immune response to hepatitis C virus infection. Cell Mol Immunol. 2014;13(1):11-35.

33. Chan YL, Chang TH, Liao CL, Lin YL. The cellular antiviral protein viperin is attenuated by proteasome-mediated protein degradation in Japanese encephalitis virus-infected cells. J Virol. 2008;82(21):10455–64.

34. Helbig KJ, Carr JM, Calvert JK, Wati S, Clarke JN, Eyre NS, Narayana SK, Fiches GN, McCartney EM, Beard MR. Viperin is induced following dengue virus type-2 (DENV-2) infection and has anti-viral actions requiring the C-terminal end of viperin. PLoS Negl Trop Dis. 2013;7(4):e2178.

35. Qiu LQ, Cresswell P, Chin KC. Viperin is required for optimal Th2 responses and T-cell receptor-mediated activation of NF-kappaB and AP-1. Blood. 2009;113(15):3520–9.

36. Takano T, Ohyama T, Kokumoto A, Satoh R, Hohdatsu T. Vascular endothelial growth factor (VEGF), produced by feline infectious peritonitis (FIP) virus-infected monocytes and macrophages, induces vascular permeability and effusion in cats with FIP. Virus Res. 2011;158(1–2):161–8.

37. Pedersen NC. An update on feline infectious peritonitis: diagnostics and therapeutics. Vet J. 2014;201(2):133–41.

38. Katakura T, Miyazaki M, Kobayashi M, Herndon DN, Suzuki F. CCL17 and IL-10 as effectors that enable alternatively activated macrophages to inhibit the generation of classically activated macrophages. J Immunol. 2004;172(3):1407–13.

39. Alferink J, Lieberam I, Reindl W, Behrens A, Weiss S, Huser N, Gerauer K, Ross R, Reske-Kunz AB, Ahmad-Nejad P, et al. Compartmentalized production of CCL17 in vivo: strong inducibility in peripheral dendritic cells contrasts selective absence from the spleen. J Exp Med. 2003;197(5):585–99.

40. Maeda S, Okayama T, Ohmori K, Masuda K, Ohno K, Tsujimoto H. Molecular cloning of the feline thymus and activation-regulated chemokine cDNA and its expression in lesional skin of cats with eosinophilic plaque. J Vet Med Sci. 2003;65(2):275–8.

41. Takano T, Azuma N, Satoh M, Toda A, Hashida Y, Satoh R, Hohdatsu T. Neutrophil survival factors (TNF-alpha, GM-CSF, and G-CSF) produced by macrophages in cats infected with feline infectious peritonitis virus contribute to the pathogenesis of granulomatous lesions. Arch Virol. 2009;154(5):775–81.

42. Giordano A, Paltrinieri S. Interferon-gamma in the serum and effusions of cats with feline coronavirus infection. Vet J. 2009;180(3):396–8.

43. Reyes M, Lund T, Lenvik T, Aguiar D, Koodie L, Verfaillie CM. Purification and ex vivo expansion of postnatal human marrow mesodermal progenitor cells. Blood. 2001;98(9):2615–25.

44. Laouar Y, Welte T, Fu X-Y, Flavell RA. STAT3 is required for Flt3L-dependent Dendritic cell differentiation. Immunity. 2003;19(6):903–12.

45. Tekes G, Hofmann-Lehmann R, Stallkamp I, Thiel V, Thiel HJ. Genome organization and reverse genetic analysis of a type I feline coronavirus. J Virol. 2008;82(4):1851–9.

46. Dinarello CA, Novick D, Kim S, Kaplanski G. Interleukin-18 and IL-18 binding protein. Front Immunol. 2013;4:289.

47. Katsikis PD, Wunderlich ES, Smith CA, Herzenberg LA, Herzenberg LA. Fas antigen stimulation induces marked apoptosis of T lymphocytes in human immunodeficiency virus-infected individuals. J Exp Med. 1995;181(6):2029–36.

Permissions

All chapters in this book were first published in VR, by BioMed Central; hereby published with permission under the Creative Commons Attribution License or equivalent. Every chapter published in this book has been scrutinized by our experts. Their significance has been extensively debated. The topics covered herein carry significant findings which will fuel the growth of the discipline. They may even be implemented as practical applications or may be referred to as a beginning point for another development.

The contributors of this book come from diverse backgrounds, making this book a truly international effort. This book will bring forth new frontiers with its revolutionizing research information and detailed analysis of the nascent developments around the world.

We would like to thank all the contributing authors for lending their expertise to make the book truly unique. They have played a crucial role in the development of this book. Without their invaluable contributions this book wouldn't have been possible. They have made vital efforts to compile up to date information on the varied aspects of this subject to make this book a valuable addition to the collection of many professionals and students.

This book was conceptualized with the vision of imparting up-to-date information and advanced data in this field. To ensure the same, a matchless editorial board was set up. Every individual on the board went through rigorous rounds of assessment to prove their worth. After which they invested a large part of their time researching and compiling the most relevant data for our readers.

The editorial board has been involved in producing this book since its inception. They have spent rigorous hours researching and exploring the diverse topics which have resulted in the successful publishing of this book. They have passed on their knowledge of decades through this book. To expedite this challenging task, the publisher supported the team at every step. A small team of assistant editors was also appointed to further simplify the editing procedure and attain best results for the readers.

Apart from the editorial board, the designing team has also invested a significant amount of their time in understanding the subject and creating the most relevant covers. They scrutinized every image to scout for the most suitable representation of the subject and create an appropriate cover for the book.

The publishing team has been an ardent support to the editorial, designing and production team. Their endless efforts to recruit the best for this project, has resulted in the accomplishment of this book. They are a veteran in the field of academics and their pool of knowledge is as vast as their experience in printing. Their expertise and guidance has proved useful at every step. Their uncompromising quality standards have made this book an exceptional effort. Their encouragement from time to time has been an inspiration for everyone.

The publisher and the editorial board hope that this book will prove to be a valuable piece of knowledge for researchers, students, practitioners and scholars across the globe.

List of Contributors

Aarti Kathrani
Veterinary Medical Teaching Hospital, School of Veterinary Medicine, University of California-Davis, Davis, CA 95616, USA
School of Veterinary Sciences, University of Bristol, Langford House, Langford, Bristol BS40 5DU, UK

Jennifer A. Larsen, Gino Cortopassi, Sandipan Datta and Andrea J. Fascetti
Department of Molecular Biosciences, School of Veterinary Medicine, University of California-Davis, Davis, CA 95616, USA

Gayeon Won, Tae Hoon Kim and John Hwa Lee
College of Veterinary Medicine, Chonbuk National University, Iksan campus, Gobong-ro 79, Iksan 54596, Republic of Korea

Hugo Saba Pereira Cardoso and Edson de Jesus Marques
Department of Exact and Earth Sciences, State University of Bahia, Campus II, Alagoinhas, BA CEP 48110-100, Brazil

Vera Lúcia Costa Vale
Department of Exact and Earth Sciences, State University of Bahia, Campus II, Alagoinhas, BA CEP 48110-100, Brazil
Immunology and Molecular Biology Laboratory, Health Sciences Institute, Federal University of Bahia, Av. Reitor Miguel Calmon s/n, Vale do Canela, Salvador, BA CEP 40110-100, Brazil

Lília Ferreira de Moura-Costa
Department of Biointeraction, Federal University of Bahia, Av. Reitor Miguel Calmon s/n, Vale do Canela, Salvador, BA CEP 40110-100, Brazil

Roberto José Meyer Nascimento and Ivana Lucia de Oliveira Nascimento
Department of Biointeraction, Federal University of Bahia, Av. Reitor Miguel Calmon s/n, Vale do Canela, Salvador, BA CEP 40110-100, Brazil
Immunology and Molecular Biology Laboratory, Health Sciences Institute, Federal University of Bahia, Av. Reitor Miguel Calmon s/n, Vale do Canela, Salvador, BA CEP 40110-100, Brazil

Soraya Castro Trindade
Department of Health, Feira de Santana State University, Avenida Transnordestina s/n, Novo Horizonte, Feira de Santana, BA CEP 44036-900, Brazil
Immunology and Molecular Biology Laboratory, Health Sciences Institute, Federal University of Bahia, Av. Reitor Miguel Calmon s/n, Vale do Canela, Salvador, BA CEP 40110-100, Brazil

Marcos da Costa Silva
Department of Life Sciences, State University of Bahia, Rua Silveira Martins 2555, Cabula, Salvador, BA CEP 41150-000, Brazil
Immunology and Molecular Biology Laboratory, Health Sciences Institute, Federal University of Bahia, Av. Reitor Miguel Calmon s/n, Vale do Canela, Salvador, BA CEP 40110-100, Brazil

Andréia Pacheco de Souza, Bruno Jean Adrien Paule and Ellen Karla Nobre dos Santos-Lima
Immunology and Molecular Biology Laboratory, Health Sciences Institute, Federal University of Bahia, Av. Reitor Miguel Calmon s/n, Vale do Canela, Salvador, BA CEP 40110-100, Brazil

Jon D. Plant
SkinVet Clinic, 15800 Upper Boones Ferry Road, Suite 120, Lake Oswego 97035, OR, USA

Moni B. Neradilek
The Mountain-Whisper-Light Statistics, 1827 23rd Avenue East, Seattle 98112, WA, USA

R. Barić Rafaj and A. Tumpa
Department of Chemistry and Biochemistry, Faculty of Veterinary Medicine, University of Zagreb, Heinzelova 55, 10 000 Zagreb, Croatia

J. Kuleš
ERA Chair team VetMedZg, Internal Diseases Clinic, Faculty of Veterinary Medicine, University of Zagreb, Heinzelova 55, 10 000 Zagreb, Croatia

A. Marinculić
Department of Parasitology and Parasitic Diseases with Clinic, Faculty of Veterinary Medicine, University of Zagreb, Heinzelova 55, 10 000 Zagreb, Croatia

A. Tvarijonaviciute and J. Ceron
Department of Animal Medicine and Surgery, Faculty of Veterinary Medicine, Regional Campus of International Excellence Campus Mare Nostrum, University of Murcia, Murcia 30100, Espinardo, Spain

Ž. Mihaljević
Veterinary Institute, Savska cesta 143, 0 000 Zagreb, Croatia

V. Mrljak
Clinic for Internal Dieaases, Faculty of Veterinary Medicine, University of Zagreb, Heinzelova 55, 10 000 Zagreb, Croatia

Barbara Kohn, Aleksandra Chirek and Sina Rehbein
FB Veterinärmedizin, Klinik für Kleine Haustiere, Freie Universität Berlin, Oertzenweg 19 b, 14163 Berlin, Germany

Abdulgabar Salama and Gürkan Bal
Institut für Transfusionsmedizin, Charité – Universitätsklinikum, Augustenburger Platz 1, 13353 Berlin, Germany

Aurore Laprais
Department of Clinical Sciences, College of Veterinary Medicine, North Carolina State University, Raleigh, NC, USA

Thierry Olivry
Department of Clinical Sciences, College of Veterinary Medicine, North Carolina State University, Raleigh, NC, USA
Comparative Medicine Institute, College of Veterinary Medicine, North Carolina State University, Raleigh, NC, USA

Gayathri Thevi Selvarajah and Farina Mustaffa-Kamal
Faculty of Veterinary Medicine, Universiti Putra Malaysia, Serdang, Selangor, Malaysia

Wang-Dong Zhang, Wen-Hui Wang, Shu-Xian Li, Shuai Jia, Xue-Feng Zhang and Ting-Ting Cao
College of Veterinary Medicine, Gansu Agricultural University, Lanzhou, Gansu 730070, China

Moeko Kohyama, Akira Yabuki and Osamu Yamato
Laboratory of Clinical Pathology, Department of Veterinary Medicine, Joint Faculty of Veterinary Medicine, Kagoshima University, 1-21-24 Kohrimoto, Kagoshima-shi, Kagoshima 890-0065, Japan

Kenji Ochiai
Laboratory of Veterinary Pathology, Department of Veterinary Medicine, Faculty of Agriculture, Iwate University, 3-18-8 Ueda, Morioka-shi, Iwate 020-8550, Japan

Yuya Nakamoto
Kyoto Animal Referral Medical Center, 208-4 Shin-arami, Tai, Kumiyama-cho, Kuse-gun, Kyoto 613-0036, Japan

Masaya Tsuboi and Kazuyuki Uchida
Laboratory of Veterinary Pathology, Graduate School of Agricultural and Life Sciences, The University of Tokyo, 1-1-1 Yayoi, Bunkyou-ku, Tokyo 113-8657, Japan

Daisuke Hasegawa
Department of Veterinary Radiology, Nippon Veterinary and Life Science University, 1-7-1 Kyouman-chou, Musashino-shi, Tokyo 180-8602, Japan

Kimimasa Takahashi
6Department of Veterinary Pathology, , Nippon Veterinary and Life Science University, 1-7-1 Kyouman-chou, Musashino-shi, Tokyo, 180-8602, Japan

Hiroaki Kawaguchi
Laboratory of Veterinary Histopathology, Department of Veterinary Medicine, Joint Faculty of Veterinary Medicine, Kagoshima University, 1-21-24 Kohrimoto, Kagoshima-shi, Kagoshima 890-0065, Japan

Dana E. Oellers, Natali Bauer and Andreas Moritz
Department of Veterinary Clinical Sciences, Clinical Pathophysiology and Clinical Pathology, Justus-Liebig University Giessen, Frankfurter Str. 126, 35392 Giessen, Germany

Melanie Ginder
IDEXX BioResearch Europe, A Division of IDEXX Laboratories, Ludwigsburg, Germany

Sigrid Johannes and Iris Pernecker
Merck Serono, Global Non-Clinical Safety, Merck KGaA, Darmstadt, Germany

Giovanni Pietro Burrai, Tiziana Cubeddu, Marta Polinas and Elisabetta Antuofermo
Department of Veterinary Medicine, University of Sassari, Via Vienna 2, 07100 Sassari, Italy

Alessandro Tanca, Marcello Abbondio and Maria Filippa Addis
Porto Conte Ricerche, S.P. 55 Porto Conte/Capo Caccia Km .400, Loc, 07041 Tramariglio, Alghero, Italy

Alicja Majewska, Małgorzata Gajewska and Adam Prostek
Department of Physiological Sciences, Faculty of Veterinary Medicine, Warsaw University of Life Sciences-SGGW, Warsaw, Poland

Kourou Dembele
Department of Small Animal Diseases with Clinic, Faculty of Veterinary Medicine, Warsaw University of Life Sciences-SGGW, Warsaw, Poland

Henryk Maciejewski
Department of Computer Engineering, Wroclaw University of Technology, Wrocław, Poland

Michał Jank
Veterinary Institute, Faculty of Veterinary Medicine and Animal Sciences, Poznań University of Life Sciences, Poznań, Poland

M. Woldemeskel, I. Hawkins and L. Whittington
Laboratory, College of Veterinary Medicine, University of Georgia, 43 Brighton Rd, Tifton, GA 31793, USA

T. C. Loh, A. Q. Sazili and A. A. Samsudin
Department of Animal Science, Faculty of Agriculture, Universiti Putra Malaysia, 43400 Serdang, Selangor, Malaysia

A. M. Dalia
Department of Animal Science, Faculty of Agriculture, Universiti Putra Malaysia, 43400 Serdang, Selangor, Malaysia
Department of Animal Nutrition, Faculty of Animal Production, University of Khartoum, Khartoum, Sudan

M. F. Jahromi
Institute of Tropical Agriculture, Universiti Putra Malaysia, 43400 Serdang, Selangor, Malaysia

Xin Jin, Man Zhang, Yan-ru Fan, Hua-er Bao, Siri-guleng Xu, Qiao-zhen Tian, Yun-he Wang and Yin-feng Yang
Veterinary Medicine College of Inner Mongolia Agricultural University, Hohhot 010018, People's Republic of China

Key Laboratory of Clinical Diagnosis and Treatment Technology in Animal Disease, Ministry of Agriculture, Hohhot 010018, People's Republic of China

Xue-min Zhu
Veterinary Medicine College of Inner Mongolia Agricultural University, Hohhot 010018, People's Republic of China
Key Laboratory of Clinical Diagnosis and Treatment Technology in Animal Disease, Ministry of Agriculture, Hohhot 010018, People's Republic of China
College of Animal Science and Technology, Henan University of Science and Technology, Luoyang 471000, People's Republic of China

Chen-guang Du
Veterinary Medicine College of Inner Mongolia Agricultural University, Hohhot 010018, People's Republic of China
Key Laboratory of Clinical Diagnosis and Treatment Technology in Animal Disease, Ministry of Agriculture, Hohhot 010018, People's Republic of China
Vocational and Technical College of Inner Mongolia Agricultural University, Baotou 014109, People's Republic of China

Thierry Olivry
Department of Clinical Sciences, College of Veterinary Medicine, North Carolina State University, Raleigh, NC 27606, USA
Comparative Medicine Institute, North Carolina State University, Raleigh, NC, USA

Keith E. Linder
Comparative Medicine Institute, North Carolina State University, Raleigh, NC, USA
Department of Population Health and Pathobiology, College of Veterinary Medicine, North Carolina State University, Raleigh, NC, USA

Frane Banovic
Department of Small Animal Medicine and Surgery, College of Veterinary Medicine, University of Georgia, Athens, GA, USA

Jorge Castro-López, Marta Planellas and Josep Pastor
Departament de Medicina i Cirurgia Animals, Universitat Autònoma de Barcelona, 08193 Barcelona, Spain
Fundació Hospital Clínic Veterinari de la Universitat Autònoma de Barcelona, 08193 Barcelona, Spain

Antonio Ramis
Servei de Diagnòstic de Patologia Veterinària, Departament de Sanitat i d'Anatomia Animals, Universitat Autònoma de Barcelona, 08193 Barcelona, Spain

Mariana Teles
Department de Biologia Cellular, Fisiologia i d'Immunologia, Universitat Autònoma de Barcelona, 08193 Barcelona, Spain

Yao Lee, Matti Kiupel and Gisela Soboll Hussey
Department of Pathobiology & Diagnostic Investigation, College of Veterinary Medicine, Michigan State University, 784 Wilson Rd, A13, East Lansing, MI 48824, USA

Perot Saelao
Integrative Genetics and Genomics Graduate Group, University of California, Davis, CA 95616, USA
Genomics to Improve Poultry Innovation Lab, University of California, Davis, CA 95616, USA
Department of Animal Science, University of California, Davis, CA 95616, USA

Ying Wang and Huaijun Zhou
Genomics to Improve Poultry Innovation Lab, University of California, Davis, CA 95616, USA
Department of Animal Science, University of California, Davis, CA 95616, USA

Terra Kelly
Genomics to Improve Poultry Innovation Lab, University of California, Davis, CA 95616, USA
6One Health Institute, University of California, Davis, CA 95616, USA

Rodrigo A. Gallardo
School of Veterinary Medicine, University of California, Davis, CA 95616, USA

Susan J. Lamont and Jack M. Dekkers
Department of Animal Science, Iowa State University, Ames, IA 50011, USA

Mohamad Zamani-Ahmadmahmudi
Department of Clinical Science, Faculty of Veterinary Medicine, Shahid Bahonar University of Kerman, Kerman, Iran

Sina Aghasharif and Keyhan Ilbeigi
Department of Clinical Science, Faculty of Veterinary Medicine, Islamic Azad University, Garmsar Branch, Garmsar, Iran

Shing Wei Ng
Institute of Bioscience, Universiti Putra Malaysia, Serdang, Selangor, Malaysia

Abdul Rahman Omar
Institute of Bioscience, Universiti Putra Malaysia, Serdang, Selangor, Malaysia
Faculty of Veterinary Medicine, Universiti Putra Malaysia, Serdang, Selangor, Malaysia

Nikoo Safi and Amin Haghani
Institute of Bioscience, Universiti Putra Malaysia, Serdang, Selangor, Malaysia
Leonard Davis School of Gerontology, University of Southern California, Los Angeles, CA, USA

Index

www.ingramcontent.com/pod-product-compliance
Lightning Source LLC
Chambersburg PA
CBHW082041190326
41458CB00010B/3429